Debates in Medicine
Volume 3

DEBATES IN MEDICINE

Editorial Board

Editor-in-Chief
Gary Gitnick, M.D.
Professor, Department of Medicine
UCLA School of Medicine
Center for Health Sciences
Los Angeles, California

Associate Editors
H. Verdain Barnes, M.D.
Professor and Chairman
Department of Medicine
Wright State University
School of Medicine
Dayton, Ohio

Thomas P. Duffy, M.D.
Professor of Medicine
Section of Hematology
Department of Internal Medicine
Yale University School of Medicine
New Haven, Connecticut

Richard P. Lewis, M.D.
Professor of Medicine
Division of Cardiology
Department of Internal Medicine
Ohio State University College of
  Medicine
Columbus, Ohio

Richard H. Winterbauer, M.D.
Head, Section of Chest and Infectious
  Diseases
Department of Medicine
Virginia Mason Clinic
Seattle, Washington

Volume 3 • 1990
Year Book Medical Publishers, Inc.
Chicago • London • Boca Raton • Littleton, Mass.

International Standard Serial Number: 0887-218X
International Standard Book Number: 0-8151-3602-1

Sponsoring Editor: Michele R. Bettis
Associate Managing Editor: Denise M. Dungey
Assistant Director, Manuscript Services: Frances M. Perveiler
Production Coordinator: Max Perez
Proofroom Supervisor: Barbara M. Kelly

This book is dedicated to those unselfish people who made it possible for me to devote the time needed to develop this text. They are my wife Cherna and my children Neil, Kim, Jill, and Tracy. This book is dedicated to them, for it belongs to them just as it does to the authors and editors who contributed to each segment.

Contributors

Garth H. Ballantyne, M.D.
Associate Professor of Surgery
Gastrointestinal Surgery Research Unit
Department of Surgery
Yale University School of Medicine
West Haven Veterans Administration Medical Center
West Haven, Connecticut

James S. Barthel, M.D.
Assistant Director
Gastrointestinal Endoscopy
Department of Gastroenterology
The Cleveland Clinic Foundation
Cleveland, Ohio

Kenneth W. Barwick, M.D.
Professor of Pathology
Department of Pathology
Baptist Medical Center
Jacksonville, Florida

Daniel E. Bechard, M.D.
Assistant Professor of Pulmonary and Critical Care Medicine
Medical College of Virginia Hospital
Richmond, Virginia

Anton J. Bilchik, M.D.
Postdoctoral Associate
Gastrointestinal Surgery Research Unit
Department of Surgery
Yale University School of Medicine
West Haven Veterans Administration Medical Center
West Haven, Connecticut

Manfred Blum, M.D.
Professor of Clinical Medicine and Radiology
Director, Nuclear Endocrine Laboratory
New York University Medical Center
New York, New York

R. D. Cohen, M.D.
Professor of Medicine
Director, Medical Unit
The London Hospital Medical College
University of London
London, England

Richard Crampton, D.M.
Professor of Medicine
Division of Cardiology
Department of Medicine
University of Virginia School of Medicine
Charlottesville, Virginia

John Dobbins, M.D.
Professor of Medicine
Director, GI Procedure Center
Department of Medicine
Yale University School of Medicine
New Haven, Connecticut

Betty J. Flehinger, Ph.D.
Manager, Statistics
Department of Mathematical Sciences
International Business Machines (IBM) Thomas J. Watson Research Center
Yorktown Heights, New York

Robert S. Fontana, M.D.
Professor of Medicine
Mayo Medical School
Rochester, Minnesota

Allen L. Ginsberg, M.D.
Professor of Medicine
George Washington University School of Medicine and Health Sciences
Washington, District of Columbia

Paul Guth, M.D.
Key Investigator
Center for Ulcer Research and Education
Professor of Medicine
University of California, Los Angeles, UCLA School of Medicine
Assistant Chief of Gastroenterology
Veterans Administration Medical Center
Los Angeles, California

Stephen Hanauer, M.D.
Associate Professor of Medicine
University of Chicago Medical Center
Chicago, Illinois

William E. Karnes, M.D.
Assistant Professor of Medicine
UCLA School of Medicine
Associate Investigator
Center for Ulcer Research and Education
Veterans Administration Medical Center
Los Angeles, California

Abbas E. Kitabchi, M.D., Ph.D.
Professor of Medicine and Biochemistry
Director, Division of Endocrinology and Metabolism and Clinical Research Center
University of Tennessee College of Medicine
Memphis, Tennessee

Simeon Margolis, M.D., Ph.D.
Professor of Medicine and Biological Chemistry
Associate Dean for Academic Affairs
Johns Hopkins University School of Medicine
Baltimore, Maryland

William H. Marks, M.D., Ph.D.
Associate Professor of Surgery
Director, Endoscopy-Surgical Service
Department of Surgery
Yale University School of Medicine
Yale-New Haven Hospital
New Haven, Connecticut

Ernest L. Mazzaferri, M.D.
Professor and Chairman
Department of Internal Medicine
Ohio State University College of Medicine
Columbus, Ohio

Myron R. Melamed, M.D.
Attending Pathologist
Memorial Sloan-Kettering Cancer Center
Professor of Pathology
Cornell University Medical College
New York, New York

David W. M. Muller, M.B., B.S.
Senior Research Fellow
Interventional Cardiology Program
Division of Cardiology
University of Michigan Medical Center
Ann Arbor, Michigan

Mary Beth Murphy, R.N., M.S.
Clinical Nurse Specialist
Division of Endocrinology and Metabolism and Clinical Research Center
University of Tennessee College of Medicine
Memphis, Tennessee

Michael F. Oliver, M.D.
Director, Wynn Institute for Metabolic Research
London, England

Gerald N. Olsen, M.D.
Professor of Medicine
Director, Division of Pulmonary and Critical Care Medicine
University of South Carolina School of Medicine
Columbia, South Carolina

Eric J. Topol, M.D.
Director of Cardiac Catheterization Laboratories
Associate Professor of Internal Medicine
University of Michigan Medical School
Ann Arbor, Michigan

Don Zwickler, M.D.
Fellow in Endocrinology
Department of Medicine
New York University Medical Center
New York, New York

Preface

Controversy traditionally has been one cornerstone of medicine. Critical analysis and the drive to challenge the basis upon which concepts have developed are essential to the scientific approach. It is no surprise that medical literature is based on the history of controversy or that controversy remains a fundamental part of the discipline of medicine. Regardless of whether a physician is discussing treatment, causation, or pathophysiology, there will be differences of opinion, conflicting data, and often contradictory concepts. Through thoughtful study of all sides of controversial issues, the astute physician or student can become a better physician.

This volume covers ten important controversies in medical science. Contributing authors are experts in the discussion topics in which they have been assigned. Each has been instructed to provide the very best case for a given point of view. As is sometimes the case with oral debates, authors may have been asked to represent views opposite to those which they actually hold. However, in most cases, the physicians present cases consistent with their own views as previously expressed in publications and public statements.

Each debate is preceded by a brief introduction and is followed by a summary statement prepared by one of the editors. These are designed to give balance to the opposing views presented. They should be taken as opinions. Many readers will find opinions in this volume with which they disagree. It is the hope of the editors that this disagreement will stimulate thought and insight, that the knowledge of all aspects of the controversy will expand basic knowledge of the diseases discussed, and that the reader will come away from this volume better educated and, to some extent, entertained. I am indebted to the contributing authors who diligently developed their arguments and their subsequent rebuttals. I am also indebted to the associate editors, Drs. H. Verdain Barnes, Thomas Duffy, Richard Winterbauer, and Richard Lewis, who made it possible to develop this book. I wish to thank Mrs. Susan Dashe for her careful, thoughtful, and diligent assistance in the development of this book.

Gary Gitnick, M.D.

Contents

Is Exercise Testing Valuable in Predicting Operative Risk?

Chapter Editor: Richard H. Winterbauer, M.D.

Affirmative: Gerald N. Olsen, M.D.
Professor of Medicine, Director, Division of
Pulmonary and Critical Care Medicine,
University of South Carolina School of
Medicine, Columbia, South Carolina

Negative: Daniel E. Bechard, M.D.
Assistant Professor of Pulmonary and
Critical Care Medicine, Medical College of
Virginia Hospital, Richmond, Virginia

Editor's Introduction

Physicians everywhere refer to "operative risk" and routinely integrate this factor into the risk/benefit analysis of an operative procedure for each individual patient. The assessment of operative risk consists of developing a mosaic of medical information which will estimate theoretically the likelihood of the patient developing serious complications and the possibility of death related to the operative procedure. Preoperative identification of comorbid conditions which enhance operative risk theoretically could lessen operative cost, morbidity, and mortality, either by allowing correction of the abnormal physiologic state preoperatively or by denying the operative procedure to high-risk groups. The types of preoperative testing used have varied greatly and include screening history and physical examination, hematocrit, electrocardiogram, serum chemistries, chest x-ray, pulmonary function tests, and, now, exercise testing. Exercise testing has an inherent appeal as a global assessment of the patient's cardiac, pulmonary, and motivational ability to handle the stress of major surgery. However, the precise role of exercise testing in predicting operative risk has been difficult to establish. The debate to come provides an excellent analysis of the pros and cons of preoperative exercise testing.

Richard H. Winterbauer, M.D.

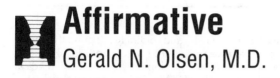

Affirmative
Gerald N. Olsen, M.D.

An ounce of prevention is worth a pound of cure.
T. C. Haliburton

Definition of Operative Risk

That surgery is associated with a risk of undesirable outcome and frequently is the basis of litigation is well accepted. In defining what is meant by the words "operative risks," a small glossary is needed.

Finding: The result of an investigation.
Complication: A difficult factor unexpectedly changing outcome, e.g., a second disease.
Postoperative morbidity: A condition in which complications produce symptoms and require additional therapy.
Postoperative mortality: A condition in which complications are of sufficient severity as to cause death.

Knowing the differences in these concepts and especially in their clinical impact will make interpretation of the literature easier. For example, a minor and asymptomatic drop in measured arterial oxygen tension (Pao_2) postcholecystectomy could be classified as a "finding," as it may not require therapy or an extended hospital stay. However, bacterial pneumonia in the remaining lung after pneumonectomy will certainly produce symptoms and could lead to disabling cardiorespiratory failure and death. This pneumonia, therefore, qualifies as a "complication." It also qualifies as "postoperative morbidity" since it will certainly require therapy. Once postoperative morbidity has occurred, two outcomes are possible. The first is that the complication will be treated successfully and the patient will survive with nothing more than a longer (and more expensive) hospital stay. The other, and most unhappy, outcome is progressive and permanent disability leading to premature death. Although effective treatment for the complication or morbidity exists, prevention would be better.

To be cost-effective, the prevention of a minor postoperative complication producing minimal morbidity requires a very inexpensive therapeutic modality. If, on the other hand, the postoperative morbidity is serious and may lead to critical illness, permanent disability, or death, then the need for prevention is profound, regardless of cost. To prevent a complication effectively, one needs to know who is at risk. This question raises the issue of not only the cost-effectiveness of the treatment, but also of who should receive it. For example, it would be impractical to give an expensive, but effective, preventive treatment to 1,000 patients at risk if only 1 were predicted to develop the complication. Therefore, a preoperative test should be designed to identify those at greatest risk of serious postoperative morbidity or mortality. To be effective, the test should be simple, relatively inexpensive, and accurate.

One also has to balance the risk of postoperative morbidity or mortality against the outcome of the disease treated without surgery. For example, it would appear to be more important to predict (and prevent) disabling or fatal cardiorespiratory failure following pneumonectomy for lung cancer than to predict a mild wound infection following liposuction for obesity. Lung cancer not successfully treated surgically has a grim prognosis; thus, surgery, though it carries risks, may be the patient's best chance for cure. However, no surgeon wishes to have a patient die in the immediate postoperative period or become disabled from cardiorespiratory insufficiency. Hence , a test which will identify those patients who are most likely to die after the surgery, while still providing high-risk patients a chance for cure, is the most desirable.

In this discussion, I will emphasize the prediction of operative risk from potentially life-threatening complications of major surgery. Those complications having the greatest potential for fatal outcome are outlined in Table 1. This obviously is not a complete list of all potentially minor complications, but rather a list of those entities which could be the result of an initially mild complication. An example would be postoperative atelectasis leading to bacterial pneumonia, leading to sepsis, leading to shock, and resulting in death. Are there any factors that might predispose a patient to enter this disastrous progression? Those clinical conditions placing patients at risk of life-threatening complications of surgery are listed in Table 2. The list in

---

TABLE 1.
Life-Threatening Postoperative Complications

Myocardial infarction
Congestive heart failure
Respiratory failure (hypoxic and hypercapnic)
Pulmonary embolism
Sepsis
Stroke
Major hemorrhage
Shock
Renal failure

TABLE 2.
Conditions of Increased
Operative Risk

Emergency surgery
Cardiovascular or cerebrovascular disease
Pulmonary (obstructive) disease
Coagulopathy
Major abdominal or thoracic procedures
Prolonged or repeated procedures
Immunocompromised?
Advanced age?
Morbid obesity??

Table 2 seems to emphasize those patients undergoing major surgical procedures who have underlying diseases. With these first two tables we have, perhaps, taken our first step in deciding who might be a candidate for a test capable of predicting an adverse postoperative outcome. For example, an elderly patient with chronic obstructive pulmonary disease and cardiovascular disease who is scheduled for a pneumonectomy for lung cancer would seem to be an ideal candidate for such testing. A young, healthy athlete scheduled to undergo an elective knee operation under local anesthesia would seem less likely to need preoperative testing.

Surgeons have been searching in perpetuity for an ideal test which, when performed preoperatively, will predict which patient will develop a serious postoperative complication. A common example of such testing is the routine preoperative measurement of hemoglobin concentration. Since surgery, anesthesia, and perioperative care have become progressively more sophisticated, more aggressive procedures can be performed on patients previously considered to be at excessively high risk. For example, an intriguing report documented successful major abdominal surgery in a group of patients with preoperative hemoglobin concentrations between 1.9 and 7.5 g/dL.[1] Prior to 1974, postoperative mortality rates in patients over 70 years of age exceeded the 5-year survival rates of lung cancer resection.[2] Currently, age alone is not considered a barrier to lung resection,[3] and a recent report also documents successful open heart surgery in octogenarians.[4] The point of this is clear: with appropriate care, more surgery can be done safely on "sicker" patients.

In summary, an "ideal" preoperative test would be one which is relatively inexpensive, accurate, and practical to perform in the appropriate population at risk. When positive, the test would warn of significant life-threatening outcome from either the procedure to be performed or those reasonably expected complications of the procedure. For example, our "ideal" test would tell us whether the patient would survive the procedure, even in the presence of complications. It would not, however, have to predict all of the myriad possible minor consequences of surgery from abscess to zoster. Such a single, all-encompassing test as I have described probably does not exist, but do any have potential?

Physiology of Exercise Testing

A common characteristic among the life-threatening complications listed in Table 1 is that they all are associated with deficient cellular respiration. The defect may be limited to one organ (e.g., renal failure) or it may be common to many (e.g., shock or sepsis). Cellular function, either at rest or with exercise, is dependent upon the adequate delivery of oxygen and metabolic substrate to the tissues and upon the subsequent removal of metabolic byproducts. Cellular respiration (viewed as cellular oxygenation) can be seen to be dependent on three "legs," as illustrated in Figure 1. Interruption of any of the three for a prolonged period without adequate compensatory mechanisms will result in cellular failure followed by organ failure. Oxygen is the ideal cellular requirement to consider, since few cells in any organ can exist long without it. The system designed to provide oxygen to all organs and cells is diagrammatically illustrated in Figure 2. This system includes the lungs, where oxygen is taken up from the atmosphere; the heart, which propels the oxygen-containing blood to the organs; the vessels (systemic and pulmonary), through which blood travels to the cells; and the mitochondria, which extract and utilize the oxygen. Severe problems with any part of this transport system may result in cellular malfunction. Because of homeostasis and compensatory mechanisms, this O_2 delivery system, even when disordered, may function adequately at rest. However, with exercise stress is applied throughout. As the exercising muscles consume more O_2, the flow of oxygen-containing blood must increase concomitantly, and ventilation to oxygenate the blood (and remove CO_2) must occur synchronously. Therefore, it is under stress that the potential for uncovering subtle defects in the O_2 delivery "chain" is the greatest. For example, with exercise one may see (1) claudication secondary to peripheral obstructive vascular disease; (2) angina or ST segment abnormality secondary to coronary artery disease; (3) dyspnea, hypercapnia, and hypoxemia due to pulmonary dysfunction; (4) hypotension due to cardiac dysfunction; and (5) severe lactate accumulation and acidosis associated with any or all of these. Standard measurements and calculations which can be made to detect defective O_2 delivery during a progressive incremental exercise test (and also in the postoperative critical care unit) are outlined in Table 3.

Of the measurements listed in Table 3, the most interesting is oxygen uptake in the lungs ($\dot{V}o_2$). During exercise, as work load is increased incrementally per unit time (for example, 25 watts each minute on a cycle ergometer), the $\dot{V}O_2$ also increases incrementally at a predictable rate (Fig 3). The rate of $\dot{V}O_2$ rise is based on the age of the patient, the type of work performed (seated cycle ergometer vs. walking on a treadmill), sex, and body weight. A useful equation[5] for estimating the exercise $\dot{V}O_2$ follows.

$$Predicted\ \dot{V}O_2 = 5.8 \times (weight\ in\ kg) + 151 + 10.1\ (W)$$

As the $\dot{V}O_2$ rises, at some point a plateau occurs which is called the maximal

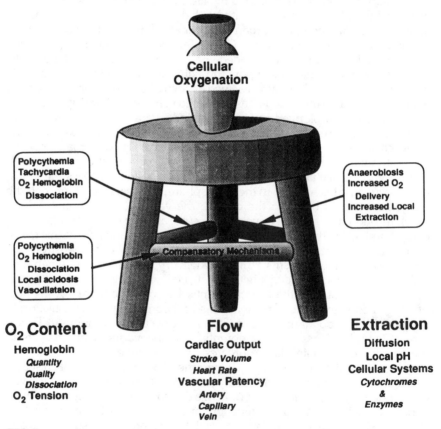

FIG 1.
Cellular oxygenation is portrayed as a fragile vase resting on a three-legged stool. The legs of the stool are O_2 content, flow, and extraction. Loss of any of the three legs could threaten cellular oxygenation. Weakness of a leg could be supported by compensatory mechanisms such as tachycardia with anemia, local vasodilation with low O_2 content, or enhanced extraction with low cardiac output.

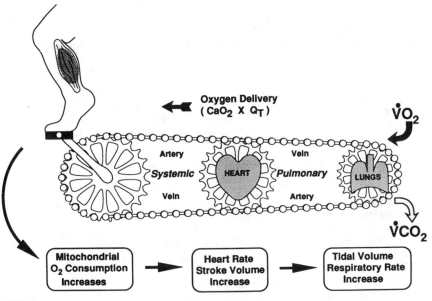

FIG 2.
Oxygen transport is illustrated as a bicycle chain which connects three coordinated systems: O_2 uptake in the lungs, cardiac output, and O_2 utilization by the mitochondria. When O_2 utilization increases, as with exercise, the entire system synchronously increases O_2 delivery. The chain connecting the three system components can also symbolize the systemic and pulmonary vasculature which must be the conduits of O_2 delivery and CO_2 removal.

$\dot{V}O_2$ or "$\dot{V}O_2$max" (see Fig 3). $\dot{V}O_2$max is the point at which further increases in work are not associated with further rises in $\dot{V}O_2$. In normal subjects, this limitation is based on age and cardiovascular limitations such as maximal heart rate rather than on abnormal vascular, mitochondrial, or lung function. In healthy normal subjects, a high $\dot{V}O_2$ max suggests "fitness." A reasonable equation[6] for predicting $\dot{V}O_2$max for a normal-weight man exercising on an ergometer follows.

Predicted $\dot{V}O_2$max (mL/min) = weight in kg $\times (50.72 - 0.372 \times$ age in years)

In subjects with disease, measured $\dot{V}O_2$max frequently is reduced. The most common abnormalities responsible for a reduced $\dot{V}O_2$max are listed in Table 4.[6] From this list it can be seen that the finding of a reduced $\dot{V}O_2$max may be relatively nonspecific and must be interpreted with other findings. These supporting data can be spirometric, blood gas, blood pressure, electrocardiographic, or others.

As work load and $\dot{V}o_2$ increase during the incremental exercise test, O_2 delivery to the exercising muscles will fall below utilization at some point, even in normal subjects. Further work beyond this point must be done anaerobically. This onset of cellular anaerobiosis is accompanied by an increase in cellular concentration, then serum lactate concentration, with a concomitant decrease in blood pH and HCO_3 levels. With the rise in serum lactate, some of the lactate will be converted to CO_2. This point is called the "AT," for anaerobic threshold, and occurs in normal subjects at or above 40% of the predicted $\dot{V}o_2$max. During the exercise study, this point is heralded by an increase in the slope of CO_2 output ($\dot{V}co_2$) (Fig 4) and, to buffer

TABLE 3.
Exercise Test Measurements

ECG (heart rate, rhythm, and R-ST architecture)
O_2 Uptake ($\dot{V}o_2$), CO_2 output ($\dot{V}co_2$), respiratory exchange ratio (R)
Minute ventilation ($\dot{V}E$)
Blood pressure (systemic, pulmonary?)
Blood gases (arterial)
Work load (watts, kilopondmeters (kpm), treadmill speed, and slope, etc.)
Oxygen transport calculations:
$\quad \dot{V}o_2$ (measured) = {inspired volume $\dot{V}I$) × inspired O_2 concentration (FIo_2)}
$\quad\quad$ – {expired volume ($\dot{V}E$) × expired O_2 concentration (FEo_2)}
$\quad \dot{V}o_2$ (calculated) = cardiac output (QT) from flow-directed thermodilution
$\quad\quad$ catheter × arteriovenous O_2 content difference
$\quad\quad$ = $QT \times (Ca - \dot{V}o_2)$
$\quad\quad$ (normal at rest = 250 mL/min)
$\quad \dot{V}co_2$ = {$\dot{V}I$ × inspired CO_2 concentration ($FIco_2$)} – {$\dot{V}E$ × expired CO_2
$\quad\quad$ concentration ($FEco_2$)}
$\quad\quad$ (normal at rest = 200 mL/min)
$\quad$ R = $\dfrac{\dot{V}co_2}{\dot{V}o_2}$
$\quad\quad$ (normal at rest = 0.8)
$\quad\quad$ (normal during exercise above anaerobic threshold [AT] = > 1.0)
$\quad O_2$ delivery = cardiac output × arterial O_2 content
$\quad\quad\quad$ = $QT \times Cao_2$
$\quad\quad$ (normal at rest = 1,000 mL/min)
$\quad O_2$ extraction = $\dfrac{\dot{V}o_2}{O_2 \text{ delivery}}$
$\quad$ or = $\dfrac{Ca - \dot{V}o_2}{Cao_2}$
$\quad\quad$ (normal at rest = 25% to 30%)

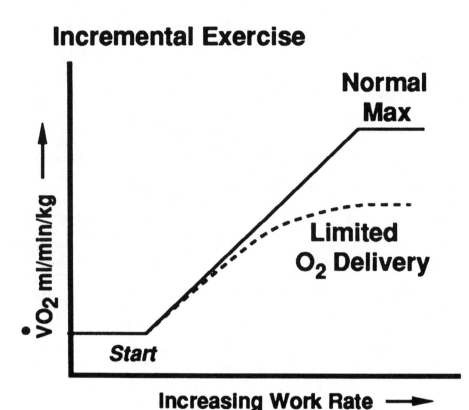

FIG 3.
Oxygen uptake ($\dot{V}_{O_2}$) is plotted on the ordinate against work rate on the abscissa. During incremental exercise, $\dot{V}_{O_2}$ increases predictably in the normal subject to a maximal level determined primarily by cardiac output. In patients with limited O_2 transport/delivery mechanisms, $\dot{V}_{O_2}$ will be limited on exercise and may never reach normal $\dot{V}_{O_2}$max. (Adapted from Wasserman K, Hansen JE, Sue DY, et al: *Principles of Exercise Testing and Interpretation.* Philadelphia, Lea & Febiger, 1987.)

the increased hydrogen ion concentration, an increase in minute ventilation ($\dot{V}_E$).

In summary, the incremental exercise study evaluates the entire O_2 delivery axis (lung-heart-tissue). This test has the potential to uncover abnormalities which may be obscure at rest unless the investigator uses a multiplicity of potentially more invasive and expensive tests.

Relationship of Exercise Physiology to the Postoperative State

In the perioperative period of any major surgical procedure, multiple physiological processes and abnormalities are seen.[7, 8] For example, a rise in $\dot{V}_{O_2}$ of 10% to 30% may be seen with just the postoperative state. With stress, such as receiving postural drainage and chest percussion, $\dot{V}_{O_2}$ can increase up to 35%. Major burns can increase energy (and O_2) requirements up to 170%. Fever produces a 7.2% increase in caloric expenditure for every degree Fahrenheit increase in temperature. Any increase in metabolism will, in general, also require more oxygen. It appears, therefore, that surgery produces stress on energy requirements and secondarily on the oxygen transport axis. Further stress would be predicted with the addition of morbid complications. Atelectasis, pulmonary edema, pneumonia, and bronchospasm may significantly increase the work and "oxygen cost" of breathing. Severe anemia and hypovolemia can complicate O_2 transport problems even further. If morbid complications are severe and progressive, they may lead to multiorgan failure when multiple O_2 transport and metabolic defects are present. In these critically ill postoperative patients, $\dot{V}_{O_2}$ and O_2 delivery rise early, but then may actually fall terminally as a manifestation of multiorgan failure and the inadequacy of oxygen delivery. Shoemaker and colleagues measured the cumulative tissue oxygen debt perioperatively in 98 consecutive high-risk patients.[9] These investigators then correlated these measurements with the development of lethal and nonlethal postoperative organ

---

TABLE 4.
Causes of Reduced $\dot{V}_{O_2}$max*

Anemia/carboxyhemoglobinemia
Heart disease
Metabolic disease
Muscular disease
Peripheral vascular disease
Pulmonary disease
Poor effort

*From Wasserman K, Hansen JE, Sue DY, et al: *Principles of Exercise Testing and Interpretation*. Philadelphia, Lea & Febiger, 1987. Used by permission.

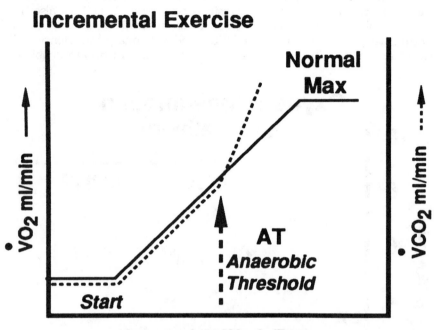

FIG 4.
Oxygen uptake ($\dot{V}o_2$) and CO_2 output ($\dot{V}co_2$) are plotted on the ordinates against an incrementally increasing work rate. As O_2 utilization by the exercising muscle exceeds O_2 delivery, $\dot{V}co_2$ from lactate metabolism will exceed $\dot{V}o_2$ ($r > 1.0$) at a point called "AT," for anaerobic threshold. (Adapted from Wasserman K, Hansen JE, Sue DY, et al: *Principles of Exercise Testing and Interpretation.* Philadelphia, Lea & Febiger, 1987.)

failure. The maximal oxygen debt was determined as the measured $\dot{V}o_2$ minus the estimated O_2 requirement. The O_2 debt was found to be highest in nonsurvivors (33.5 ± 36.9 L/m²), intermediate in survivors with organ failure (26.6 ± 32.1 L/m²), and lowest in survivors without organ failure (8.0 ± 10.9 L/m²). This strongly suggests that those postoperative patients unable to provide O_2 transport to meet their O_2 requirements may sustain single or multiorgan failure.

Recently, a relationship has been described between reductions in oxygen delivery and oxygen consumption. This relationship between $\dot{V}o_2$ and O_2 delivery is illustrated in Figure 5. At some point, oxygen consumption ($\dot{V}o_2$) appears to become dependent upon O_2 delivery. This suggests that a limitation of O_2 delivery to the tissue (associated with a failure of compensatory mechanisms [see Fig 1]) may result in a reduction of cellular O_2

consumption and then in organ failure. This phenomenon is reported most frequently in the adult respiratory distress syndrome (ARDS) but also has been described in other entities such as sepsis, hypovolemic shock, chronic obstructive pulmonary disease (COPD), and pulmonary hypertension. It would appear possible, therefore, that those patients who are unable to

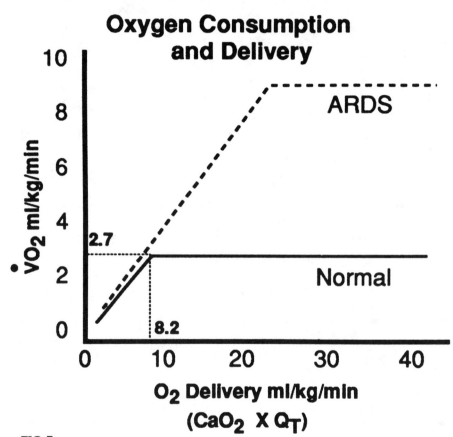

FIG 5.
Oxygen uptake ($\dot{V}O_2$) is plotted on the ordinate against O_2 delivery on the abscissa. In normal subjects at rest, $\dot{V}O_2$ of the tissues is not compromised until O_2 delivery falls below 8.2 mL/kg/min. This point has been called the "critical threshold." In patients with systemic O_2 transport problems such as the adult respiratory distress syndrome (ARDS), $\dot{V}O_2$ may become directly dependent upon O_2 delivery at a much higher point (e.g., 21 mL/kg/min). (Adapted from Shibutani K, Komatsu T, Kubal K, et al: *Crit Care Med* 1983; 11:640, Danek SJ, Lynch JP, Weg JD, et al: *Am Rev Respir Dis* 1980; 122:387, and Mosenifar Z, Goldbach P, Tashkin DP, et al: *Chest* 1983; 84:267.)

sustain an elevated cardiac output and O_2 delivery may be susceptible to single- or multiorgan failure postoperatively. A reasonable hypothesis would suggest that those who are limited in generating a high $\dot{V}O_2$ (O_2 delivery) on the stress of preoperative exercise also may be those unable to do so in response to the stress of the (complicated) postoperative period.

Preoperative Exercise Testing and Postoperative Complications

Monitoring of the electrocardiogram (ECG) during treadmill exercise has been used for decades to predict the presence of coronary artery disease. In populations at an increased risk for coronary artery disease, a J-point and ST-segment depression, ventricular ectopy, or hypotension can be highly sensitive and predictive of the disease. Predictive accuracy, however, decreases in populations who are at lower risk (e.g., young women). An association between preoperative cardiac abnormalities and postoperative cardiac events and mortality has been shown.[10,11] Exercise testing usually is not required to assess cardiac risk preoperatively, but it has been used. Gerson and coworkers[12] found that the inability to perform 2 minutes of supine cycle ergometer exercise to raise the heart rate to over 99 beats per minute was more predictive of postoperative cardiac complications than were clinical findings or exercise radionuclide ventriculography in elderly subjects. This study suggests that a limited cardiac reserve on exercise may portend an adverse outcome of noncardiac surgery.

Preoperative pulmonary function evaluation to predict pulmonary complications of nonthoracic, thoracic, and cardiovascular surgery has been reviewed recently.[13] It is in the area of preoperative evaluation for lung resection that the most interesting exercise data reside.[14] These studies can be roughly divided into those assessing (1) the simple accomplishment of a fixed exercise challenge (e.g., stair climb of x flights), (2) the prediction of post-resectional pulmonary hypertension, and (3) the measurement of exercise $\dot{V}O_2$ to predict postoperative morbidity and mortality.

Exercise Accomplishment

The first such study was published by Gaensler and co-investigators in 1955.[15] They found little predictive value in measuring minute ventilation during a level walk of 180 feet in 1 minute. For a 70-kg man, this mild exercise is equal to about 25 W on an ergometer and would require a $\dot{V}O_2$ of 800 mL/min or 12 mL/kg/min.

Positive results, however, were reported in 1972 by Reichel.[16] In his study, 31 of 75 preoperative patients were exercised using an incremental treadmill protocol. The exercise was terminated with severe symptoms or when the patient reached 3 mph at 10% grade for a total exercise time of 14 minutes. Those reaching this pinnacle suffered no complications or mortality. This level of exercise equates to approximately 100 W on a cycle ergometer and a $\dot{V}O_2$ of 1,750 mL/min or 25 mL/kg/min for a 70-kg man. The results of the exercise test were more accurate in predicting post-resectional complications (24% mortality, 17% major morbidity) than were the resting ECG, blood gases, diffusing capacity, lung volumes, spirometry, or measurements of intrapulmonary gas (helium) mixing.

In 1987, Bolton and coworkers[17] reported an association between stairs climbed and spirometric pulmonary function. They found that those elderly men able to climb 127 steps successfully demonstrated a forced vital capacity (FVC) $\geq$ 2.5 L and a forced expiratory volume in 1 second (FEV_1) > 1.75 L. A climb of 5 flights (127 steps, each 17.4 cm high) by a 70-kg man at 60 steps/min would be a work rate of about 120 W and would require a $\dot{V}O_2$ of approximately 1,759 mL/min or 25 mL/kg/min. No specific association with postoperative outcome was sought in this study, but surgeons have been using this test preoperatively for many years.

Prediction of Postoperative Pulmonary Hypertension

Early clinicians were concerned about pulmonary hypertension and cor pulmonale following lung resection. This complication occurs secondary to the resection of functioning lung and vascular bed in patients with parenchymal abnormality in the remaining lung. Right heart catheterization was combined with exercise to test the compliance of the pulmonary vasculature to the increased cardiac output. Some workers added an inflatable balloon to the catheter tip to occlude the pulmonary artery of the lung to be resected. This unilateral pulmonary artery occlusion tested vascular compliance further by forcing all cardiac output through the lung destined to remain. Severe pulmonary hypertension and hypoxemia during this procedure portended a poor outcome following resection.[18] This balloon occlusion technique is expensive and technically difficult, and generally has been discarded.

In 1975, Fee and co-investigators[19] reported their findings using treadmill exercise with a flow-directed right-heart catheterization prior to lung resection. They divided their 45-patient population into two groups based on spirometric and Pao_2 criteria. Both groups of patients were then exercised at two workloads: 2 mph at 4% grade, then 4 mph at 4% grade. These exercise rates equate, in a 70-kg man, to 27 and 54 W on a cycle ergometer with predicted $\dot{V}O_2$ levels of 830 mL/min (12 mL/kg/min) and 1.1 L/min (16 mL/kg/min), respectively. In the study, cardiac outputs and pulmonary vascular pressures were measured every minute during exercise and were used in the calculation of pulmonary vascular resistance (PVR). Thirty of the 45 patients received a thoracotomy and 5 died. All the deaths occurred in the patients whose PVR was more than 190 dyne·seconds·cm^{-5} and 4 of the 5 had been in the group with the "better" spirometric function and higher Pao_2. Thus, in this study, it appears that pulmonary vascular disease, and probably defects in O_2 transport as well, were limiting factors in survival. Unfortunately, $\dot{V}O_2$ levels were not measured.

Measurement of $\dot{V}o_2$ on Exercise

This newest area of investigation appears to be the most exciting, yet also the most perplexing. Following the description of quantitative lung scanning to predict spirometric lung function after lung resection in the mid-1970s,[13] there were few new ideas proposed until the brief publication by Eugene in 1982.[20] In this study of 19 patients with a range of spirometric function, an incremental exercise test to "maximum" was performed. In some studies, the word "maximum" is substituted for "maximal" if the $\dot{V}o_2$max plateau (see Fig 3) was not sought and the patients were exercised to their symptomatic limit. These workers found that following lung resection, there were 3 postoperative deaths. All 15 survivors demonstrated a measured $\dot{V}o_2$max with exercise of > 1L (1.299 ± .048 L/min) and all 3 nonsurvivors had a $\dot{V}o_2$ of < 1L (.821 L ± 0.34 L/min). No suggestion was offered as to how the low $\dot{V}o_2$max predicted the postoperative mortality.

Smith and co-investigators reported their results in 1984.[21] Those workers studied 22 patients prior to thoracotomy with routine pulmonary function tests, quantitative scintillation lung scanning, and incremental exercise testing. They found that a low $\dot{V}o_2$max was predictive not only of failure to survive resection but also of nonfatal complications as well. These nonfatal complications included transient respiratory failure, pneumonia, myocardial infarction, atelectasis, and cardiac arrthythmias requiring therapy. The lung scan prediction of post-resection spirometric lung function failed to identify the patients with complications. These investigators noted that 6 of 6 patients experiencing complications demonstrated an exercise $\dot{V}o_2$max < 15 mL/kg/min, whereas only 1 of 10 patients with a $\dot{V}o_2$max > 20 mL/kg/min suffered a nonfatal complication. Again, no pathophysiological mechanism was proposed to explain how $\dot{V}o_2$max predicted morbidity or mortality.

In 1987, Bechard and Wetstein[22] reported their findings on 50 consecutive thoracotomy patients studied with incremental exercise to exhaustion or dyspnea. They sought and reported the same nonfatal complications (see Smith et al.[21]) in 6 of the 50 patients (12%). Two fatalities and 5 patients suffering survivable morbidity had preoperative $\dot{V}o_2$max levels < 10 mL/kg/min (P < .001). Anaerobic threshold also was significantly lower in the group with complications. These workers also did not propose a hypothesis to explain their results.

Miyoshi and colleagues[23] also published positive results in 1987. These workers studied 33 patients using routine pulmonary function studies and incremental exercise testing. Rather than simply measuring $\dot{V}o_2$ alone, these investigators also assessed exercise-induced anaerobiosis. They measured serum lactate concentrations during the last 30 seconds of each work rate. They compared the $\dot{V}o_2$ to the lactate levels and corrected for body surface area (BSA). They measured the $\dot{V}o_2$ per meter of BSA at a submaximal exercise lactate level of 20 mg/dL (2.2 mM/L or mEq/L) and called it the "$\dot{V}o_2$/BSA at La-20." This $\dot{V}o_2$ measurement at a specific lactate level

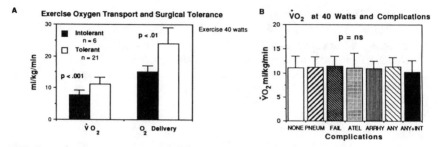

FIG 6.
A, oxygen transport ($\dot{V}o_2$ and O_2 delivery) during 40 W of steady-state exercise is compared in those patients who tolerated lung resection (*open bars*) to those who were intolerant of the resection (*closed bars*). There is a statistically significant difference in O_2 transport parameters between these two groups. **B**, oxygen uptake ($\dot{V}o_2$) is plotted on the ordinate against the various nonfatal complications found in the tolerant group. *NONE* = no complications (41% of the tolerant patients); *PNEUM* = pneumonia (23%); *FAIL* = transient respiratory failure (27%); *ATEL* = atelectasis requiring bronchoscopy (27%); *ARRHY* = arrhythmia requiring therapy (41%); *ANY* = any complications (59% of the tolerant group); *ANY + INT* = the $\dot{V}o_2$ of the "any" complication subgroup combined with the intolerant group. The $\dot{V}o_2$ failed to reveal a statistically significant difference between any of these subgroups. (Data from Olsen GN, Weiman DS, Bolton JWR et al: *Chest* 1989; 95:267–273.

discriminated those patients who survived complications after lung resection from those who succumbed. However, these workers found that nonfatal complications were higher in the group with the worst spirometric lung function, but were not predicted by the exercise $\dot{V}o_2$.

Our own experience is similar to that of Miyoshi et al.[23] We reported the results of preoperative submaximal exercise testing in 29 lung resection patients.[24] Seven of our patients failed to tolerate lung resection (intolerant group), with 5 dying perioperatively and 2 requiring prolonged (300 days) mechanical ventilation. All 29 patients were elderly and had severe preoperative pulmonary dysfunction ($FEV_1 < 2$ L). Our patients were studied at 25 and 40 W using nonincremental "steady-state" cycle ergometer exercise, and systemic arterial and flow-directed pulmonary artery catheterization was performed. These invasive procedures provided systemic arterial and pulmonary artery blood gases and thermal dilution cardiac output so that multiple O_2 transport parameters could be assessed. These exercise findings then were compared to clinical and lung function data obtained at rest. The results illustrated in Figure 6 suggest that the "intolerant" patients had significantly lower cardiac outputs, $\dot{V}o_2$, and O_2 delivery at 40 W of submaximal exercise than did the tolerant group. The pH decrement with exercise in our patients was similar to that which would have accompanied the lactate levels reported by Miyoshi and coworkers.[23] The data obtained at rest failed to predict the intolerant group. No relationship was demonstrated between exercise $\dot{V}o_2$ and the occurrence of survivable complications, however.

The results of these studies[20-24] are in sharp contrast to two reports published thus far not to find exercise $\dot{V}o_2$ predictive of risk. Colman and colleagues[25] reported a prospective study of 59 patients evaluated with routine pulmonary function tests and incremental exercise to maximum $\dot{V}o_2$. In addition to the physiological complications normally associated with lung resection (see Smith et al.[21] earlier), these investigators also looked for "technical" complications such as excess blood loss, air leak, empyema, and wound infection. They were unable to detect a difference in $\dot{V}o_2$max between the group sustaining complications and the group free of complications. Other than this difficulty in associating $\dot{V}o_2$max with technical postoperative complications such as an air leak, the reason this study's results are negative is not clear. Similar results were recently reported by Markos and coworkers.[26] They found the lung scan prediction more accurate than exercise $\dot{V}o_2$.

Conclusion

A review of these studies, especially those reported in the last several years, provides a compelling case for a relationship between failure of O_2 delivery ($\dot{V}o_2$) during exercise and operative risk. What is yet to be established are the pathophysiological mechanisms to explain the association.

Most important in providing an "ounce of prevention" is knowing how to identify those at the highest risk. If noninvasive exercise testing can predict postoperative single- or multiorgan failure in the patients at the greatest clinical risk, then two benefits accrue: (1) surgery can be offered to more patients who were previously thought to be physiologically inoperable, and (2) surgery can be withheld from those at the very highest risk of postoperative disabling morbidity or mortality.

References

1. Tremper KK, Friedman AE, Levine EM, et al: The preoperative treatment of severely anemic patients with a perfluorochemical oxygen-transport fluid, Fluosol-DA. *N Engl J Med* 1982; 307:277–283.
2. Weiss W: Operative mortality and five year survival rates in patients with bronchogenic carcinoma. *Am J Surg* 1974; 128:799–804.
3. Sherman S, Guidot CE: The feasibility of thoracotomy for lung cancer in the elderly. *JAMA* 1987; 258:927–930.
4. Edmonds LH, Stephenson LW, Edie RN, et al: Open-heart surgery in octogenarians. *N Engl J Med* 1988; 319:131–136.
5. Wasserman K, Whipp BJ: Exercise physiology in health and disease. *Am Rev Respir Dis* 1975; 112:219–259.

6. Wasserman K, Hansen JE, Sue DY, et al: *Principles of Exercise Testing and Interpretation.* Philadelphia, Lea & Febiger, 1987.
7. Rehder K, Sessler AD, March HM: General anesthesia and the lung. *Am Rev Respir Dis* 1975; 112:541–563.
8. Gump FE, Martin P, Kinney JM: Oxygen consumption and caloric expenditure in surgical patients. *Surg Gynecol Obstet* 1973; 137:499–513. *This paper reviews those factors which affect the body's metabolic response to the stress of major surgery.*
9. Shoemaker WC, Appel PL, Kram HB: Tissue oxygen debt as a determinant of lethal and non-lethal postoperative organ failure. *Crit Care Med* 1988; 16:1117–1120. *This interesting report suggests that the inability to meet the high oxygen consumption requirements induced by the severe complications of surgery correlates with survival and organ failure.*
10. Goldman L, Caldera DL, Nussbaum SR, et al: Multifactorial index of cardiac risk in non-cardiac surgical procedures. *N Engl J Med* 1977; 297:845–850. *This classic study established many of the now-standard cardiac risk factors for surgery.*
11. Goldman L: Cardiac risks and complications of non-cardiac surgery. *Ann Intern Med* 1983; 98:504–513. *This recent report reviews and updates the previous findings on cardiac risk.*
12. Gerson MC, Hurst JM, Hertzberg VS, et al: Cardiac prognosis in non-cardiac geriatric surgery. *Ann Intern Med* 1985; 103:832–837. *The premise of this report is that exercise may be more predictive of postoperative cardiac risk than some of the "Goldman" criteria.*
13. Gass GD, Olsen GN: Preoperative pulmonary function testing to predict postoperative morbidity and mortality. *Chest* 1986; 89:127–135. *A review article on preoperative pulmonary function testing.*
14. Olsen GN: The evolving role of exercise testing prior to lung resection. *Chest* 1989; 95:218–225. *A recent review of exercise testing in evaluating lung resection patients.*
15. Gaensler EA, Cogell DW, Lindgren I, et al: The role of pulmonary insufficiency in mortality and invalidism following surgery for pulmonary tuberculosis. *J Thorac Cardiovasc Surg* 1955; 29:16–87. *This "classic" paper was one of the first to suggest that preoperative pulmonary function testing could predict postoperative mortality.*
16. Reichel J: Assessment of operative risk of pneumonectomy. *Chest* 1972; 62:570–576. *This retrospective analysis suggested that the completion of a treadmill exercise protocol was associated with low mortality and morbidity in lung resection.*
17. Bolton JWR, Weiman DS, Haynes JL, et al: Stair climbing as an indicator of pulmonary function. *Chest* 1987; 92:783–788. *A study relating the completion of stair climbing to measured resting pulmonary function test results.*
18. Uggla LG: Indications for and results of thoracic surgery with regard to respiratory and circulatory function tests. *Acta Chir Scand* 1956; 111:197–213. *One of the few studies suggesting that balloon occlusion of the pulmonary artery plus exercise may predict post–lung resection mortality or cardiopulmonary "crippling."*
19. Fee JH, Holmes EC, Gerwitz HS, et al: Role of pulmonary resistance measurement in preoperative evaluation of candidates for lung resection. *J Thorac*

Cardiovasc Surg 1975; 75:519–524. *This study suggests that high preoperative pulmonary vascular resistance on exercise predicts postoperative mortality.*

20. Eugene J, Brown SE, Light RW, et al: Maximum oxygen consumption: A physiologic guide to pulmonary resection. *Surg Forum* 1982; 33:260–262. *The first brief report linking reduced exercise maximum oxygen consumption to postoperative mortality in lung resection.*

21. Smith TO, Kinasewitz GT, Tucker WY, et al: Exercise capacity as a predictor of post-thoracotomy morbidity. *Am Rev Respir Dis* 1984; 129:730–734. *This study suggests that a reduced preoperative exercise maximum oxygen consumption can predict not only postoperative mortality, but also morbidity.*

22. Bechard D, Wetstein L: Assessment of exercise oxygen consumption as preoperative criteria for lung resection. *Ann Thorac Surg* 1987; 44:344–349. *A study of 50 consecutive lung resection patients also showing that a low preoperative exercise maximum oxygen consumption predicts postoperative mortality and morbidity.*

23. Miyoshi S, Nakahara K, Ohno K, et al: Exercise tolerance test in lung cancer patients; the relationship between exercise capacity and post-thoracotomy hospital mortality. *Ann Thorac Surg* 1987; 44:487–490. *This study suggests that a low exercise oxygen consumption at a fixed lactate production is predictive of postoperative mortality, but not morbidity, in lung resection patients.*

24. Olsen GN, Weiman DS, Bolton JWR, et al: Submaximal invasive exercise testing and quantitative lung scanning in the evaluation for tolerance of lung resection. *Chest* 1989; 94:267–273. *This recent study suggests that a low calculated submaximal exercise oxygen consumption and delivery preoperatively is associated with postoperative mortality but is not predictive of morbidity.*

25. Colman NC, Schraufnagel DE, Rivington RN, et al: Exercise testing in evaluation of patients for lung resection. *Am Rev Respir Dis* 1982; 125:604–606. *This is one of the few studies published that found no relationship between exercise oxygen consumption and postoperative mortality or morbidity.*

26. Markos J, Mullan BP, Hillman DR, et al: Preoperative assessment as a predictor of mortality and morbidity after lung resection. *Am Rev Respir Dis* 1989; 139:902–910. *Calculations of predicted postoperative lung function using data for quantitative lung scans were better predictors than exercise oxygen consumption.*

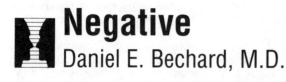

Negative
Daniel E. Bechard, M.D.

With the improvement in anesthetic and surgical techniques, surgical intervention is now being offered to patients of increased age and with significant systemic disease. The decision to operate requires weighing the risks and benefits of medical and surgical therapy against the natural history of the disease process. The eventual success of the surgical procedure requires accurate diagnosis and operative risk assessment, proper preoperative preparation, correct timing, proper surgical technique, and appropriate postoperative care. Of these, improved operative risk assessment offers the greatest hope for significantly lowering operative morbidity and mortality.

Many modalities of risk assessment have been examined, and the determination of exercise capacity is currently in vogue. Exercise stress testing has been studied extensively and utilized for predicting coronary artery disease. However, over the past 10 years, exercise testing has gained increased interest as a means of assessing operative risk, not only for cardiac surgery but also for general surgery and, more specifically, for thoracotomy. This explosive interest in exercise testing is the result of several factors. With the increasing life span of our population and the maturation of the "baby boom" generation, operative procedures are being offered to an increasing number of patients with advanced age, which is a well-recognized operative risk factor. In an attempt to offer surgical therapy (which in most cases is life-prolonging) to the broadest group of patients, physicians are actively seeking more sensitive and specific means of preoperative assessment. Escalating health care costs compel the physician to identify those patients at increased risk for postoperative complications. Once identified, the institution of specific measures theoretically could lessen postoperative morbidity, mortality, and hospitalization costs. Finally, operative intervention remains the only proven curative option in the treatment of lung cancer, a leading cause of death in the United States. Unfortunately, many lung cancer patients suffer from comorbid diseases such as chronic obstructive lung disease and cardiovascular diseases, complicating the assessment of operative risk.

Determining a patient's exercise capacity as a means of ascertaining operative risk is not a novel concept. It is postulated that the increase in cardiac output and myocardial oxygen consumption generated by exercise reproduces the cardiovascular stresses of a major surgical procedure. If this were true, patients at increased risk for postoperative complications could be identified. Most exercise testing in the past has concentrated on identifying ischemic changes in response to stress using the well-known cardiac stress test. Few studies have addressed the cardiovascular and pulmonary physiological responses to exercise. Despite the obvious appeal of assessing the physiological exercise capacity as an indicator of operative risk, it has not been applied routinely to the clinical setting due to the unwieldy equipment that is required (Douglas bags, Tissot spirometers, pneumotachometers, gas analyzers, etc.). However, with the advent of microprocessor technology and its incorporation into clinical medicine, exercise physiology testing has become a less cumbersome process. The manufacturers claim that minimal space is required to run the equipment and technical expertise is developed easily. All of this increases the appeal of an office-based setup. The equipment is smartly packaged with a variety of software programs and is readily available in the marketplace today.

This new accessibility to exercise physiology testing has raised concerns that its clinical application will be justified by the "newness" of the technology, rather than by its "soundness" and actual clinical benefit. This is no trivial matter when one considers the number of patients undergoing preoperative assessment per year. Thus, it is appropriate that our topic of debate addresses this very issue. I have been asked to determine whether *exercise testing is valuable in predicting operative risk*. Please note that I am not debating whether exercise testing predicts operative risk, but rather whether it is valuable in predicting operative risk. To be of value in predicting operative risk, I submit that exercise physiology testing satisfy the following criteria:

1. The test must offer a unique, more specific, and more sensitive method of assessing operative risk than that currently offered by "standard" techniques. The information obtained must be useful in determining the therapeutic course.

2. The test must be reliable and reproducible.

3. The test must be readily available and cost-effective.

4. The appropriate group of patients requiring the study must be clearly defined.

The type of exercise testing I will examine involves the incorporation of gas exchange analysis into the exercise protocol, specifically oxygen uptake (Vo_2) and carbon dioxide production (Vco_2). This method of testing has many labels: cardiopulmonary exercise testing, exercise physiology testing, exercise with gas exchange analysis, etc. The underlying principle is the same, however. The patient exercises, usually on a treadmill or cycle ergometer, while exhaled gases are analyzed and the Vo_2 and Vco_2 are determined. This methodology also allows for the detection of the anaerobic threshold, although this parameter has had little impact on preoperative assessment due to the debilitated state of the majority of patients.

Exercise Physiology Testing Offers a More Sensitive Means of Assessing Operative Risk

In order to examine this all-important point, it is necessary to group the available studies on the basis of the nature of the surgery performed. There is a marked disparity in the number of studies and their findings based on the type of surgery performed.

Nonthoracic Surgery

Very few well-controlled studies are available which address the role of exercise physiology studies in assessing the operative risk of nonthoracic surgery (i.e., abdominal, peripheral vascular, orthopedic, etc.). These studies are limited primarily to estimating the risk for cardiac complications. Carliner et al[1] found no benefit from routine exercise testing in predicting cardiac complications in patients undergoing major noncardiac surgery. This and other studies have found no added benefit of exercise studies over the physical status scale of the American Society of Anesthesiologists (ASA)[2] or Goldman's multifactorial risk analysis[3] in assessing operative risk. Thus, in nonthoracic surgery, there is no evidence that exercise physiology testing is of any value in assessing operative risk compared to standard clinical physical and cardiac status assessment. Therefore, the application of exercise physiology testing to assess operative risk in the general surgery population is not justified at this time. However, more controlled studies utilizing maximal exercise testing are necessary to fully evaluate this large operative group.

Cardiac Surgery

Surprisingly, there are few studies examining the role of exercise physiology testing in assessing the operative risks, other than mortality, in patients undergoing coronary artery bypass surgery. Two studies found no correlation between exercise performance and postoperative survival.[4,5] One study reported that peak exercise performance correlated with survival, though no better than clinical or angiographic assessment.[6] The standard cardiac stress test has been the exercise study commonly employed to assess the extent of ischemic disease. However, this exercise modality has fallen into clinical disfavor with the multicenter Coronary Artery Surgery Study (CASS), which reported dipyridamole thallium-201 reperfusion radionuclide testing to be more specific and sensitive in assessing the extent of ischemia than the standard exercise stress test.[7] In addition, identifying patients at increased risk for morbidity becomes a relatively moot point in patients with life-threatening three-vessel or left main coronary disease. Most of these patients will be considered for life-prolonging surgery regardless of their underlying condition. It comes down to the question of what is an acceptable risk for surgery in patients with a life-threatening disease.

In summary, exercise physiology testing has not been evaluated adequately in assessing patients for coronary surgery. There are no substantial data to support exercise physiology testing as a risk assessment tool in cardiac surgery. Even if these data were available, it is unlikely that they would dramatically alter the decision to operate, given the life-threatening nature of the underlying condition. There are a few preliminary studies advocating the use of exercise physiology testing to aid in the timing of surgery in patients with aortic stenosis or ventricular-septal defects. If these initial studies are supported by well-planned and well-executed multicenter trials, it may represent a defined and limited application of exercise physiology testing in patients with cardiovascular disorders.

Noncardiac Thoracic Surgery

I have limited this surgical category to thoracotomy with lung resection performed primarily in an attempt to cure lung carcinoma, which is a uniformly fatal disease. In this respect, the clinical condition is similar to that of coronary artery disease, although the life expectancy is somewhat longer in the case of lung carcinoma. However, we are faced again with the question of determining what represents an acceptable surgical risk (morbidity and mortality) in patients who will die of their disease if not cured surgically. To complicate matters further, this group of patients is extremely difficult to assess for operative risk due to the existence of comorbid diseases and the fact that pulmonary function will be directly affected by the surgical resection. Thus, the physician has to be concerned that the patient may be cured of lung cancer only to end up as a pulmonary cripple. In assessing these patients, physicians must determine their ability to tolerate resection as well as the general stress of surgery.

Faced with these problems, it is not surprising that the bulk of exercise physiology studies are found in this group of extremely complicated patients. The rationale for using exercise studies in assessing these patients is complex, but seems to reside in the purported ability of exercise testing to accomplish one or more of the following: (1) predict pulmonary function test (PFTs) results; (2) predict operability; (3) predict postoperative morbidity; and (4) predict postoperative mortality.

Predicting PFTs.—Exercise testing, primarily in the form of stair climbing, has been advocated by our surgical colleagues for many years as a means of assessing operability.[8] Though few clinical trials have investigated this practice, it is considered a "time-honored" method of preoperative assessment and commonly is passed down from house officer to house officer. The rationale for this practice is that stair climbing predicts static pulmonary function, which in turn reflects operability.[9] Bolton et al.[10] reported a significant correlation ($r = .69$) between standard PFTs and stair climbing. The authors suggest that this correlation indicates that stair climbing may be helpful in preoperative assessment. However, multiple studies have shown no correlation between exercise testing and preoperative PFTs. A recent study by Bechard and Wetstein prospectively examined the predictive value of preoperative PFTs in 59 patients undergoing thoracotomy and found no correlation between PFTs and postoperative complications.[11] Furthermore, no prospective studies on stair climbing performance and postoperative complications are available to determine whether this form of exercise testing has any role in preoperative assessment. A preliminary study by this author examined the ability of stair climbing performance to predict postoperative complications in 27 patients and found no predictive value. Thus, there is little, if any, correlation between exercise capacity and PFTs, and even less correlation between PFTs and postoperative complications.

Predicting Operability.—The determination of resectability (i.e., adequate postoperative pulmonary reserve) is based primarily on PFTs combined with split-function lung perfusion studies. However, several studies have incorporated exercise physiology studies in an attempt to enhance the assessment of resectability. The determination of pulmonary vascular resistance by flow-directed pulmonary catheters and balloon occlusion has been reported to aid in determining operability. However, identifying the patients who would benefit from these invasive studies has proven difficult. Brundler et al. reported that 59% of patients evaluated preoperatively with a flow-directed pulmonary artery (PA) catheter during exercise had evidence of pulmonary hypertension, and they found standard preoperative evaluation to be of little help in differentiating these patients.[12] Thus, preoperative exercise testing with invasive hemodynamic monitoring would need to be applied to all patients, given the current state of knowledge. Since this is obviously impractical, should we evaluate only those patients undergoing pneumonectomy? If so, should we evaluate all pneumonectomy candidates or only those with "borderline" pulmonary function? Certainly these questions must be answered before widespread clinical application of this type of exercise assessment can be advocated.

Others have suggested monitoring exercise performance during balloon occlusion of the pertinent bronchus as a method of determining resectability.[13] Though this method offers the advantages of noninvasiveness and strict anatomical evaluation, the study consisted of only six patients and assessed only survival. Certainly it is too early to recommend that such testing be applied clinically. Thus, although there are a few studies reporting enhancement in the determination of resectability through the application of exercise studies, well-designed prospective clinical trials are necessary to fully assess their utility and to define the patient group most likely to benefit from these additional studies.

Predicting Postoperative Morbidity.—Perhaps the greatest application of exercise testing in lung resection candidates has been in predicting postoperative morbidity. The studies are balanced fairly evenly between those that report benefit and those that do not. However, attempts at critically evaluating these studies are hampered by differences in exercise formats, definitions of complications, lengths of time studied, and endpoint determinations. If we limit our evaluations to those studies with similar designs and definitions, the conclusions are still contradictory. Two studies of very similar design found exercise performance to be highly predictive of postoperative morbidity. Expressing exercise performance as maximal O_2 consumption per minute per kilogram of body weight ($\dot{V}o_2$max), Smith et al.[14] reported that 92% of postoperative complications occurred in patients with a $\dot{V}o_2$max of less than 20 mL/min/kg, and that morbidity occurred in all patients with a $\dot{V}o_2$max of less than 15 mL/min/kg. Using identical exercise parameters, Bechard and Wetstein[11] reported an even lower cutoff value for the development of postoperative morbidity. Patients with a $\dot{V}o_2$max of less than 10 mL/min/kg had a 71% complication rate, whereas patients with a $\dot{V}o_2$max of greater than 10 mL/min/kg had only a 7% complication rate. However, Colman et al.[15] and Miyoshi et al.[16] reported that preoperative exercise performance yielded no added predictive value for postoperative morbidity compared to standard assessment strategies. It should be noted that these contradictory studies utilized different complication criteria and exercise designs. Thus, their findings may not truly contradict those of Smith and Bechard.

Even if we accept that exercise performance predicts postoperative morbidity (which I feel it does), will it alter our overall therapeutic approach? Will we deny a patient the opportunity of a curative resection because he is at risk for atrial fibrillation, atelectasis, or pneumonia? What added interventions will we employ? All patients are followed acutely postoperatively, usually in surgical intensive care units (ICUs), with intensive nursing and respiratory therapy intervention. What else can we add to those patients "at risk" for complications? I will even concede that exercise performance is more sensitive than standard preoperative PFTs in predicting postoperative morbidity, but so what? It has been well established that PFTs are insensitive indicators of the postoperative course. What needs to be addressed is how exercise performance compares to more sensitive indicators of the postoperative course (i.e., ASA physical status, Goldman's multifactorial risk analysis). None of the studies to date have examined this. It may well be that the highly technical and expensive exercise studies are no better than the physical examination in predicting postoperative complications.

Thus, I submit that even though exercise performance seems to be a more sensitive predictor of postoperative complications based on two studies, it is clinically of no added value in assessing operative risk. Exercise performance has not been assessed adequately against the more sensitive clinical predictors of operative risk. In addition, the ability to predict postoperative morbidity has limited clinical value in and of itself. Due to the terminal nature of lung cancer, we are not about to deny a curative procedure on the basis of increased risk for atelectasis or pneumonia. As in coronary artery disease, postoperative morbidity is a relatively moot point when confronted with a uniformly fatal disease process.

Predicting Postoperative Mortality.—This represents the crucial aspect of assessing operative risk. If we could reliably identify those patients unable to survive the proposed surgical intervention, we could avoid the needless suffering, stress, operative time, and cost generated by a hopeless surgical venture. It is well established that as a patient's exercise capacity deteriorates, the risk for postoperative death increases. However, is there a level of exercise impairment that accurately predicts a fatal outcome? To address this question, we will look at three recent studies comparing exercise performance with postoperative mortality.

Smith et al.[14] reported a mortality rate of 9% (2 of 22), and the patients with fatal outcomes had Vo_2max values of 14 and 19 mL/min/kg. Thus, on the basis of this study, we would have had to deny surgery to all patients with a Vo_2max of less than 20 mL/min/kg in order to have prevented a fatal outcome. This would have represented 55% of the patients studied by Smith's group! Obviously, this cutoff is too high. Bechard and Wetstein[11] reported a mortality rate of 4% (2 of 50), and the patients with fatal outcomes had Vo_2max values of 5 and 7 mL/min/kg. If a cutoff Vo_2max value of 7 mL/kg/min was applied, three patients would have been denied a curative procedure. Though group statistics would accept such a value, it is difficult to apply group statistics to individuals, as I am sure those three patients would agree! Miyoshi et al.[16] report a mortality rate of 12% (4 of 33). However, it is impossible to determine the Vo_2max from the data given. If we assume a body surface area of 1.4 m² and a weight of 70 kg, the Vo_2max averages 7 mL/kg/min for the patients who died. Thus, a Vo_2max of less than 10 mL/min/kg would seem to represent a level of exercise impairment associated with increased mortality. However, clinical application of this value would deny a curative procedure to 60% of the patients in Bechard's study with this level of exercise impairment. Thus, although exercise impairment appears to be directly proportional to postoperative mortality, there is no clear cutoff that reliably separates those who can tolerate the surgery from those who cannot. Without such a specific cutoff value, the results of exercise testing are of no benefit in the preoperative assessment of patients.

Does exercise testing offer a more sensitive means of assessing operative risk? The data presented would argue that it does not. More prospective standardized studies are necessary, particularly in those patients undergoing nonthoracic surgery, before we can adequately judge the merits of exercise testing. There are no exercise studies comparing risk stratification based on the ASA criteria or other well-established clinical criteria. Is the highly technical exercise physiology testing any better at assessing risk than clinically evaluating the patient and seeing the "glint in the eye and the spring in the step?" The ability of exercise testing to predict postoperative morbidity is of little clinical value when addressing coronary artery disease or lung cancer.

Exercise Testing Is Reliable and Reproducible

Obviously, for a clinical test to be applied universally in the preoperative assessment of patients, it is crucial that such a test be standardized, reliable, and reproducible from hospital to hospital. Currently there is no standardized method of exercising patients. Should they be exercised on a treadmill or a cycle ergometer? The choice is extremely important, because the method of exercise can directly influence the $\dot{V}o_2$max. Reliability is another crucial factor. Although the incorporation of microchip technology has enhanced the reliability of exercise testing, there is evidence of marked disparity in the interpretation of these studies.[17] In addition, inadequate technical training can seriously affect the reliability of the test. Reproducibility also needs to be ensured. Exercise testing by definition is effort dependent. The physicians and technicians must be fully trained in exercise physiology and in the assessment of patient effort to ensure reproducible results. Multiple factors (i.e., time of day, medications, humidity, temperature, etc.) may alter a patient's exercise performance and interfere with obtaining reliable and reproducible results. Thus, before exercise testing can be considered for clinical application, a standardized protocol must be developed.

Exercise Testing Is Readily Available and Cost-effective

The problem is that exercise testing equipment is all too readily available. One cannot look through a medical journal or attend a medical meeting without being inundated by advertisements or salespeople hawking their wares. This easy accessibility, combined with the promise of enhancing our diagnostic acumen, makes it difficult to refuse. For an initial outlay of $30,000 to $50,000, it is possible to outfit your office with the latest in exercise technology and software. However, until the clinical utility of exercise testing is soundly established, this may be money poorly invested. Proof that the routine use of preoperative exercise assessment is cost-effective is sorely lacking. As shown earlier, the only true clinical value of exercise assessment in patients undergoing coronary or lung resection surgery would be if it could reliably predict mortality. If a sensitive and specific value could be identified (which I doubt), every patient considered for surgery would require a $300 to $500 screening test in an attempt to identify the 4%

to 12% of patients who would not survive the surgery. This cost to the health care system would need to be weighed against the possible savings realized.

Exercise Testing Is Applicable to a Select Subgroup of Patients

The data currently available reveal no clinical factor which would identify those patients who would benefit from the preoperative assessment of exercise capacity. Thus, we are left with the cost-containment problem generated by the indiscriminate testing of all patients being considered for surgical procedures.

In summary, there are no data to support the contention that exercise testing is of value in assessing operative risk. Exercise testing represents a fascinating investigation into the relationship of exercise physiology and operative stress, but too little is known to recommend widespread application of this new technology into the clinical field. It is imperative that large, multicenter, prospective studies be established to effectively evaluate the possible roles and indications of exercise testing in patient care. Only through properly designed and executed clinical trials will we discover the true value of exercise physiology testing. I eagerly await such trials.

References

1. Carliner N, Fisher N, Plotnick G, et al: Routine preoperative exercise testing in patients undergoing major noncardiac surgery. Am J Cardiol 1985; 56:51–57. This is a prospective study finding no correlation between preoperative exercise performance and postoperative cardiac complications.
2. Owens WD, Felts JA, Spitznagel EL: ASA physical status classifications: A study of consistency of ratings. Anesthesiology 1978; 49:239–246. A review of the ASA classification system based on preoperative activity level is given.
3. Goldman L, Caldera DL, Nussbaum SR, et al: Multifactorial index of cardiac risk in noncardiac surgical procedures. N Engl J Med 1977; 297:845–850. This is the classic retrospective analysis which identified independent risk factors for cardiac complications following noncardiac surgery.
4. Hammermeister KE, Kennedy JW: Predictors of surgical mortality in patients undergoing direct myocardial revascularization. Circulation 1974; 49(suppl II):112–118. These authors found no correlation between functional aerobic impairment or the presence of ischemic ST-segment depression and 6-week perioperative mortality in 122 patients undergoing cardiac bypass surgery.
5. Bruce RA, DeRouen TA, Hammermeister KE: Noninvasive screening criteria for enhanced 4-year survival after aortocoronary bypass surgery. Circulation

1979; 60:638–644. *Derived from data of the Seattle Heart Watch, this study reported that exercise-induced ST-segment depression or angina did not correlate with the 4-year survival rate post-bypass.*

6. Weiner DA, Ryan TJ, McCabe CH, et al: The value of preoperative exercise testing in predicting long-term survival in patients undergoing aortocoronary bypass surgery. *Circulation* 1984; 70(suppl I):226–231. *This report examines 7-year survival of patients in the Coronary Artery Surgery Study (CASS) registry, noting that left ventricular score was the most potent predictor of survival, followed by peak exercise performance and number of diseased vessels.*

7. Weiner DA, Ryan TJ, McCabe CH: Exercise stress testing. Correlation among history of angina, S-T segment response and prevalence of coronary artery disease in the coronary-artery surgery study. *N Engl J Med* 1979; 301:230–235. *This is a large multicenter study reporting that exercise stress testing contributed little in predicting the extent of coronary vessel disease compared to clinical history alone.*

8. Sonders CR: The clinical evaluation of the patient for thoracic surgery. *Surg Clin North Am* 1961; 41:545–558. *This is an outdated review of the clinical approach to evaluating patients for thoracic surgery.*

9. Gass CD, Olsen GN: Preoperative pulmonary function testing to predict postoperative morbidity and mortality. *Chest* 1986; 89:127–135. *This is an excellent review of standard techniques for the preoperative assessment of surgical candidates; it highlights the "pulmonary function criteria" suggesting increased operative risk.*

10. Bolton JWR, Weiman DS, Haynes JL, et al: Stair climbing as an indicator of pulmonary function. *Chest* 1987; 92:783–788. *This prospective study in 70 men correlated the number of stairs climbed to standard pulmonary function tests (PFTs). However, no data are presented on the postoperative course.*

11. Bechard DE, Wetstein L: Assessment of exercise oxygen consumption as preoperative criterion for lung resection. *Ann Thorac Surg* 1987; 44:344–349. *This is a prospective study in 50 surgical candidates reporting oxygen consumption at peak exercise to be highly predictive of postoperative morbidity and mortality.*

12. Brundler H, Chen S, Perruchoud AP: Right heart catheterization in the preoperative evaluation of patients with lung cancer. *Respiration* 1985; 48:261–268. *This fascinating retrospective study reports a high incidence of clandestine left ventricular (LV) dysfunction in patients evaluated for thoracotomy. The authors derived a discriminative function which accurately predicted precapillary pulmonary hypertension in a follow-up group of patients.*

13. Pierce RJ, Pretto JJ, Rochford PD, et al: Lobar occlusion in the preoperative assessment of patients with lung cancer. *Br J Dis Chest* 1986; 80:27–36. *This is an interesting approach to preoperatively evaluating the effects of lung resection on postoperative exercise tolerance utilizing temporary balloon occlusion of the lobar bronchus, but it suffers from a small number of patients.*

14. Smith TP, Kinasewitz GT, Tucker WY, et al: Exercise capacity as a predictor of post-thoracotomy morbidity. *Am Rev Respir Dis* 1984; 129:730–734.

This is a well designed prospective study reporting exercise tolerance to be a sensitive predictor of postoperative complications.

15. Colman NC, Schraufnagel DE, Rivington RN, et al: Exercise testing in evaluation of patients for lung resection. *Am Rev Respir Dis* 1982; 125:604–606. *This prospective study examines postoperative complications, reporting no prognostic value from preoperative exercise performance. The study is flawed by exclusion bias, use of "technical" complications, and failure to account for body mass.*

16. Miyoshi S, Nakahara K, Ohno K, et al: Exercise tolerance test in lung cancer patients: The relationship between exercise capacity and postthoracotomy hospital mortality. *Ann Thorac Surg* 1987; 44:487–490. *These authors reported that preoperative exercise capacity (expressed as O_2 consumption at an arterial lactate level of 20 mg/dL, La-20) predicted postoperative mortality, but not morbidity. The sensitivity of exercise testing was limited by submaximal exercise testing.*

17. Gladden LB: Current anaerobic threshold controversies. *Physiologist* 1984; 27:312–318. *This fascinating article reviews other factors responsible for the "anaerobic threshold" (AT) and questions the accuracy of the noninvasive methods for determining its development. It presents some interesting data showing the development of the AT in patients with McArdle's disease!*

Rebuttal: Affirmative
Gerald N. Olsen, M.D.

"The absence of proof is not the same as the proof of absence."

Author Unknown

A debate is an interesting way of examining a subject since it "forces" antagonist and protagonist into polarized positions to present both sides of a question. Outside this format, the authors themselves are rarely so polarized in their actual concepts and so it probably is with Dr. Bechard and myself. As a latecomer to the exercise field, I have great respect for his important contribution in this area and am looking forward to the publication of his negative study on stair climbing.

In reviewing Dr. Bechard's antagonist position, he appears to be taking a stringent view of the Bayesian concepts of value, sensitivity, specificity, etc. He concludes that there are insufficient data to recommend exercise testing as valuable. However, he fails to provide us with a reasonable alternative except for Goldman's multivariate analysis of risk [1] and the American Society of Anesthesiologists (ASA) rating [2] (Table 5). The former is fairly complicated and primarily rates cardiac risk, which is not the only cause of postoperative morbidity and mortality. On the other hand, the ASA criteria are simple enough, but they are incredibly subjective and vague. With millions of surgical procedures performed annually in the United States, potentially serious complications occur with great regularity in some procedures (e.g., 88% of upper abdominal procedures[3]) and rarely, if ever, in others (e.g., cataract extraction under local anesthesia). The cost of identifying all preoperative risks in healthy asymptomatic patients is extremely high.[4] This mandates a closer look at selected higher clinical risk patients. This point is very important when considering a complete cardiopulmonary exercise test which would not be cost-effective if done on all patients preoperatively.

In his review of the topic, Dr. Bechard proposes the following criteria that exercise testing must satisfy to qualify as "valuable": (1) specificity and sensitivity above "standard techniques" and usefulness in directing therapy, (2) reliability and reproducibility, (3) availability and cost-effectiveness, and (4) the ability to define appropriate subjects. He then qualifies his review of the literature to exercise testing with gas exchange ($\dot{V}O_2 + \dot{V}CO_2$) analysis. Dr. Bechard divides his analysis of sensitivity into nonthoracic, cardiac, and noncardiac thoracic surgery.

TABLE 5.
Preoperative Screening Methods*

Multivariate Analysis of Risk[†]		Points	ASA Physical Status Classification	
History	Over age 70 years	5	Class 1	Normally healthy patient
	Infarction < 6 months	10	Class 2	Patient with mild systemic disease
Examination	Jugular venous distention or S_3	11	Class 3	Patient with severe, not incapacitating, systemic disease
	Significant aortic stenosis	3	Class 4	Patient with incapacitating systemic disease not constant threat to life
Electrocardiogram	Any rhythm but sinus or PACs	7		
	> 5 PVCs/min	7	Class 5	Moribund patient not expected to survive > 24 hours with or without operation
General	Po_2 < 60 mm Hg or Pco_2 > 50 mm Hg	3		
	K^+ < 3 mEq/L or HCO_3 < 20 mEq/L Creatinine > 3 mg/dL or BUN > 50 mg/dL SGOT[†] or chronic liver disease Bedridden			
Operation	Emergency	4		
	Aortic, intra thoracic, intra peritoneal	3		

Scale vs. Outcome

Total Points	Life-Threatening Complications	Cardiac Death
0–5	0.7%	0.2%
6–12	5%	2%
13–25	11%	2%
>26	22%	56%

*Adapted from Goldman L, Caldera DL, Nussbaum SR, et al: *N Engl J Med* 1977; 297:845–50 and Owens WD, Fetts JA, Spitnagel GL: *Anesthesiology* 1978; 49:239–46.
[†]PACs = premature atrial contractions; PVCs = premature ventricular contractions; BUN = blood urea nitrogen; SGOT = serum glutamic oxaloacetic transaminase.

Nonthoracic Surgery

Here Dr. Bechard and I agree on the paucity of controlled studies (if any) of gas exchange–type preoperative exercise studies in this type of surgery. However, Dr. Bechard quotes the negative study of Carliner and coworkers[5] which only evaluated electrocardiographic (ECG) criteria of coronary insufficiency vs. postoperative cardiac risk. The Carliner study did not use gas exchange measurements. I favor the study of Gerson and coworkers [6] which, although it did not use $\dot{V}o_2$, specifically, did use a related parameter of exercise duration. "Other studies" are purported to have found no added benefit of (gas exchange?) exercise tests over ASA and Goldman. We are not given these references on which to comment.

Cardiac Surgery

It is in this area that careful reading and review are needed. Dr. Bechard's negative analysis of the literature again seems to concentrate on ECG-oriented exercise testing rather than on gas exchange–type testing. This is true of the study of Hammermeister and Kennedy,[7] who found angiocardiographic criteria of ventricular dysfunction more predictive of perioperative mortality than ECG ST segments on maximal exercise. However, $\dot{V}o_2$ was not measured. Furthermore, the other studies he quotes[8–10] emphasize the criterion of long-term survival rather than perioperative risk. I concede that the data relating preoperative exercise ECG ST segments to even the existence of coronary artery disease is tenuous in asymptomatic patients, and probably is not very predictive of long-term survival of coronary artery bypass grafting (CABG). That is not strictly the issue, however. With the overall perioperative mortality of coronary artery bypass grafting surgery already extremely low,[11] exercise testing may play little additional role in reducing the mortality further. This is especially true if one considers the intensity of even routine CABG postoperative care.[12] One must also consider the fact that the surgery itself is performed (A) to improve cardiac function in the postoperative period, and (B) to prevent subsequent myocardial infarction. However, one of the many causes of a reduced $\dot{V}o_2$ on exercise is cardiac dysfunction. Studies with gas exchange analysis during exercise in the highest risk subpopulation of CABG patients have not been published, to my knowledge. There is little question, however, that cardiac surgery does produce pulmonary sequelae, but these seem to be poorly predicted or influenced by spirometric pulmonary function testing.[12,13,14]

Noncardiac Thoracic Surgery

Dr. Bechard and I agree in many areas on the assessment of risk for lung resection. One area in which we differ is in the prediction of morbidity vs. mortality by exercise ($\dot{V}o_2$) testing. I do agree with him that survivable postoperative atelectasis is (perhaps) predictable, but to what avail? We differ, however, in our interpretation of the importance of the prediction. He criticizes the predictive accuracy of a low $\dot{V}o_2$max value as including too many patients who could still undergo successful (and lifesaving) lung resection for carcinoma. Applying an overly stringent cutoff may not be practical when dealing with a uniformly fatal disease like lung cancer unresected. However, the patient, his family, and his surgeon may come to a better therapeutic decision if the patient knows preoperatively that the risk is very high (e.g., 25% to 50% mortality) vs. accepting surgical therapy naively expecting the mortality risk to be only 1% to 10%. Interposing a hard and fast numerical cutoff may actually interfere with this crucially important individual decision (e.g., the risk of early postoperative mortality vs. later, but almost certain, mortality with nonsurgical therapy).

In reviewing the reliability and reproducibility of exercise testing, I direct the reader to a study showing very stable $\dot{V}o_2$max readings in repeated studies on chronic obstructive pulmonary disease (COPD) patients.[15] A study by Matthews and coworkers[16] found comparable data obtained from automated microprocessor systems vs. "traditional" methods in 12 normal men exercised in random sequence. There is no question, however, that a learning curve probably exists for those doing and interpreting the testing using complicated or simplified equipment, and comparison to normal "standards" can be somewhat difficult.

As far as availability is concerned, many well-equipped hospitals already have automated, packaged "metabolic carts." Perhaps the use of these in preoperative assessment will simply enhance the utility of this already purchased (and underutilized?) equipment.

The cost-effectiveness of gas exchange–type exercise testing, in my opinion, is not yet established for any disease, much less for preoperative evaluation. This is where simpler studies are attractive. For example, Dr. Bechard's unpublished negative study of stair climbing achieves major importance if it has the power to avoid type II (β) error. If it is carefully and systematically performed, stair climbing should be extremely inexpensive, but it also may be somewhat nonspecific if the patient is limited. One can estimate the $\dot{V}o_2$ accomplished, however, using the following equations[17,18]:

(1) Workload in watts = (step height in meters) × (steps per minute) × (body weight in kilograms)

(2) Predicted $\dot{V}o_2 = 5.8 \times$ (weight in kilograms) $+ 151 + (10.1 \times$ workload in watts)

Another study estimated $\dot{V}o_2$max from clinical data, but not preoperatively.[19] Further studies will be needed to put this into perspective.

Group Selection

In previous studies on exercise testing prior to lung resection, the patient selection criteria varied greatly from young to old age and from good to poor cardiopulmonary function. Our study[20] involved only highly selected patients with severe pulmonary dysfunction ($FEV_1 < 2$ L). We concluded that at 40 W of steady state–type exercise $\dot{V}o_2$ was predictive of postoperative intolerance (mortality) but not of survivable morbidity. My personal bias is clearly that gas exchange–type exercise testing may not be recommended for all preoperative patients. Clearly, lung resection patients are good research candidates because their cardiopulmonary function is not likely to be improved by the surgery. Perhaps future studies should include selected patients following a screening stair climb, using specific cardiac or pulmonary function criteria, or maybe even having a low ASA or Goldman score.

Summary

In looking back over my shoulder at what has been proposed before (and failed) as preoperative predictors, I hold out the hope that an ideal test can be found that satisfies sufficient criteria to be useful. I still maintain that the studies on gas exchange–type cardiopulmonary exercise testing published thus far cannot be dismissed as "proof of absence" of benefit until we have more and larger studies to overcome the "absence of proof" problem.

References

1. Goldman L, Caldera DL, Nussbaum SR, et al: Multifactorial index of cardiac risk in non-cardiac procedures. *N Engl J Med* 1977; 297:845–850.
2. Owens WD, Fetts JA, Spitnagel EL: ASA physical status classifications: A study of consistency of ratings. *Anesthesiology* 1978; 49:239–246.
3. Celli BR, Rodriguez KS, Snider GL: A controlled trial of intermittent positive pressure breathing, incentive spirometry, and deep breathing exercises in preventing pulmonary complications after abdominal surgery. *Am Rev Respir Dis* 1984; 130:12–15.
4. Robbins JA, Mushlin AI: Preoperative evaluation of the healthy patient. *Med Clin North Am* 1979; 63:1145–1156.
5. Carliner NH, Fisher ML, Plotnick GD, et al: Routine preoperative exercise

testing in patients undergoing major non-cardiac surgery. *Am J Cardiol* 1985; 56:51–58.

6. Gerson MC, Hurst JM, Hertzberg VS, et al: Cardiac prognosis in non-cardiac geriatric surgery. *Ann Intern Med* 1985; 103:832–837.

7. Hammermeister KE, Kennedy JW: Predictors of surgical mortality in patients undergoing direct myocardial revascularization. *Circulation* 1974; 49(suppl II):112–118.

8. Bruce RA, DeRouen TA, Hammermeister KE: Noninvasive screening criteria for enhanced 4-year survival after aortocoronary bypass surgery. *Circulation* 1979; 60:638–644.

9. Weiner DA, Ryan TJ, McCabe CH, et al: The value of preoperative exercise testing in predicting long-term survival in patients undergoing aortocoronary bypass surgery. *Circulation* 1984; 70(suppl I):226–231.

10. Weiner DA, Ryan TJ, McCabe CH: Exercise stress testing: Correlation among history of angina, S-T segment response and prevalence of coronary artery disease in the coronary artery surgery study. *N Engl J Med* 1979; 301:230–235.

11. Wright JG, Pifarré R, Sullivan HJ, et al: Multivariate discriminant analysis of risk factors for operative mortality following isolated coronary artery bypass graft. *Chest* 1987; 91:394–399.

12. Matthay MA, Wiener-Kronish JP: Respiratory management after cardiac surgery. *Chest* 1989; 95:424–434.

13. Braun SR, Birnbaum ML, Chopra PS: Preoperative and postoperative pulmonary function abnormalities in coronary artery revascularization surgery. *Chest* 1978; 73:316–320.

14. Cain HD, Stevens PM, Adaniya R: Preoperative pulmonary function and complications after cardiovascular surgery. *Chest* 1979; 76:130–135.

15. Brown SE, Fischer CE, Stansbury DW, et al: Reproducibility of Vo_2max in patients with chronic air-flow obstruction. *Am Rev Respir Dis* 1985; 131:435–438.

16. Matthews JI, Bush BA, Morales FM: Microprocessor exercise physiology systems vs a non-automated system. *Chest* 1987; 92:696–703.

17. Gupta S, Fletcher CM, Edwards RHT: A progressive exercise step test. *J Assoc Physicians India* 1973; 21:555–564.

18. Wasserman K, Whipp BJ: Exercise physiology in health and disease. *Am Rev Respir Dis* 1975; 112:219–259.

19. Lee TH, Shammash JB, Ribeiro JP, et al: Estimation of maximum oxygen uptake from clinical data: Performance of the specific activity scale. *Am Heart J* 1988; 115:203–204.

20. Olsen GN, Weiman DS, Bolton JWR, et al: Submaximal invasive exercise testing and quantitative lung scanning in the evaluation for tolerance of lung resection. *Chest* 1989; 95:267–273.

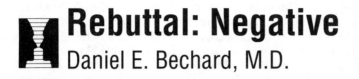

Rebuttal: Negative
Daniel E. Bechard, M.D.

I would like to compliment Dr. Olsen on his succinct overview of the theory and application of exercise testing. However, after reading his argument, I find myself asking the age-old question: "Where's the beef?" Though Dr. Olsen has presented an up-to-date review of the recently published exercise studies, he has not confronted the issue at hand, that being: Is exercise testing of *value* in predicting operative risk? We are not deliberating the ability of exercise testing to identify patients at risk for postoperative complications, or the underlying physiological basis for exercise limitation. Rather, we are trying to weigh the relative merits of this new microchip technology against readily available risk assessment protocols to determine whether exercise testing is of any added value in selecting patients for surgical intervention. I maintain that the data currently available are insufficient to justify the widespread application of exercise testing as a definitive preoperative assessment modality.

The prevention of postoperative complications, especially mortality, certainly represents a crucial goal in improving the delivery of health care to our patients. However, in order to prevent a complication, we first must be able to identify those at risk and then institute appropriate prophylactic therapy. I will not address the role and efficacy of prophylactic therapy, as that is a subject for a future debate. What we need to critically examine is whether exercise testing can identify patients at risk for complications *in a cost-effective manner* which offers increased sensitivity, specificity, and applicability over standard preoperative evaluation.

Operative Risk

The determination of operative risk represents the crux of the problem. How can we identify patients who will benefit from preoperative exercise assessment in a cost-effective manner? I have wrestled with this question ever since I became interested in preoperative assessment and have yet to answer it adequately. Dr. Olsen proposes a partial listing of conditions which he contends will help identify this group of patients (see Table 2). From a practical point of view, however, which of these conditions is truly helpful in identifying patients likely to benefit from exercise assessment? Several of these conditions are not applicable to the question at hand. *Emergency surgery* is a well-established risk for postoperative complications; however, it can hardly be used as a criterion for scheduling exercise assessment. The presence of a *coagulopathy* calls for correction of the underlying deficit, rather than exercise testing. The need for *prolonged* or *repetitive procedures* is often appreciated only after the procedure has begun or when the patient has not fully recovered from the initial surgery. These represent times when exercise assessment is impractical. The *immunocompromised state* is definitely an inherent risk factor, but I am confused as to how exercise testing will assess risk in this patient group. If we remove these conditions and add other putative risk factors (i.e., diabetes mellitus), we are left with a smaller, but no less overwhelming set of criteria. Applying these criteria to preoperative candidates would necessitate exercise testing in most patients over the age of 45 years (due to the high incidence of cardiovascular and/or pulmonary disease) undergoing major abdominal or thoracic surgery! Conservatively, this represents over 80% of adults undergoing surgery. If we are going to subject this large group of patients to preoperative risk assessment, it is imperative that the assessment tool(s) be specific and cost-effective, owing to the large number of patients reportedly at risk. Any new method of risk assessment also must be shown to be more sensitive than the method(s) of risk appraisal currently available.

Rationale For Exercise Testing

Exercise testing definitely has a certain physiological appeal for use as an assessment tool. In theory, the systemic stresses of the perioperative state are mimicked by exercise testing. Thus, weaknesses within the oxygen transport chain may become apparent and alert the physician to potential problems. I have no problem with this assumption. However, one glaring deficiency with the current practice of exercise testing is its lack of standardization. How do we properly stress the patient's oxygen transport mechanism? Do we exercise the patient via a treadmill, a stairway, a walk around the block, an arm ergometer, a rowing machine, and/or a cycle? The method of testing will dramatically affect the observed $\dot{V}o_2$, the ability to monitor the patient closely, and the ability to obtain invasive hemodynamic parameters. How do we account for the variety of factors (time of day, diet, humidity, medications, etc.) capable of affecting $\dot{V}o_2$? For example, a recent study reported that heart rate response alone is capable of directly altering the $\dot{V}o_2$.[1] The choice of monitoring techniques during exercise will affect the predictive potential of the test also. Dr. Olsen argues that with exercise testing, angina or ST-segment abnormalities may be detected. However, in a recently published study, the patients were monitored with only a single-lead electrocardiogram (ECG).[2] Although this monitoring setup provides for patient safety, it is inadequate for monitoring ST segments for ischemic changes and will not alert the physician to potential cardiovascular problems. This is one example of the discrepancy between the theory and the application of exercise physiology testing. I mention this to underscore the need for standardization of exercise protocols. Without well-designed, uniform protocols, we are left with a potpourri of interesting but disparate studies.

The diversity in the level of exercise also restricts inter-study comparisons. I have divided the more commonly cited exercise studies arbitrarily into three main categories, similar to those outlined by Dr. Olsen.

Minimal Achievement

This method of testing usually is based on an arbitrary threshold of exercise performance, an "all or none" approach. Stair-climbing performance and the 12-minute walk are two examples. Over the years, studies repeatedly have shown this method to be insensitive in predicting postoperative complications.[3-5] Though a recent study claimed a correlation between stair climbing and pulmonary function tests (PFTs), no correlation with postoperative outcome was presented.[6] I feel it is safe to say that "minimal achievement" or "exercise accomplishment" testing, despite its availability and ease of application, has no predictive value in assessing operative risk.

Submaximal Exercise

Supporters of submaximal exercise testing argue that the test is better tolerated by patients with poor cardiopulmonary reserve. However, if our primary supposition is that the perioperative period produces *intense physiological stress* on the O_2 delivery system, how sensitive can a submaximal test be? Two recent studies found that submaximal exercise predicted only postoperative mortality, not morbidity.[2,7] By not fully stressing the cardiopulmonary systems, significant physiological derangements were overlooked. Accepting that mortality is the critical complication to identify preoperatively, is submaximal exercise performance specific enough to warrant the cancellation of surgery (see later)?

Maximal Exercise

As stated earlier, the bulk of the data addressing exercise capacity as a preoperative assessment tool has been generated by maximally exercising candidates for thoracotomy. Submaximal testing predicts only mortality, whereas maximal symptom-limited exercise testing appears to identify patients at risk for morbidity as well as mortality. From the studies supporting a correlation between maximal exercise performance and postoperative complication,[8-10] it appears that a maximal $\dot{V}o_2$ of less than 10 mL/kg/min is associated with a high degree of morbidity and mortality. However, before we accept this as a definitive parameter, several questions remain to be answered:

1. Is this parameter ($\dot{V}o_2$) any more sensitive than standard clinical assessment profiles of the patient?

2. If so, are we able to identify the subgroup of patients that would benefit from exercise testing?

3. Is this finding specific enough to exclude patients with a $\dot{V}o_2$ of less than 10 mL/kg/min from surgical consideration?

To gain some clinical insight, let us apply these questions to the study performed at my institution.[10] Were the exercise data more sensitive than the standard preoperative assessment modalities? Exercise testing was certainly better than standard PFTs and resting ECG tracings. However, we did not compare the exercise results directly to a more subjective scale, such as the physical status scale of the American Society of Anesthesiologists[11] or to the "gut reaction" of the physicians caring for the patients. Could it be that the predictive value of the computerized exercise test is no better than the subjective evaluation based on the "spring in the step and the glint in the eye"? A preliminary study along this line is currently underway at our institution, though a much larger study is necessary to address this question adequately.

In addition, claims that the diffusing capacity of the lung for carbon monoxide represents the most important predictor of mortality and pulmonary morbidity in patients undergoing lung resection have appeared recently.[12] I feel that more controlled studies are required before we can state definitively that exercise testing is more sensitive than the standard assessment protocols. However, for the sake of argument, let us assume that exercise performance is more sensitive than currently available assessment tools. Can we identify those patients who would benefit from a preoperative assessment of exercise capacity? In my study, the two patients with a $\dot{V}o_2$ of less than 10 mL/kg/min who suffered a fatal outcome had normal pulmonary function and resting ECGs.[10] There was no clinical "flag" to alert the physician to the disastrous outcome. Our coveted criteria in Dr. Olsen's Table 2 were of no help! Thus, I would have to conclude that every potential candidate for thoracotomy would require preoperative exercise assessment, hardly a cost-effective measure given the current cost of equipment, time, and qualified personnel. Concerning the application of these criteria to patients undergoing major, nonthoracotomy surgery, there are not enough data available to venture a recommendation. Finally, would I recommend that surgery be canceled on a patient who is unable to achieve a $\dot{V}o_2$max greater than 10 mL/kg/min? As Dr. Olsen states, a goal of preoperative exercise testing is to identify patients likely to die as a result of the operative stress, thus avoiding futile surgical intervention. By applying a minimal $\dot{V}o_2$max of 10 mL/kg/min as a cutoff for surgical consideration, seven patients in my study would have been denied surgery.[10] Two patients (29%) would have been spared futile surgery. However, 5 patients (71%) would have been denied a curative resection! If we apply the same criteria to the patients reported in Dr. Olsen's recent study[2] (with the understanding that this represents O_2 consumption at 40 W), 11 patients would have been denied surgery. This would have prevented futile surgery in 5 patients (45%), but denied curative resection to the remaining 6 (55%)! In dealing with a uniformly fatal disease, denying a curative procedure to 55% to 71% of the patients identified as "high-risk" hardly qualifies as *primum non nocere*. With the limited data available, the maximal Vo_2, though sensitive, has not been shown to be specific enough to allow one to approve or cancel major surgery.

Besides O_2 consumption, are there other exercise parameters which may aid in identifying high-risk patients? Dr. Olsen argues that hypercapnia and hypoxemia may be uncovered with exercise testing. However, in his recent study[2] as well as in mine,[10] the development of hypercapnia and/or hypoxemia had no predictive value as a prognosticator of perioperative complications. Measurement of the anaerobic threshold (AT) also has been proposed as a prognostic factor. Of the 50 patients in my study, only 29 (58%) attained the AT.[10] Of the 8 patients experiencing complications, the AT was detected in only 4! Due to the presence of comorbid and debilitating diseases in these patients, a large percentage are unable to reach their AT, limiting the usefulness of this measure. In addition, Dr. Olsen refers to the value of monitoring the pulmonary vascular pressure response to exercise in assessing operative risk. Yet, in reporting the results of exercise testing in 29 thoracotomy patients, Dr. Olsen concludes that "pulmonary vascular pressures and calculated resistance did not predict [surgical] intolerance."[2] Thus, despite the mass of physiological data which can be obtained from formal exercise testing, there is no convincing evidence that it is of any added value in predicting postoperative morbidity and mortality.

In conclusion, I feel the current data available on exercise testing do not support its widespread application into the realm of preoperative assessment. The current studies suffer from a lack of standardization and critical comparison to standard methods of assessing operative risk. Exercise testing represents an exciting application of physiology to the clinical field and has value in assessing dyspnea, disability, and response to therapeutic interventions. However, it is too early to recommend its use in operative risk assessment. We need well-planned, multi center studies using a unified exercise protocol to assess the value of exercise testing adequately. I would welcome cooperating with Dr. Olsen on such a project.

References

1. Casaburi R, Spitzer S, Haskell R, et al: Effect of altering heart rate on oxygen uptake at exercise onset. *Chest* 1989; 95:6–12.
2. Olsen G, Weiman D, Bolton J, et al: Submaximal invasive exercise testing and quantitative lung scanning in the evaluation for tolerance of lung resection. *Chest* 1989; 95:267–273.
3. Gaensler E, Cugell D, Lindgren I, et al: The role of pulmonary insufficiency in

mortality and invalidism following surgery for pulmonary tuberculosis. *J Thorac Cardiovasc Surg* 1955; 29:163–187.

4. Bagg L: The 12 minute walking distance; its use in the preoperative assessment of patients with bronchial carcinoma before lung resection. *Respiration* 1984; 46:342–345.

5. Van Nostrand D, Kjelsberg M, Humphrey E: Pre-resectional evaluation of risk from pneumonectomy. *Surg Gynecol Obstet* 1968; 127:306–310.

6. Bolton J, Weiman D, Haynes J, et al: Stair climbing as an indicator of pulmonary function. *Chest* 1987; 92:344–349.

7. Miyoshi S, Nakahara K, Ohno K, et al: Exercise tolerance test in lung cancer patients: The relationship between exercise capacity and postthoracotomy hospital mortality. *Ann Thorac Surg* 1987; 44:487–90.

8. Eugene J, Brown SE, Light RW, et al: Maximal oxygen consumption: A physiologic guide to pulmonary resection. *Surg Forum* 1982; 33:260–262.

9. Smith TO, Kinasewitz GT, Tucker WY, et al: Exercise capacity as a predictor of post-thoracotomy morbidity. *Am Rev Respir Dis* 1984; 129:730–734.

10. Bechard D, Wetstein L: Assessment of exercise oxygen consumption as preoperative criterion for lung resection. *Ann Thorac Surg* 1987; 44:344–349.

11. Owens WD, Felts JA, Spitznagel EL: ASA physical status classifications: A study of consistency of ratings. *Anesthesiology* 1978; 49:239–246.

12. Ferguson MK, Little L, Rizzo L, et al: Diffusing capacity predicts morbidity and mortality after pulmonary resection. *J Thorac Cardiovasc Surg* 1988; 96:894–900.

Editor's Comments
Richard H. Winterbauer, M.D.

The debate by Drs. Olsen and Bechard focuses on exercise testing but, equally important, it nicely develops the logic behind preoperative testing, offers a definition of the "ideal test," and emphasizes the need to identify the patient group that would best benefit from extensive preoperative evaluation. The hypothetical ideal test should be not only predictive of complications and mortality, but also inexpensive and able to be performed with minimal discomfort to the patient. The factor of cost has to be weighed carefully these days. For the readers' perspective, a multistage pulmonary exercise test measuring $\dot{V}E$, $\dot{V}O_2$, and $\dot{V}CO_2$ will cost \$450 to \$650. Unfortunately, no test distinctly divides the operative population into those patients with no mortality and those with 100% mortality. Instead, a continuum of increasing risk is defined. Thus, the potential benefit from surgery becomes a major dictate of acceptable risk. For example, in a patient with an asymptomatic inguinal hernia, surgery should be canceled in the face of a test predictive of major operative mortality. However, in a patient with a life-threatening disease such as lung cancer, for which there is no nonoperative therapeutic option, a major operative risk is justified. Preoperative testing may be more appropriate in the former patient than in the latter. Defining the group of patients who would best benefit from a specific level of preoperative testing remains a challenge for future clinical investigation.

Exercise testing with gas exchange analysis has been with us for years. Although it has its proponents, it has not been adopted as a community standard. Much greater clinical experience is needed to provide a sharper definition of who should be tested, how results should be interpreted, and how the test compares with other forms of preoperative assessment. Until such experience is available, preoperative cardiopulmonary exercise testing might best be considered still in the investigational phase.

Should Thrombolytic Therapy Be Used in Suspected Cases of Myocardial Infarction by Appropriately Trained Paramedics?

Chapter Editor: Gary Gitnick, M.D.

Affirmative: Richard Crampton, D.M.
Professor of Medicine, Division of
Cardiology, Department of Medicine,
University of Virginia School of Medicine,
Charlottesville, Virginia

Negative: David W. M. Muller, M.B., B.S.
Senior Research Fellow, Interventional
Cardiology Program, Division of Cardiology,
University of Michigan Medical Center, Ann
Arbor, Michigan

Eric J. Topol, M.D.
Director of Cardiac Catheterization
Laboratories, Associate Professor of Internal
Medicine, University of Michigan Medical
School, Ann Arbor, Michigan

Editor's Introduction

Heart disease is one of the leading causes of death in the United States and Europe and we have witnessed a variety of advances in the past decade clearly designed to save the lives of those suffering from it. Among these has been the concept that thrombolytic therapy will be efficacious if administered early in the course of a myocardial infarction. Having advanced to this point, the question now arises whether the medication should be administered immediately on a routine basis by appropriately trained paramedics or whether it should be administered according to the needs of each individual patient after arrival in a hospital emergency room. The following debate reveals the advantages and disadvantages of the administration of thrombolytic therapy by appropriately trained paramedics.

Gary Gitnick, M.D.

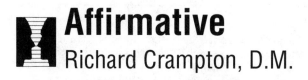

Affirmative
Richard Crampton, D.M.

To attain the highest level of physical capacity and psychological tranquility, the patient suffering an acute coronary attack depends most heavily upon competent prehospital care. The first priority of this care is the prevention and treatment of cardiac arrest. The prompt relief of symptoms, stress, and attendant autonomic dysfunction, and the early prevention and minimization of damage to heart muscle tissue augment the patient's chance for a longer, better life after the episode.[1] Because it is essential for survival and for achieving a high quality of life, advanced technology must be humanely employed in each patient.[2] Modern treatment now includes the prehospital infusion of thrombolytic agents. Coronary reperfusion is then followed in the hospital by further intensive care and often by diagnostic testing with simultaneous stress electrocardiography and radionuclide myocardial perfusion scanning to assess the risk of a recurrent coronary attack. Coronary angiography and angioplasty frequently ensue, as does surgical revascularization. Each crucial element of these diagnostic and therapeutic technologies has implicit benefits and risks for the patient which must be ascertained for potential merit and harm case by case.

Five thrombolytic drugs are now approved for clinical use or are undergoing carefully devised prospective clinical trials in patients with acute myocardial infarction. These agents are streptokinase (SK), urokinase (UK), recombinant tissue plasminogen activator (rt-PA), acylated plasminogen streptokinase activator complex (APSAC), and single chain urokinase plasminogen activator (scu-PA, prourokinase). Moreover, 160 mg of crushed aspirin given immediately and continued daily for a month was shown to significantly reduce 5-week vascular mortality. When aspirin was given in conjunction with an infusion of SK, the combination was more effective than either agent alone.[3] The resumption of coronary flow with consequent primary salvage of heart muscle probably constitutes the major impact of early thrombolytic treatment, and aspirin apparently plays an important part in this process. Benefits may accrue to the patient from the maintenance of collateral blood flow, the cessation of propagation of thrombus, the lowering of plasma fibrinogen content, the rise in breakdown products of fibrinogen, the impaired adhesive activity of platelets, and, possibly, the vasodilation by SK. Other hypothetical and potential benefits include the reduction of damage to the myocardial cell wall, the dissolution of microthrombi, and the diminution of the frequency of complications such as rupture of myocardium, mural thrombus, expansion of infarction, heart failure, and malignant primary and secondary dysrhythmias. In general, treating clinicians should be prudent in the use of thrombolysis because good prognostic early results favoring treated groups over placebo groups indicate some erosion of sustained benefit.[4] The synergistic action of relatively low doses of paired thrombolytic agents such as saruplase, single and 2-chain alteplase, rt-PA, and scu-PA may permit safer recanalization of coronary arteries in acute myocardial infarction, but the comparative efficacy of various combinations awaits further investigation.[5]

Compelling clinical evidence dictates the initiation of thrombolytic therapy before hospital arrival.[6-16] Table 1 displays the remarkable benefit gained by 1,342 patients who received early thrombolysis (mean gain, 47.5 minutes of therapeutic time) in 11 prospective assessments of prehospital vs. hospital therapy. No treatment was given in one study which was limited to feasibility and potential therapeutic time relations.[13] From eight investigations,[6-13] it was possible to calculate and compare weighted means of prehospital and hospital time intervals for 814 patients from the onset of ischemic symptoms to the initiation of thrombolytic treatment. The result was a mean time gain of 51.2 minutes for the 401 patients who received early therapy. Three other investigations reported only the mean time gained,[14-16] but when included with the first eight reports as weighted means, the mean therapeutic time gained for 595 patients given prehospital thrombolytic treatment was 47.5 minutes as compared to 747 patients whose thrombolytic therapy was deferred until hospitalization. Patients treated preflight by helicopter teams received an infusion of rt-PA within 28 ± 9 minutes of arrival of the team. In contrast, patients not treated preflight both experienced a transport delay and did not receive an infusion of rt-PA until 41 ± 18 minutes after arrival at the hospital.[12]

Table 2 portrays the superior patency rate of prehospital thrombolysis in the infarct-related coronary artery. Five reports relate the mean prehospital thrombolytic time gain to the superior coronary patency rate of early treatment. With the mean time gained ranging from 30 minutes to 55 minutes to initiation of coronary thrombolytic treatment, this prehospital group with a 50-minute mean time gain had a 75% coronary patency rate, significantly greater than the 64% rate for the hospital-treated group. Coronary patency rates also were greater for those patients who received thrombolytic therapy before helicopter transfer from a community hospital to a tertiary care center than for those who did not.[17]

The apparent quantifiable advantage of a 32% smaller enzymatic size of anterior wall myocardial infarction with prehospital streptokinase treatment[9] must be weighed against two reports of no differences in infarct size between prehospital and hospital groups.[10,18] One investigation involved treatment with the combination of rt-PA and heparin[10] and the other involved streptokinase.[18] The prehospital streptokinase cohort had both superior QRS scores by electrocardiogram (ECG) and better left ventricular function as defined by lower end diastolic pressure and higher global and infarct regional ejection fractions.[18] In contrast, no difference was found in

TABLE 1.
Prehospital Time Gain in Coronary Thrombolysis

| | Mean Time From the Onset of Symptoms to the Initiation of the Thrombolytic Agent | | | | | |
| | Prehospital | | Hospital | | Mean Time Gain | |
Prehospital Treatment*	Minutes	Number of Patients	Minutes	Number of Patients	Minutes	Number of Patients
Streptokinase heparin[6]	60	29	114	84	54	113
Streptokinase[7]	155	41	219	37	64	78
Streptokinase heparin to prehospital controls[8]	84†	17	124†	19	40	36
Streptokinase[9] rt-PA	70	40	125	36	55	76
Heparin[10]	93	56	137	44	44	100
APSAC[11]	91	13	137	13	46	26‡
rt-PA[12]	165	109	201	84	36	193
None§[13]	72	96	140	96	68	192‡
Streptokinase[14]	NA¶	39	NA	27	30	66
APSAC[15]	NA	54	NA	56	54	110
rt-PA[16]	NA	101	NA	251	40	352
Totals	108.8‖	595	151.7‖	747	47.5	1,342‖

*APSAC = acylated plasminogen streptokinase activator complex; rt-PA = recombinant tissue plasminogen activator.
†60 minutes added for mean duration of symptoms of entire group before arrival of mobile coronary care unit.
‡Time gain to hospital admission calculated from hospital arrival of prehospital-treated group.
‖Proportionately weighted mean of means.
§Myocardial infarction, triage, and intervention project: phase 1.
¶NA = not available; therefore, not included in the proportionately weighted mean of means.

regional wall motion between other prehospital-treated and hospital-treated groups, with the French patients receiving APSAC and the Israelis receiving rt-PA.[10,15]

No morbidity or mortality occurred in a prehospital group treated with the combination of streptokinase and heparin.[18] The hospital group included 2 early deaths (3.7%), with 1 patient dying of cardiogenic shock within 30 minutes and 1 dying of cerebral hemorrhage, possibly attributable to streptokinase. Two groups found no complications in their prehospital group.[9,15] One team successfully countershocked 2 patients who developed ventricular fibrillation in the ambulance during prehospital treatment out of 56 patients who received the combination of rt-PA and heparin,[10] underscoring the need for skilled prehospital coronary care including prompt resuscitation.[1] No ventricular fibrillation occurred in the 44 patients in whom the rt-PA–heparin therapy was randomly deferred until hospitalization. Mortality was not significantly different at 60 days, with 3 deaths out of 56 patients in the prehospital treatment group and 3 out of 44 in the hospital treatment group.[10]

Another investigation encountered no serious bleeding problems, but described 1 case of ventricular fibrillation and 1 of hypotension after the prehospital initiation of streptokinase. The hospital streptokinase group that had received heparin in the prehospital phase included 1 patient with ventricular fibrillation, 1 with ventricular tachycardia, and 1 with complete heart block.[8] More hypotension and more need for atropine treatment of bradycardia during helicopter flight was encountered in 1 group receiving prehospital rt-PA. However, hemorrhagic complications in the first 24 hours were less common in the prehospital group. Neither group had any deaths during flight and the occurrence of serious dysrhythmias was similar in each group.[12] In summary, the risks and complications encountered in patients started on

TABLE 2.
Superior Coronary Patency After Prehospital Initiation of Thrombolysis

| Thrombolytic Agent Used | Mean Time Gain Over Hospital Treatment | | Patency of Infarct-Related Coronary Artery by Site of Thrombolysis Initiation | | | |
| | | | Prehospital | | Hospital | |
	Minutes	Number of Patients	Open	Closed	Open	Closed
Streptokinase[6]	54	113	25	4	71	13
Streptokinase[14]	30	66	32	7	19	8
Streptokinase[8]	40	36	16	1	12	7
Streptokinase[9]	55	76	27	17	6	30
APSAC*[15]	54	110	39	15	34	22
Totals	50.0[†]	401	135[‡]	44	142	80

*APSAC = acylated plasminogen streptokinase activator complex.
[†]Proportionately weighted mean of means.
[‡]$\chi^2 = 6.01$, 1 df, $P = .014$.

prehospital thrombolysis very precisely resemble those of patients who receive inhospital treatment. Therefore, the benefits of prehospital thrombolytic therapy (see Tables 1 and 2) clearly outweigh its risks and adverse complications.

Is prehospital thrombolysis worthwhile? There is always the risk of a persistent, tight coronary stenosis after successful thrombolytic therapy. There is some anticipated reocclusion construed as failure of treatment, a limited improvement of left ventricular performance, a high frequency of acute ischemic episodes after acute myocardial infarction, and a limited effect on mortality.[4] Nevertheless, one cannot dismiss the fact that early thrombolysis leads to the dissolution of clot in the coronary artery, thereby converting the patient's hopeless, full-blown infarction into a potentially remedial early and long-term situation. The high-risk, recently thrombolysed coronary patient should be evaluated carefully with a conservative, low-level exercise stress test and then with a higher-level exercise stress test with monitoring of blood pressure responses, heart rate, and ST segment of the ECG, and a radionuclide perfusion scan of the myocardium. Pending the results of a stratification of risk based on these noninvasive data, coronary angiography can then be employed to determine which patients are suitable for further treatment with beta adrenergic or calcium channel blockade and nitrates and which are suitable for coronary angioplasty and coronary bypass surgery. Thus, the patient clearly receives a better overall chance for appropriate diagnostic and therapeutic interventions and a resultant higher quality of life when thrombolysis is administered early.

Traditionally, the remote emergency physician served both as a direct medical controller of paramedics by radio, telephone, and cellular radio telephone[19-21] and as an indirect supervisor through education, training, and protocols for treatment.[22] Thus, before thrombolytic treatment was available for acute myocardial infarction, paramedics provided early, specific emergency treatment in the field and during ambulance transport, augmenting the good results historically achieved by the pioneering mobile intensive care units staffed by physicians and nurses.[22-24]

The advent of cellular radio-telephone transmission of a 12-lead ECG of high quality has made feasible the prehospital thrombolytic treatment of acute myocardial infarction by paramedics.[13,19,20,25] Transmitted ECGs clearly showed epicardial injury meriting thrombolytic treatment by standard clinical criteria of 1 or more millimeters (0.1 mV) of ST segment elevation in two or more contiguous leads.[13]

The same complications previously identified with inhospital treatment occur with the prehospital administration of thrombolytic therapy. These include hypotension and reperfusion bradydysrhythmias, including complete heart block, and reperfusion ventricular tachycardia and fibrillation. For the latter complication, since prophylactic lidocaine has proved marginally effective, paramedics must continue to be prepared for the management of dangerous complex dysrhythmias, resuscitation, dc cardioversion, and dc countershock. Bleeding and hemorrhagic stroke occur no more often than with hospital-initiated thrombolytic treatment, but may be more difficult to manage in the field. In the acute, clinically induced, thrombolysed anticoagulative state, the mechanical trauma of resuscitation remains a potential clinical liability, but no more so than for patients managed in the hospital. Emergency treatment in the field and transportation to hospital-level intensive care in the emergency department and coronary care unit have risks and benefits clearly resembling those of inpatient thrombolytic treatment.

What constitutes the standard for appropriate training for paramedics for the prehospital initiation of thrombolytic treatment? Contemporary paramedics interpret dysrhythmias and manage them with intravenous drug therapy, resuscitation, dc cardioversion, and dc countershock. However, paramedics neither interpret the standard 12-lead ECG nor routinely pursue a differential diagnosis of the patient's cause of chest pain among musculoskeletal causes, hyperventilation, dissection of the aorta, and pericarditis. Moreover, a prehospital assessment for the initiation of thrombolysis must comprise a history and review of systems designed to elucidate relative or absolute contraindications.[17]

Is a major change in the education and training of paramedics necessary or desirable for the practice of prehospital thrombolysis? While a change is probably not crucial for 12-lead ECG interpretation, it certainly is for the collection of relevant historical information from and about the patient. Appropriately trained and supervised on-line by the remote physician, the paramedic can collect more historical details and transmit by cellular telephone the 12-lead ECG for analysis of the ST segments. Thus, the paramedic may competently and safely initiate prehospital thrombolytic treatment. As this practice develops among paramedics, the impetus will almost certainly emerge for some paramedics to learn to interpret the 12-lead ECG for the acute features relevant to initiating or denying thrombolysis. Clinical research performed in the field by paramedic units may even establish a new minimal ECG using fewer leads for future standard practice. For example, the six frontal plane leads combined with lead V_2 and the large monitor-defibrillator electrode pad at the cardiac apex, a rough V_5 equivalent, might provide valid samples of ST segment elevation for identifying those patients who qualify for the initiation of thrombolytic treatment. Further time spent in the field must be weighed against the availability of suitable emergency departments and critical care beds in the community and the significant delays (see Table 1) and their consequences (see Table 2) encountered with hospital initiation of thrombolysis. The clinical data (see Tables 1 and 2) now available indicate that the additional time spent in the field is worthwhile in terms of achieving favorable short- and long-term outcome.[6-16]

Appropriately trained paramedics can use the technology of the cellular telephone in concert with a remote supervising physician to add thrombolytic treatment to their prehospital armamentarium. This type of collaboration will permit the identification of those patients with acute myocardial infarction suitable for thrombolytic treatment before arrival at a hospital.[13] Paramedics will continue to obtain an appropriate limited history and physical examination and the 1 mm (0.1 mV) of ST elevation in two or more contiguous ECG leads accepted as the standard criterion for epicardial injury will be transmitted by cellular telephone to the remote physician as is current practice.[13] In addition to starting intravenous infusions, administering pain-relieving narcotics, and dealing with primary life-threatening dysrhythmias, paramedics will also treat the identical dysrhythmias that can be associated with the reperfusion induced by a thrombolytic drug.

Since the risks and complications associated with prehospital thrombolytic treatment are identical to those of therapy in the hospital, the many advantages of early thrombolysis militate for the timely initiation of treatment by paramedics. Therefore, it is an inescapable and irrefutable conclusion that the administration of thrombolytic treatment by appropriately trained and supervised paramedics before hospital arrival will significantly reduce both acute and long-term morbidity and mortality from acute coronary attacks.

References

1. Pantridge JF, Adgey AAJ, Geddes JS, et al: *The Acute Coronary Attack.* Tunbridge Wells, Kent, England, Pitman Medical Publishing, 1975. *This classic work summarizes prehospital coronary care and its clinical impact before thrombolytic therapy became available.*
2. Julian DG: Quality of life after myocardial infarction. *Am Heart J* 1987; 114:241–244. *This perceptive overview adds the early use of fibrinolytic agents to basic contemporary prehospital therapy and relates skilled early care to a better, longer life after an acute coronary attack.*
3. Second International Study of Infarct Survival (ISIS-2) Collaborative Group: Randomized trial of intravenous streptokinase, oral aspirin, both or neither among 17187 cases of suspected acute myocardial infarction: ISIS-2. *Lancet* 1988; 2:349–360. *This report indicates that intravenous streptokinase, potentiated by oral aspirin, improved survival after acute myocardial infarction.*
4. Chamberlain DA: Unanswered questions in thrombolysis. *Am J Cardiol* 1989; 63:34A–40A. *A skeptic asserts that no thrombolytic agent can be risk-free because none distinguishes between hemostatic and pathologic clot, although rates of reocclusion may vary among present and future methods of attaining the fibrinolytic state.*
5. Tranchesi B Jr, Bellotti G, Chamone DF, et al: Effect of combined administration of saruplase and single-chain alteplase on coronary recanalization in acute myocardial infarction. *Am J Cardiol* 1989; 64:229–232. *This report discusses the advantages and disadvantages of the combined use of various fibrinolytic drugs.*
6. Weiss AT, Fine DG, Applebaum D, et al: Prehospital coronary thrombolysis. A new strategy in acute myocardial infarction. *Chest* 1987; 92:124–128. *A*

clinical investigation is described which randomly assessed prehospital time gained after the onset of symptoms of acute myocardial ischemia over hospital time of initiation of thrombolysis. Coronary patency rates are also compared for prehospital and hospital fibrinolysis.

7. Villemant D, Barriot P, Riou B, et al: Achievement of thrombolysis at home in cases of acute myocardial infarction. *Lancet* 1987; 1:228–229. *As above, except patency rates are not compared.*

8. Bippus PH, Storch WH, Andresen D, et al: Thrombolysis started at home in acute myocardial infarction: Feasibility and time-gain (abstract). *Circulation* 1987; 76(suppl IV):122. *As above, with comparison of patency rates.*

9. Oemrawsingh PV, Bosker HA, Vander Laarse A, et al: Early reperfusion by initiation of intravenous streptokinase infusion prior to ambulance transport (abstract). *Circulation* 1988; 78(suppl II):110. *As above.*

10. Roth A, Barbash GI, Hod H, et al: Should rt-Pa be administered by the mobile intensive care unit teams (abstract)? *Circulation* 1988; 78(suppl II):187. *As above, except patency rates are not compared.*

11. Bossaert LL, Demey HE, Colemont LJ, et al, Huisartsengroep Regio Mortsel: Prehospital thrombolytic treatment of acute myocardial infarction with anisoylated plasminogen streptokinase activator complex. *Crit Care Med* 1988; 16:823–830. *As above.*

12. Spangler DE Jr, MacLean WA, Rogers WJ, et al: Is delivery of rt-PA by helicopter transport teams safe and time effective (abstract)? *J Am Coll Cardiol* 1989; 13:192A. *As above.*

13. Weaver WD, Eisenberg MS, Martin JS, et al: Myocardial infarction, triage and intervention project: Phase 1. Characteristics of patients and feasibility of prehospital initiation of thrombolytic therapy. *J Am Coll Cardiol* 1990, in press. *This investigation examines the feasibility of prehospital thrombolysis initiated by appropriately trained and supervised paramedics in the world's finest community prehospital emergency cardiac care system.*

14. Martens U, Lange-Braun P, Langer R, et al: Systemische frühlyse des akuten myokardinfarkts. Vergleich zwischen klinik und prähospitalplase. *Dtsch Med Wochenschr* 1987; 112:910–914. *This investigation provides the mean time gained by the prehospital initiation of thrombolysis without the duration of ischemic symptoms in either the prehospital or the hospital group. Coronary patency rates are also compared for prehospital and hospital fibrinolysis.*

15. Dubois Rande JL, Duval AM, Herve C, et al: At home thrombolysis in acute myocardial infarction (abstract). *Circulation* 1988; 78 (suppl II):276. *As above.*

16. Holmberg S, Hartford M, Herlitz J, et al: Very early thrombolysis with rt-PA in acute myocardial infarction (abstract). *Circulation* 1988; 78 (suppl II):276. *As above, except patency rates are not compared.*

17. Sternbach G, Tintinalli JE: Myocardial salvage: Thrombolytic therapy. *Emerg Med Clin North Am* 1988; 6:351–359. *This good review emphasizes that although interhospital thrombolysis is acceptable, prehospital thrombolysis remains inadequately assessed despite potential beneficial effects and because of great adverse risks.*

18. Koren G, Weiss AT, Hasin Y, et al: Prevention of myocardial damage in acute myocardial ischemia by early treatment with intravenous streptokinase. *N Engl*

J Med 1985; 313:1384–1389. *This report was among the earliest to assess and establish the favorable influence of prehospital thrombolytic treatment upon coronary patency rate, infarct size, and regional and global function of the left ventricle.*

19. Grim P, Feldman T, Martin M, et al: Cellular telephone transmission of 12-lead electrocardiograms from ambulance to hospital. *Am J Cardiol* 1987; 60:715–720. *This report addresses and establishes the feasibility of radio–cellular phone transmission of high-quality ECGs for the initiation of out-of-hospital thrombolysis by physician-supervised paramedics.*

20. Grim PS, Feldman T, Childers RW: Evaluation of patients for the need of thrombolytic therapy in the prehospital setting. *Ann Emerg Med* 1989; 18:483–488. *As above.*

21. Greenberg H, Sherrid MV, Lynn S, et al: Out-of-hospital, paramedic administered streptokinase for acute myocardial infarction. *Lancet* 1988; 2:1187. *As above.*

22. Committee on Emergency Medical Services: *Medical Control in Emergency Medical Services Systems.* Washington, DC, National Academy Press, 1981. *The principles and standards of the out-of-hospital extension of emergency care by the remote physician via protocols and radio-telephone medical command to paramedics are described with important observations upon interactions.*

23. Pozen MW, D'Agostino RB, Sytkowski PA, et al: Effectiveness of a prehospital medical control system: An analysis of the interaction between emergency room physician and paramedic. *Circulation* 1981; 63:442–447. *As above.*

24. Crampton RS: Impact of the mobile coronary care unit in the USA, in Geddes JS (ed): *The Management of the Acute Coronary Attack.* London, Academic Press Inc, 1986, pp 9–22. *This chapter examines quantifiable and unquantifiable clinical and epidemiologic aspects of prehospital coronary care in the prethrombolytic era in the United States.*

25. European Myocardial Infarction Project (EMIP) Subcommittee: Potential timesaving with pre-hospital intervention in acute myocardial infarction. *Eur Heart J* 1988; 9:118–124. *This report also addresses and establishes the feasibility of radio–cellular phone transmission of high-quality ECGs for the initiation of out-of-hospital thrombolysis by physician-supervised paramedics.*

Negative

David W. M. Muller, M.B., B.S.
Eric J. Topol, M.D.

The recent demonstration of an unequivocal reduction in the mortality of acute myocardial infarction by intravenous streptokinase, tissue-type plasminogen activator (tPA), and anisoylated plasminogen streptokinase activator complex (APSAC) [1-4] has initiated calls for broadening of the indications for the use of these agents and for increasing their availability to community hospitals and local physicians. In order to augment myocardial salvage further, it has been advocated that appropriately trained paramedics administer thrombolytic therapy for suspected myocardial infarction. More recently, attempts have been made to fashion stable analogues of these agents for intramuscular use to allow self-administration by suitably educated patients. [5]

It is clear that the use of fibrinolytic agents is continuing to increase and will become first-line therapy for patients with acute myocardial infarction in whom there are no contraindications to thrombolysis. [6] What is not clear, however, is whether it is appropriate to extend the indications for thrombolytic therapy to include suspected infarction and unstable angina and whether the prehospital administration of these potent therapies by paramedical staff or patients themselves is safe or desirable. Since these issues have not yet been systematically evaluated, one can only draw conclusions indirectly by considering the question from three viewpoints. First, is such an approach necessary and of benefit to the patient? Second, is it safe? And, finally, are there better alternatives?

Is the Administration of Thrombolytic Therapy by Paramedics Beneficial?

Several recent studies[7-9] have shown that, under optimal conditions, thrombolytic therapy can be administered by intensive care ambulance physicians an average of 30 to 40 minutes earlier than if given on arrival in the emergency room. Is there evidence that a delay of this magnitude is critical to the extent of myocardial salvage? Few studies have addressed this question directly. Weiss et al.[9] compared the outcomes of 29 patients treated with intravenous streptokinase prior to transportation with those of 84 consecutive patients treated after arrival in the emergency room. The time from the onset of symptoms to the initiation of streptokinase infusion was 1.0 ± 0.4 hours for those patients treated out of the hospital compared with

1.9 ± 0.9 hours for those treated in the hospital. Vessel patency at follow-up angiography 6 days after admission was the same in each group, but preservation of left ventricular function, particularly following anterior infarction, was significantly greater in the paramedic-treated patients. A similar benefit was also suggested by the Gruppo Italiano per lo Studio della Streptochinasi nell Infarto miocardico (GISSI) study,[1] which showed a greater reduction in mortality in those patients treated with streptokinase during the first hour of symptoms compared with those treated less than 3 hours and 3 to 6 hours later (47% vs. 23% and 18%, respectively). In contrast, no such hour-by-hour time dependence was apparent in the larger Second International Study of Infarct Survival (ISIS-II)[2] using streptokinase and aspirin or in the APSAC Intervention Mortality Study (AIMS) study[4] using APSAC in acute infarction.

The time from symptom onset to the initiation of therapy appears to be even less critical for the relatively fibrin-selective thrombolytic agents such as tPA. Roth et al.[7] for example, showed no reduction in infarct size or improvement in left ventricular function for a group of 56 patients treated at home with intravenous tPA 44 minutes earlier than a similar group transported rapidly to an emergency room prior to the initiation of therapy. The larger trials of tPA for acute infarction have shown similar findings. The recently reported Anglo-Scandinavian Study of Early Thrombolysis (ASSET),[3] for example, showed an overall reduction in 5-week vascular mortality of 26% for patients treated with tPA within 5 hours of the onset of symptoms. No significant difference in outcome was discernible, however, for those treated in under or over 3 hours (25.7% vs. 24.4%). Similarly, the Thrombolysis and Angioplasty in Myocardial Infarction (TAMI) study group[10] showed no difference in the extent of tPA-mediated recovery of left ventricular function between those patients treated less than 2 hours from symptom onset compared with those treated from 2 to 4 hours from symptom onset (Table 3). It appears, therefore, that although the ability of thrombolytic therapy to preserve myocardial function and enhance survival following acute infarction undoubtedly does become attenuated with delays of several hours from symptom onset, the small delays inherent in patient transportation may not be of critical importance.

The alternative approach is to consider each minute vital to the extent of myocardial salvage. If this "time is muscle" approach is adopted, it could be argued that a more reasonable strategy would be to minimize prehospital care and to provide rapid transport to the nearest hospital, as has been recommended for the management of major trauma.[11,12] While several studies have demonstrated a reduction in the mortality of high-risk patients transported by mobile intensive care units,[13,14] some have suggested that the conventional prehospital care currently performed by paramedics is already unnecessarily protracted.

A recently reported study from Salt Lake City,[15] for example, compared the outcome of 134 patients with acute infarction who received conventional

TABLE 3.
**Relationship Between Left Ventricular Function and Time
to Therapy***

Time From Chest Pain to rt-PA[†]	n	Acute Ejection Fraction		7-Day Ejection Fraction	
		Mean ± SD	Median	Mean ± SD[†]	Median[§]
0 – <2	40	0.55 ± 0.11	0.55	0.56 ± 0.11	0.59
2 – <3	62	0.53 ± 0.10	0.55	0.53 ± 0.11	0.54
3 – <4	49	0.53 ± 0.10	0.52	0.54 ± 0.11	0.53
≥ 4	25	0.53 ± 0.10	0.55	0.55 ± 0.08	0.55

*From Topol EJ, Califf RM, Kereiakes DJ, et al: *J Am Coll Cardiol* 1987;
109:65B–74B. Used by permission.
[†]rt-PA = recombinant tissue plasminogen activator.
[†]For 0 to 2 hours vs. > 2 hours, 7-day ejection fraction: $P = .12$, t test.
[§]For 0 to 2 hours vs. > 2 hours, 7-day ejection fraction: $P = .08$, Wilcoxon test.

prehospital care from a mobile paramedic unit with that of a comparable group who chose alternate means of transportation. In this study, medical care was initiated 5 minutes after it was sought by the group transported by paramedics. Prehospital care included a brief history and physical examination; the establishment of intravenous access; the administration of oxygen, intravenous fluids, analgesia, and prophylactic lidocaine; and continuous electrocardiographic (ECG) monitoring. The mean time to hospital arrival was 44 minutes from the time medical care was sought. In contrast, the mean time to hospital arrival and initiation of medical care for patients choosing other means of transport was only 15 minutes. No difference was demonstrable in the survival of the two groups or in the incidence of adverse outcomes. The authors concluded that the time required for conventional care, all of which would be necessary prior to the initiation of thrombolytic therapy, is already substantial. The additional time required to more thoroughly exclude conditions which would contraindicate fibrinolytic therapy, to obtain and transmit a 12-lead ECG, to confer with medical personnel, and to prepare the thrombolytic agent for infusion may indeed be detrimental to the outcome of the patient.

In reality, the major delay which occurs in the conventional management of acute infarction generally is not related to ambulance response and transport time, but rather to delays from symptom onset to the initiation of the call for medical assistance. It is this much greater delay that is critical and requires urgent public education to increase both awareness of the symptoms of acute infarction and the availability of and access to appropriate resources for early acute intervention.

When examining the need for paramedic-initiated thrombolytic therapy, it is important also to consider the size of the population which may benefit from such an approach. A recent feasibility study from Seattle[16] determined the proportion of patients treated by a mobile intensive care ambulance crew who fulfilled conventional criteria for eligibility for thrombolytic therapy. Of 757 patients transported during the study period, 209 (27.6%) were considered candidates for thrombolytic therapy on the basis of symptoms, age, and absence of contraindications to fibrinolysis. Of these, only 30 (or 4.0% of the total group) had ECG changes of acute infarction. If these figures are valid nationally, it is doubtful whether the additional manpower and training required to operate such a program is justifiable in view of the arguable benefit for a relatively small population of patients. If, on the other hand, the need for ECG changes of acute infarction was eliminated from the criteria for eligibility and thrombolytic therapy was given on the basis of clinical suspicion alone, a much greater proportion of the above population would have been eligible for treatment.

Is there any evidence that this is a reasonable approach? Only two of the large thrombolytic therapy trials, ISIS-II[2] and ASSET,[3] have included patients with clinically suspected acute infarction without diagnostic ECG changes. Each of these trials showed a very low mortality in patients with "normal" ECGs and a nonsignificant trend towards a reduction in mortality (1.9% vs. 3.9% for ISIS-II and 1.6% vs. 3.0% for ASSET). In the subgroup of patients in ISIS-II with ST segment depression on the admission ECG, 5-week vascular mortality was significantly higher than in those without ECG changes and was unaffected by the administration of thrombolytic therapy (18.7% vs. 18.5%). Therefore, while the benefits of giving thrombolytic therapy to patients without electrocardiographically confirmed acute myocardial infarction currently appear to be small, the potential hazards of such an approach may be substantial.

Can Thrombolytic Therapy Be Administered Safely by Paramedics?

Many studies have now demonstrated the feasibility of transporting patients with acute myocardial infarction following the initiation of thrombolytic therapy. Early concerns about the increased risks of bleeding, reperfusion arrhythmias, and allergic reactions during transportation appear to have been largely dispelled. In a study by Topol et al.[17] of 55 patients who received physician-initiated thrombolytic therapy prior to or during helicopter transport, no deaths occurred and no patient experienced hemorrhagic or allergic complications. Ventricular tachycardia and third-degree atrioventricular (AV) block occurred more frequently in the treated patients than in a comparable group not receiving thrombolytic therapy (12.7% vs. 1.1%; P=.005). None of these episodes was sustained, however, and none required cardioversion, temporary pacing, or antiarrhythmic therapy in addition to the intravenous lidocaine given prophylactically prior to commencement of the tPA infusion.

Of much greater concern than these apparently benign side effects is the potential hazard of misdiagnosis and the subsequent administration of thrombolytic therapy to patients with noncardiac pain due to conditions such as acute aortic dissection, acute pericarditis, and peptic ulcer disease. This is of particular concern when ECG changes are not considered a necessary prerequisite for eligibility. In the ASSET study, for example, 17.5% of the total population treated had normal entry ECGs. Of the 5,011 patients enrolled in the study, 554 (11%) were later recognized to have had noncardiac pain after being exposed to the potential hazards and unnecessary costs of thrombolytic therapy (Table 4). Thirteen patients were shown to have acute aortic dissections. Five of the 8 such patients treated with tPA died within 48 hours of admission. Similarly, in the Swedish Thrombolysis in Early Acute Heart Attack Trial (TEAHAT) of tPA in acute infarction,[18] no ECG criterion was required for eligibility to receive thrombolytic therapy. Of the 479 patients fulfilling the inclusion criteria, 8 were excluded by the treating physicians because of suspected and subsequently confirmed acute aortic dissections. Two patients with unrecognized aortic dissection, however, received tPA and died soon after admission. Thus, a total of 10 patients

TABLE 4.
Hospital Discharge Diagnostic Categorizaton*

Diagnosis	rt-PA[†] (2,512)	Placebo (2,493)
Myocardial infarction	1,811 (72.1%)	1,783 (71.5%)
Definite	1,420 (56.5%)	1,464 (58.7%)
Probable	233 (9.2%)	191 (7.6%)
Possible	158 (6.3%)	128 (5.1%)
Ischemic heart disease	429 (17.0%)	426 (17.0%)
Chest pain of unknown cause	198 (7.8%)	202 (8.1%)
Other diagnosis	73 (2.9%)	81 (3.2%)
Missing data	1	1

*From Anglo-Scandinavian Study of Early Thrombolysis (ASSET): *Lancet* 1988; 2:525–530. Used by permission.
[†]rt-PA = recombinant tissue plasminogen activator.

with aortic dissection fulfilled the clinical inclusion criteria and were eligible for treatment with thrombolytic therapy. In each of these studies, the patients were questioned carefully and examined by experienced clinicians. It is highly likely that the incidence of potentially fatal misdiagnosis would have been higher without this careful screening.

It is important to note that the inappropriate administration of lytic therapy may occur even when ECG changes are mandatory for eligibility. Of 865 consecutive patients enrolled in five multicenter TAMI studies, acute myocardial infarction was incorrectly diagnosed by emergency room physicians in 12 patients (1.4%).[19] The final diagnoses in these patients included acute pericarditis, prior myocardial infarction with persisting ST segment elevation, and atypical chest pain with left bundle branch block or left ventricular hypertrophy. While this incidence of misdiagnosis is acceptably low, the error was made in each case by an experienced clinician working under optimal conditions. No data are yet available on the diagnostic accuracy of appropriately trained paramedical staff attending patients in the more difficult, out-of-hospital environment.

What is the cost of the inappropriate administration of thrombolytic therapy? Apart from the substantial economic cost, the major hazard is life-threatening hemorrhage. This risk has been well documented and recently summarized.[20] Major bleeding events are most commonly related to arterial puncture sites, but the potential for retroperitoneal, gastrointestinal, and genitourinary hemorrhage is significant (Table 5). Although the risk of intracranial hemorrhage is very low (approximately 0.5% with current dosage regimens), the prognosis for these patients has been uniformly poor. Furthermore, the risk of intracranial hemorrhage appears to be dose-dependent, rising to 1.6% in patients treated with 150 mg of tPA.[21] This is highly relevant to this discussion because of the inevitable difficulties in monitoring intravenous infusion rates during transportation and the possibility of accidental bolus dosing of potent fibrinolytic drugs. Even the small possibility of such a devastating complication represents an unacceptable risk.

Are There Better Alternatives to Paramedic-Initiated Thrombolysis?

The optimal approach to the prehospital management of acute myocardial infarction would consist of the rapid deployment of medical teams including appropriately trained physicians equipped with facilities for performing 12-lead ECGs to the site of first contact, with a crew available to establish intravenous access and to prepare and administer medications, including thrombolytic therapy, while the patient is being promptly loaded and transported to the nearest community hospital. Radio contact would

TABLE 5.
Incidence of Hemorrhagic Events After
Intravenous Recombinant Tissue
Plasminogen Activator*

Event	rt-PA[†] (%) (n = 143)	SK[†] (%) (n = 147)
Type of blood loss		
Major	15.4	15.6
Minor	17.5	15.6
Site		
Intracranial	0	0
Of catheterization	27.3	27.2
Of other puncture	4.9	4.1
Gastrointestinal	4.9	6.8
Genitourinary	6.3	3.4
Retroperitoneal	0.7	0.7
Transfusion	22.4	19.7
Fibrinogen <100 mg/dL	3.0	30.0

*From Faxon DP: *J Am Coll Cardiol* 1988; 12(suppl A):
52A–57A. Used by permission.
[†]rt-PA = recombinant tissue plasminogen activator; SK =
streptokinase.

then allow the emergency room to be bypassed and direct admission to the coronary care unit to be expedited, thereby eliminating the often considerable delays associated with hospital triage and patient reevaluation. Although this has been achieved in some centers,[9] in the absence of unlimited resources and medical manpower, this approach is clearly not universally feasible.

The alternative to physician-operated mobile intensive care units is a physician-supervised system. This necessitates ready contact between the field team and the hospital-based physician and the ability to obtain and transmit high-fidelity 12-lead ECGs. Several systems capable of achieving this are currently under investigation, including radiotelemetry units which are limited by poor frequency response and suboptimal signal-to-noise ratio, and cellular telephones which are limited by the possibility of emergency calls being "blocked" during times of heavy commercial communications traffic.[22] Although this approach has been shown to be feasible in preliminary studies,[23] the necessary increase in out-of-hospital triage time may well prevent any substantial reduction in the time to the initiation of thrombolytic therapy.

In any given community, the recommended strategy will vary according to its geography and budgetary considerations. In most communities, transportation times are short and the most appropriate strategy is to load and transport the patient as rapidly as possible. Rather than spending time at the scene, early notification of the emergency room is appropriate, thereby allowing staff to act promptly on arrival. Twelve-lead electrocardiography can be performed immediately and, if possible, compared with already obtained copies of old ECGs to confirm changes of acute infarction. Clinical assessment can be performed quickly by experienced medical personnel and noncardiac causes can be excluded. This strategy is the most universally applicable. Its major limitation is the triage and reevaluation delay which often occurs in the emergency room. It is imperative that emergency room staff be cognizant of the importance of promptly confirming the suspected diagnosis, efficiently initiating therapy, and transferring the patient to a unit with monitoring facilities and skilled nursing care as rapidly as possible.

The widespread use of thrombolytic therapy already has had a substantial impact on the natural history of coronary artery disease, but its value can be realized only for those patients who seek and receive medical care during the early hours of acute infarction. It is important to recognize, however, that many patients remain ineligible for thrombolytic therapy. Although the optimal management of this subgroup is not as well defined, they too require prompt evaluation and triage to immediate angiography and, if necessary, coronary angioplasty or alternative pharmacotherapy.

The in-hospital mortality rate for patients who are treated with thrombolytic therapy has now fallen to the very low level of approximately 5%. Further reductions in the mortality of this group will be more difficult to achieve. The proportion of patients dying before receiving medical care, however, is still substantial. It is this issue which is critical and can be affected only by widespread public education programs urging the early presentation of individuals with symptoms suggestive of acute infarction.

The preceding risk-benefit analysis does not support the proposition to allow paramedics to administer thrombolytic therapy for suspected acute infarction. The potential for the inadvertent administration of potent fibrinolytic agents to patients with noncardiac pain is not insignificant and would have complex medicolegal implications. Apart from these considerations, the substantial costs of recruiting and training additional paramedical staff, providing and maintaining additional communications equipment, and using these agents inappropriately represent a drain on the budget of an already compromised health care system. The funds allocated to such a program could be more usefully employed to educate the public and encourage very early presentation following the onset of symptoms of acute infarction, thereby maximizing the impact of acute intervention on the early mortality of this very prevalent disease.

References

1. Gruppo Italiano per lo Studio della Streptochinasi nell Infarto miocardico (GISSI): Effectiveness of intravenous thrombolytic treatment in acute myocardial infarction. *Lancet* 1986; 1:397–402. *This was the first trial with the statistical power to demonstrate a substantial improvement in mortality following thrombolytic therapy.*
2. Second International Study of Infarct Survival: Randomised trial of intravenous Streptokinase, oral aspirin, both, or neither among 17,187 cases of suspected acute myocardial infarction: ISIS-II. *Lancet* 1988; 2:349–360. *Similar to reference 1, this trial confirmed the impact of intravenous streptokinase therapy on survival following acute myocardial infarction and, for the first time, demonstrated a potentiation of its efficacy by concomitant aspirin therapy.*
3. Anglo-Scandinavian Study of Early Thrombolysis (ASSET): Trial of tissue plasminogen activator for mortality reduction in acute myocardial infarction. *Lancet* 1988; 2:525–530. *This recently published study was the first to demonstrate a statistically significant improvement in survival following tPA administration.*
4. AIMS Trial Study Group: Effect of intravenous APSAC on mortality after acute myocardial infarction: Preliminary report of a placebo-controlled trial. *Lancet* 1988; 2:545–549. *This study showed that the reduction in postinfarction mortality is not limited to streptokinase and tPA. The 47% reduction in mortality is the largest of any acute intervention trial.*
5. Sobel BE, Safnitz JE, Fields LE, et al: Intramuscular administration of human tissue-type plasminogen activator in rabbits and dogs and its implications for coronary thrombolysis. *Circulation* 1987; 75:1261–72. *This is an early report of ongoing investigations designed to develop fibrinolytic agents with optimal pharmacokinetic profiles.*
6. Hlatky MA, Cotugno H, O'Connor C, et al: Adoption of thrombolytic therapy in the management of acute myocardial infarction. *Am J Cardiol* 1988; 61:510–514. *A national survey of 1,065 physicians, this study documents current patterns of use of thrombolytic therapy for acute infarction and compares the findings with those of a similar survey conducted in 1979.*
7. Roth A, Barbash GI, Hod H, et al: Should rt-PA be administered by the Mobile Intensive Care Unit teams (abstract)? *Circulation* 1988; 78 (suppl 2):II–186. *This is a small study examining the safety of intravenous tPA given during the prehospital phase by mobile intensive care units.*
8. Rande JLD, Duval AM, Herve C, et al: At home thrombolysis in acute myocardial infarction (abstract). *Circulation* 1988; 78 (suppl 2):II–276. *As above.*
9. Weiss AT, Fine DG, Applebaum D, et al: Prehospital coronary thrombolysis. A new strategy in acute myocardial infarction. *Chest* 1987; 92:124–128. *This small study examines the feasibility of physician-operated paramedic teams administering intravenous streptokinase and compares its efficacy with that of hospital-delivered streptokinase.*
10. Topol EJ, Califf RM, Kereiakes DJ, et al: Thrombolysis and Angioplasty in Myocardial Infarction (TAMI) trial. *J Am Coll Cardiol* 1987; 109:65B–74B.

This large study prospectively examined changes in left ventricular function following early tPA administration and showed no significant time dependence for the recovery of left ventricular function.

11. Smith JP, Bodai BI, Hill AS, et al: Pre-hospital stabilization of critically injured patients: A failed concept. *J Trauma* 1985; 25:65–70. *One of several studies which critically examined the widespread practice of cardiopulmonary stabilization prior to transportation and highlighted the potentially adverse impact of this practice on survival following multiple trauma.*

12. Trunkey DD: Is ALS necessary for pre-hospital trauma care? *J Trauma* 1984; 24:86–87. *As above.*

13. Pressley JC, Severance HW, Raney MP, et al: A comparison of paramedic versus basic emergency medical care of patients at high and low risk during acute myocardial infarction. *J Am Coll Cardiol* 1988; 12:1555–61. *This is one of several studies critically evaluating the impact of mobile intensive care units on early mortality from acute infarction.*

14. Crampton RS, Aldrich RF, Gascho JA, et al: Reduction of prehospital, ambulance and community coronary death rates by the community-wide emergency cardiac care system. *Am J Med* 1975; 58:151–65. *As above.*

15. Dean NC, Haug PJ, Hawker PJ: Effect of mobile paramedic units on outcome in patients with myocardial infarction. *Ann Emerg Med* 1988; 17:1034–1041. *In contrast to references 13 and 14, this recent study questions the effectiveness of mobile paramedic units and highlights potential delays which may actually adversely affect patient outcome by interfering with therapies that are necessarily hospital-based.*

16. Weaver WD, Martin JS, Litwin PE, et al: Prehospital thrombolytic therapy: Preliminary report on feasibility (abstract). *Circulation* 1988; 78(suppl 2):II–110. *This is a preliminary report of important ongoing studies examining the role of paramedical staff in the prehospital management of acute infarction. The results of these studies will be critical to many currently unanswered questions.*

17. Topol EJ, Fung AY, Kline E, et al: Safety of helicopter transport and out-of-hospital intravenous fibrinolytic therapy in patients with evolving myocardial infarction. *Cathet Cardiovasc Diagn* 1986; 12:151–155. *This study documenting the safety of ambulance transport following thrombolytic therapy has important implications for the early use of thrombolytic therapy by community hospitals.*

18. Holmberg S, Hartford M, Herlitz J, et al: Very early thrombolysis with rt-PA in acute myocardial infarction (abstract). *Circulation* 1988; 78 (suppl 2):II–276. *This abstract is a preliminary report from a large study which highlights some of the potential difficulties of accurate diagnosis of acute infarction in the prehospital phase of therapy.*

19. Chapman GD, O'Connor CM, Kereiakes DJ, et al: Consequences of misdiagnosis of acute myocardial infarction leading to thrombolytic therapy: A multicenter experience (abstract). *J Am Coll Cardiol* 1990; 15:227. *This is one of a few studies which examines diagnostic accuracy in large teaching hospitals and emphasizes the potential hazards of the indiscriminate use of thrombolytic therapy.*

20. Faxon DP: The risk of reperfusion strategies in the treatment of patients with acute myocardial infarction. *J Am Coll Cardiol* 1988; 12 (suppl A):52A–57A.

This paper from a recent symposium concisely summarizes the known hazards of fibrinolytic therapy.

21. Braunwald E, Knatterud GL, Passammani EP, et al: Announcement of a critical change in thrombolysis in myocardial infarction trial (letter). *J Am Coll Cardiol* 1987; 9:467. *Following the demonstration of an unacceptably high incidence of hemorrhagic stroke, the investigators of the Thrombolysis in Myocardial Infarction Study elected to reduce the dose of tPA from 150 mg to 100 mg and subsequently showed a reduction in the incidence of this side effect.*

22. Grim P, Feldman T, Martin M, et al: Cellular telephone transmission of 12 lead electrocardiograms from ambulance to hospital. *Am J Cardiol* 1987; 60:715–720. *This study provides early data on the use of battery-powered cellular telephones to transmit 12-lead ECGs to the parent hospital and highlights some of the potential problems associated with their use.*

23. Greenberg H, Sherrid MV, Lynn S, et al: Out-of-hospital paramedic administered streptokinase for acute myocardial infarction (letter). *Lancet* 1988; 2:1187. *As above.*

Rebuttal: Affirmative
Richard Crampton, D.M.

As evidenced by the clinical investigations summarized by Dr. Muller, Dr. Topol, and me, thrombolytic agents emphatically have joined narcotics and beta adrenergic blocking drugs as standard first-line early therapy for appropriately selected patients with acute myocardial infarction. Like pre-hospital relief of ischemic chest pain with narcotics and relief of dysrhythmo-genic autonomic stress with acute beta blockade to prevent ventricular fibrillation and cardiac rupture,[1,2] acute prehospital fibrinolysis has produced a significant decrement in mortality and morbidity by reperfusing otherwise doomed ischemic heart muscle. The benefit of prehospital thrombolysis derives from its superior coronary patency rate achieved by significantly earlier administration, as outlined in the tables I presented previously. An essential, new third arm of early treatment, it is relatively safe and its benefits clearly outweigh its risks.[3-10] The combination of thrombolysis and aspirin added to early intravenous beta blockade has significantly enhanced the 15% reduction of early deaths attributable to beta blockade alone.

No superior alternative now exists to the earliest possible dissolution of the clot in the coronary artery causing an acute myocardial infarction. Yet, Drs. Muller and Topol argue an approach designed "to minimize prehospital care and to provide rapid transport to the nearest hospital, as has been recommended for the management of major trauma." Acute myocardial infarction and major trauma differ so greatly that the attempted analogy erodes this argument. They cite the Salt Lake City report in which paramedic treatment of acute myocardial infarction caused a 29 minute median delay (44 minutes longer) in entering the hospital for 134 patients when compared to 101 patients who used other conventional transportation.[11] The results of this study differ remarkably from cumulative experience with prehospital intensive care by paramedics or physicians.[1,2,12,13] Thus, before it can be used to refute the value of prehospital thrombolysis by paramedics, closer examination is mandatory.

The reality of the Salt Lake City study is that 10 of 134 patients with acute myocardial infarction seen by paramedics a median of 5 minutes after the call for aid were resuscitated from ventricular fibrillation before or during transport and, therefore, presented alive at the hospital. Four had arrested before the arrival of paramedics. Eighty percent of the 134 patients received intravenous lidocaine a median of 88 minutes after the onset of symptoms. Thus, although prevention of ventricular tachycardia and fibrillation oc-curred, it is unquantifiable. In contrast, these investigators recorded no patients arresting before nonparamedic arrival; yet 5 of the 101 patients died during contact with conventional ambulance personnel. Using Fisher's exact test, two-sided, these data significantly favored paramedic prehospital care (P = .03). Thus, procrastination of on-the-spot emergency treatment in favor of antiquated "scoop and run" ambulance service remained fatal.

Although the patients not attended by paramedics received treatment a median of 15 minutes after the call for help, they received lidocaine a median of 133 minutes after the onset of symptoms. Thus, paramedic treatment with lidocaine was given 45 minutes earlier, a time gain with a favorable outcome similar to the superiority of prehospital initiation of thrombolysis (see my previous Tables 1 and 2). By prehospital life-saves alone, 44 minutes of paramedic treatment time clearly outweighed "horizontal taxi" ambulance service accompanied by 45 minutes of deferred and delayed hospital treatment of acute myocardial infarction. Finally, before Drs. Muller and Topol continue to advocate a reversion to the "scoop and run" ambulance era, ethical and practical considerations of such a misguided step backward must be examined. Like Wilson's group in Northern Ireland,[12] the Salt Lake City investigators at least recognized that the investigation of randomized provision of paramedic vs. conventional ambulance service was both unethical and impractical.

Should the criteria,[1,2,12,14,15] of acceptable treatment with narcotics, beta blockers, aspirin, lidocaine, and ventricular defibrillation be applied to prehospital thrombolytic treatment by appropriately trained and supervised paramedics? By analogy, yes. It is very doubtful that prehospital delays will tip the scales against paramedics as long as the care rendered is crucial, as in the earliest possible initiation of thrombolysis, and of the highest quality, as is ensured by the supervising remote physician. First, the rapid recognition of acute myocardial infarction is mandatory to initiate the salvage of jeopardized heart muscle with thrombolytic therapy. Like patients with early acute anterior myocardial infarction, patients with early and large threatened inferior infarctions stand to benefit substantially from reduced morbidity and mortality. The possibly superior patency rates associated with the use of recombinant tissue plasminogen activator (rt-PA) may make this agent practicable in a broader prehospital time frame. Finally, since thrombolytic treatment in acute myocardial infarction has virtually achieved the level of first-line standard of care in hospitals, its prehospital use as a standard of care treatment is inevitable.

Will some patients with causes of chest pain other than early acute myocardial infarction receive thrombolytic treatment inappropriately? Most certainly, some patients will receive such treatment to their detriment, but probably no more than the small number now receiving physician-mandated hospital thrombolysis for unrecognized aortic dissection, acute pericarditis, and musculoskeletal chest pain. The ethical problem of withholding prehospital thrombolysis until arrival at the hospital has already arisen. In at least one study in which there was a significant hospital delay in starting treatment, patients randomized to prehospital placebo treatment received thrombolytic treatment at home at the insistence of a caring, but code-breaking, research physician in a mobile intensive care unit.[16]

Will an adequate number of patients be seen early enough to justify providing prehospital thrombolysis by paramedics? Educating the public about coronary attacks is problematic, as evidenced by a recent study in which no change was found in the time from symptom onset to the call for help in cases of acute chest pain despite a community-wide media blitz.[17] Providing paramedic prehospital thrombolysis has a potential benefit for over one third of all patients with acute myocardial infarction determined by hospital criteria.[18] The time consumed for the longer out-of-hospital contact is reasonable, and delaying therapy costs lives and heart muscle. In the study cited by Drs. Muller and Topol, the interval from the time it took to reach the patient to performing the electrocardiogram (ECG) and discussing the findings and treatment with a physician was 18 ± 10 (SD) minutes, 7 minutes of which was for the ECG component.[18]

How much distinction will there be between the physician-initiated thrombolytic experience[19] and the proposed physician-initiated and supervised prehospital thrombolysis carried out by paramedics? Very little, because the adverse dysrhythmic and hemorrhagic effects to date are well recognized to occur with equal frequency in both groups. The very real risk remains of inadvertently using thrombolysis for aortic dissection, pericarditis, and musculoskeletal chest pain. Life-threatening hemorrhage is a problem with treatment administered both in and out of the hospital. Traditional, but untested, objections such as the difficulty of monitoring intravenous infusion rates during transport may soon be obviated by the use of acylated plasminogen streptokinase activator complex (APSAC), since a single injection over 5 minutes makes it an ideal agent for prehospital administration.

From a societal or community viewpoint, paramedic services to patients in the field might be augmented by redistributing surplus American physicians into the prehospital emergency system as is common in health services in the Soviet Union and other European nations. Certainly, greater physician involvement has already made inroads on hospital delays by expediting prehospital treatment with thrombolysis (see Table 1). Despite early technical problems, paramedics in a recent study successfully transmitted 522 of 677 ECGs (77%). Emergency services and their logistics vary from community to community. Transport time, level of care, and efficacy of service are profoundly affected by municipal traffic jams and greater rural distances, particularly when coupled with emergency department and other hospital delays. A return to "horizontal taxi" emergency service would deny adequate care for the substantial proportion of patients at risk of dying from or experiencing severe morbidity from an undissolved clot in a coronary artery.

The risk-benefit analysis suggested by Drs. Muller and Topol to preclude prehospital thrombolysis by physician-supervised paramedics actually strongly supports this treatment when examined closely in the light of present-day clinical reality. Despite the appropriate concerns regarding inadvertently administering potent fibrinolytic agents, raising new medical-legal issues, and raising health-care costs, the future practice of prehospital thrombolysis by paramedics will further minimize the morbidity and mortality of many patients suffering acute myocardial infarction. Ultimately, prehospital thrombolysis will reduce the number of individuals dying of or debilitated by coronary disease. Thus, the community's financial burden in caring for these potential invalids or their destitute dependents will be substantially lessened. Therefore, can our society afford not to provide prehospital thrombolytic treatment by paramedics?

Remote physician-directed out-of-hospital therapy need not be and has not been limited to paramedics. In both the presence or absence of people trained in venipuncture, complimentary systems employing basic and advanced telephonic technologies have extended high-quality intensive care supervised by the remote physician to the patient's emergency environment anywhere: in homes, extended-care facilities, office blocks, factories, stadia, and nonmedical civic and emergency systems.[20–24] Contemporary cellular telephonic technology has provided high-quality ECGs for the diagnosis and monitoring of dysrhythmias,[18,25,26] thereby permitting the informed remote physician to supervise lay persons such as patients, family members, bystanders, civic personnel, and a variety of different health care providers. The remote, telephonically linked physician can now supervise the administration of rt-PA by autoinjector[27] and can perform resuscitation with cardioversion and countershock if reperfusion ventricular tachycardia or fibrillation occurs.[20,21] Using the latter type of telephonic emergency care system, an informed remote ICU nurse recently terminated ventricular tachycardia by a telephonically activated defibrillator after the patient's spouse had applied monitor/defibrillator electrode pads to the chest.[23,24] A lidocaine autoinjector can be used to prevent recurrent or reperfusion ventricular dysrhythmias.[28]

In summary, prehospital thrombolysis by paramedics under the conventional supervision of a remote physician has arrived to stay as standard, first-line treatment for appropriately selected patients. In addition, the prehospital autoinjection of thrombolytic treatment by lay persons and less sophisticated health care or civic personnel telephonically supervised by a remote physician is feasible and merits investigation.

Acknowledgment

The author thanks Doctors D. G. Julian and D. A. Chamberlain for the opportunity to participate in the British Heart Foundation's Conference on the Management of Acute Myocardial Ischaemia, at the Royal College of Physicians in London from May 31 to June 2, 1989.

References

1. Crampton RS: Impact of the mobile coronary care unit in the USA, in Geddes JS (ed): *The Management of the Acute Coronary Attack*. London, Academic Press Inc, 1986, pp 9–22.
2. Geddes JS: Twenty years of prehospital coronary care. *Br Heart J* 1986; 56:491–495.
3. Gruppo Italiano per lo Studio della Streptochinasi nell Infarto miocardico (GISSI): Effectiveness of intravenous thrombolytic treatment in acute myocardial infarction. *Lancet* 1986; 1:397–402.
4. Second International Study of Infarct Survival: Randomised trial of intravenous Streptokinase, oral aspirin, both, or neither among 17,187 cases of suspected acute myocardial infarction: ISIS-II. *Lancet* 1988; 2:349–360.
5. Anglo-Scandinavian Study of Early Thrombolysis (ASSET): Trial of tissue plasminogen activator for mortality reduction in acute myocardial infarction. *Lancet* 1988; 2:525–530.
6. AIMS Trial Study Group: Effect of intravenous APSAC on mortality after acute myocardial infarction: Preliminary report of a placebo-controlled trial. *Lancet* 1988; 2:545–549.
7. Hlatky MA, Cotugno H, O'Connor C, et al: Adoption of thrombolytic therapy in the management of acute myocardial infarction. *Am J Cardiol* 1988; 61:510–514.
8. Roth A, Barbash GI, Hod H, et al: Should rt-PA be administered by the Mobile Intensive Care Unit teams (abstract)? *Circulation* 1988; 78 (suppl 2):II–186.
9. Rande JLD, Duval AM, Herve C, et al: At home thrombolysis in acute myocardial infarction (abstract). *Circulation* 1988; 78 (suppl 2): II–276.
10. Weiss AT, Fine DG, Applebaum D, et al: Prehospital coronary thrombolysis. A new strategy in acute myocardial infarction. *Chest* 1987; 92:124–128.
11. Dean NC, Haug PJ, Hawker PJ: Effect of mobile paramedic units on outcome in patients with myocardial infarction. *Ann Emerg Med* 1988; 17:1034–1041.
12. Mathewson ZM, McCloskey BG, Evans AE, et al: Mobile coronary care and community mortality from myocardial infarction. *Lancet* 1985; 1:441–444.
13. Pressley JC, Severance HW, Raney MP, et al: A comparison of paramedic versus basic emergency medical care of patients at high and low risk during acute myocardial infarction. *J Am Coll Cardiol* 1988; 12:1555–61.
14. Pantridge JF, Adgey AAJ, Geddes JS, et al: *The Acute Coronary Attack*. Tunbridge Wells, Kent, England, Pitman Medical Publishing, 1975.
15. Julian DG: Quality of life after myocardial infarction. *Am Heart J* 1987; 114:241–244.
16. Castaigne AD, Herve C, Duval-Moulin A-M, et al: Prehospital use of APSAC: Results of a placebo-controlled study. *Am J Cardiol* 1989; 64:30A–33A.
17. Herlitz J, Hartford M, Holmberg S, et al: Effects of a media campaign on delay time and ambulance use in acute chest pain (abstract). *Circulation* 1988; 78 (suppl II):188.
18. Weaver WD, Eisenberg MS, Martin JS, et al: Myocardial infarction, triage and intervention project: Phase 1. Characteristics of patients and feasibility of prehospital initiation of thrombolytic therapy. *J Am Coll Cardiol* 1990, in press.

19. Topol EJ, Fung AY, Kline E, et al: Safety of helicopter transport and out-of-hospital intravenous fibrinolytic therapy in patients with evolving myocardial infarction. *Cathet Cardiovasc Diagn* 1986; 12:151–155.
20. Gessman LJ, Li J K-J, Lewandowski J, et al: Transtelephonic resuscitation — a new approach to sudden death (abstract). *Am J Cardiol* 1979; 43:422.
21. Dalzell GWN, Cunningham SR, Prouziara S, et al: Assessment of a device for transtelephonic control of defibrillation. *Lancet* 1988; 1:695–697.
22. Capone RJ, Stablein D, Visco J, et al: The effects of a transtelephonic surveillance and prehospital emergency intervention system on the 1-year course following acute myocardial infarction. *Am Heart J* 1988; 116:1606–1615.
23. Associated Press: Phone link heart device rescues woman. *New York Times* July 9, 1989, p 25.
24. Ruffy R, Smith P: Remote site termination of life-threatening tachyarrhythmia by transtelephonic cardioversion. *JAMA* 1990, in press.
25. Grim P, Feldman T, Martin M, et al: Cellular telephone transmission of 12-lead electrocardiograms from ambulance to hospital. *Am J Cardiol* 1987; 60:715–720.
26. Grim PS, Feldman T, Childers RW: Evaluation of patients for the need of thrombolytic therapy in the prehospital setting. *Ann Emerg Med* 1989; 18:483–488.
27. Sobel BE, Saffitz JE, Fields LE, et al: Intramuscular administration of human tissue-type plasminogen activator in rabbits and dogs and its implications for coronary thrombolysis. *Circulation* 1987; 75:1261–1272.
28. Koster RW, Dunning AJ: Intramuscular lidocaine for prevention of lethal arrhythmias in the prehospitalization phase of acute myocardial infarction. *N Engl J Med* 1985; 313:1105–1110.

Rebuttal: Negative

David W. M. Muller M.B., B.S.
Eric J. Topol, M.D.

In his presentation of the protagonist's perspective, Dr. Crampton has provided compelling evidence to support the prehospital initiation of thrombolytic therapy for suitable patients with evolving acute myocardial infarction. His discussion is both comprehensive and well focused, and we agree with many of his statements. We acknowledge, for example, that several studies have now demonstrated that a dedicated, well-trained, physician-operated ambulance crew is able to initiate early, pretransport intravenous thrombolytic therapy safely and that this may result in an increased 90-minute patency of the infarct-related artery with some thrombolytic agents. Ideally, every ambulance crew should include a physician, a critical-care nurse, and several experienced paramedics. Unfortunately, these resources are not universally available and this approach will apply to only a very few, well-funded centers. For the remaining majority of community hospitals and for many tertiary referral centers, the question remains whether appropriately trained paramedics should be responsible for the initiation of a potent, potentially life-threatening therapy in situations in which they suspect a patient is suffering from an acute myocardial infarction. Dr. Crampton's arguments have not adequately addressed this issue.

To date, no randomized trials examining the impact of paramedic-initiated thrombolysis on definitive end points such as left ventricular function and mortality have been reported. It is not possible, therefore, to be dogmatic about these questions. However, as we noted previously, several conclusions can be drawn from the available data. First, there are no data in the current literature to support the use of thrombolytic therapy by paramedics or physicians for suspected, as opposed to confirmed, myocardial infarction. Indeed, in the Gruppo Italiano per lo Studio della Streptochinasi nell Infarto miocardico (GISSI) study, the mortality of the subgroup of patients with ST segment depression was somewhat higher both during the initial in-hospital phase (20.5 vs. 16.3%)[1] and at long-term follow-up (19.1 vs. 12.6%).[2] While neither of these differences reached statistical significance, the suggestion that thrombolysis may be harmful in this group with definite myocardial ischemia is of concern. When one considers that a proportion of patients with suspected myocardial infarction will actually have conditions such as aortic dissection, peptic ulcer disease, or pericarditis in which fibrinolytic therapy is relatively or absolutely contraindicated, the use of thrombolytic agents by paramedics for anything but unequivocal myocardial infarction cannot be condoned.

Given, then, the need for diagnostic accuracy and electrocardiographic documentation of acute changes of myocardial infarction, is it likely that a team of "appropriately trained" paramedics will be able to evaluate patients with ischemic-sounding chest pain rapidly, obtain and transmit a high-fidelity 12-lead electrocardiogram, and confer with a supervising physician prior to initiating thrombolytic therapy and transporting the patient? It is probable that a great proportion of the documented 40 to 50 minutes saved by physician-operated crews will be eroded. Will the remaining minutes saved justify the additional time spent in the field away from the facilities for hemodynamic monitoring, cardiac pacing, and endotracheal intubation provided by the emergency room or coronary care environment? These questions will require controlled evaluation before this approach can be recommended. In the meantime, attention needs to be drawn to delays occurring in emergency rooms and coronary care units which, at present, are often considerable. The study by Spangler and colleagues [3] referred to by Dr. Crampton highlights this problem. The time from the onset of symptoms to the initiation of thrombolytic therapy was 201 ± 34 minutes in the group treated posttransport compared with 165 ± 38 minutes in the group treated prior to helicopter transport. Importantly, however, the time taken for the initiation of therapy after arrival at the tertiary care facility was 41 ± 18 minutes in the former group compared with 28 ± 9 minutes in the helicopter team–treated group. There is no reason for a delay of this magnitude if the emergency room is notified prior to arrival and the patient is evaluated rapidly upon arrival by a dedicated and experienced medical team.

On the basis of currently available data, the prehospital initiation of thrombolytic therapy for suspected myocardial infarction by paramedics, suitably trained and supervised by a remote physician, cannot be condoned. Investigations currently being performed may show an improvement in myocardial salvage and early mortality for physician-initiated prehospital thrombolytic therapy for unequivocal myocardial infarction. If so, careful evaluation of paramedic-initiated therapy may be warranted. Before this approach can be advocated for the wider community, however, it must be shown that such a strategy results in a time savings comparable to that of physician-initiated therapy, that this time savings results in increased myocardial salvage, and that prehospital therapy can be given by paramedics without increasing the frequency of misdiagnosis and the morbidity of such therapy. Until then, efforts by both community hospitals and referral centers should be made to maximize the efficiency of the transport system, the emergency room, and the coronary care unit to avoid unnecessary delays in the transport, evaluation, and initiation of therapy for patients with evolving acute myocardial infarction.

References

1. Gruppo Italiano per lo Studio della Streptochinasi nell Infarto miocardico (GISSI): Effectiveness of intravenous thrombolytic treatment in acute myocardial infarction. *Lancet* 1986; i:397–402.
2. Rovelli F, De Vita C, Feruglio GA, et al: GISSI trial: Early results and late follow-up. *J Am Coll Cardiol* 1987; 10:33B–9B.
3. Spangler DE Jr, MacLean WA, Rogers WJ, et al: Is delivery of rtPA by helicopter transport teams safe and time effective (abstract)? *J Am Coll Cardiol* 1989; 13:192A.

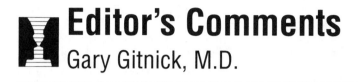

Editor's Comments
Gary Gitnick, M.D.

Drs. Crampton, Muller, and Topol provide cogent arguments and exceptional literature to document their points of view. Dr. Crampton points out that five thrombolytic drugs are now approved for clinical use or are undergoing prospective clinical trials. He contends that the resumption of coronary artery blood flow following thrombolytic therapy results in the salvage of significant amounts of heart muscle. He provides a variety of hypothetical or potential benefits and cites a series of studies offering "compelling clinical evidence" for the early initiation of thrombolytic therapy. He cites one report which documents a quantifiable advantage of a 32% smaller myocardial infarction with the prehospital administration of streptokinase, but also admits that two other reports failed to confirm these results. No morbidity or mortality occurred in the prehospital group treated with streptokinase and heparin, while the hospital-treated group included two deaths. He points out that the risks involved in prehospital thrombolysis are the same as those involved with in-hospital treatment. He maintains that the benefits outweigh the risks and makes the strong point that "one cannot dismiss the fact that early thrombolysis leads to the dissolution of a clot in the coronary artery, thereby converting the patient's hopeless, full-blown infarction into a potentially remedial early and long-term situation." Finally, he cites the extensive training offered to paramedics and notes that currently they are allowed to start intravenous infusions, administer pain-relieving narcotics, and handle primary life-threatening dysrhythmias. He asserts that if they are allowed to undertake these life-preserving measures, they should be allowed to administer thrombolytic agents.

Drs. Muller and Topol agree that prehospital thrombolysis administered by paramedics enables patients to receive this therapy 30 to 40 minutes earlier than they would with in-hospital administration. However, they question whether this delay is of clinical significance and they cite several published studies in support of their argument. They argue that the time it takes to transport patients to the emergency room should be reduced rather than devoting resources and efforts to the prehospital administration of drugs. They point out that the major delay is not related to ambulance response or transport time, but to the failure of patients to recognize the need for urgent care. They further argue that the relatively small population of patients who might benefit from prehospital thrombolytic therapy does not justify the costs involved in training additional paramedics and developing additional resources. Furthermore, they maintain that the administration of thrombolytic therapy to patients without electrocardiographically confirmed acute myocardial infarction is potentially dangerous.

They argue that a better approach would be to send trained teams including physicians equipped with 12-lead electrocardiographic equipment to the site of first contact with the patient, with a crew available to establish intravenous access and administer medications, including thrombolytic therapy, if it is confirmed that the patient is suffering a myocardial infarction. Thus, they favor the development of physician-operated mobile intensive care units. Overall they maintain that the risk-benefit analysis does not support the use of paramedics to administer thrombolytic therapy.

After reviewing both sides of this argument, it appears that the current data base is inadequate to resolve the question. I suspect that those communities that have taken the lead in paramedic-administered medical care will experiment with this approach and a rational decision can be made from future evidence.

Should Hypercholesterolemia Be Treated Aggressively?

Chapter Editor: H. Verdain Barnes, M.D.

Affirmative: Simeon Margolis, M.D., Ph.D.
Professor of Medicine and Biological
Chemistry, Associate Dean for Academic
Affairs, Johns Hopkins University School of
Medicine, Baltimore, Maryland

Negative: Michael F. Oliver, M.D.
Director, Wynn Institute for Metabolic
Research, London, England*

*Formerly The Duke of Edinburgh Professor of Cardiology, University of Edinburgh,
Department of Medicine, Edinburgh, Scotland.

Editor's Introduction

Health maintenance and disease prevention have gained increasing national attention in the past 5 years. With this new impetus, physicians increasingly are being asked by their patients for help in defining and instituting more healthy lifestyles and habits. On the forefront of this new enthusiasm is the national priority for identifying and treating hypercholesterolemia. Hence, the thrust of this debate between Dr. Simeon Margolis of Johns Hopkins School of Medicine and Dr. M. F. Oliver of the University of Edinburgh is whether and when aggressive therapy of hypercholesterolemia is justified.

In addressing whether a national priority to reduce cholesterol in the population is justified, our debaters agree that current data support a strong association between elevated cholesterol levels and atherosclerosis and that there is a decrease in nonfatal coronary events in persons whose cholesterol has been lowered. Unfortunately, the data are applicable only to males 30 to 60 years old. Our debaters do not agree as to whether these data can be extrapolated to younger and older males and to women. The issue as to which patients are at greatest risk and at what level of cholesterol is also addressed. The use of LDL_{ch} and HDL_{ch} levels in addition to total cholesterol as well as the reliability of the various lipid ratios for predicting risk are critically reviewed.

Should physicians be evangelistic in advocating a therapy more aggressive than simply a prudent diet? You will find substantial "food for thought" (low-cholesterol of course) in the papers of these two scholars.

H. Verdain Barnes, M.D.

▼ Affirmative
Simeon Margolis, M.D., Ph.D.

A number of epidemiological studies have shown a clear association between cholesterol levels and the risk of coronary artery disease (CAD). Also well documented is the development of CAD before the age of 20 years in homozygotes for familial hypercholesterolemia who have extreme elevations of cholesterol. This association between high blood cholesterol levels and accelerated atherosclerosis observed in humans is buttressed by experiments in animals, including nonhuman primates, showing that cholesterol-raising diets provoke CAD and that subsequent cholesterol-lowering diets can cause regression of the lesions. Taken together, these studies indicate that low-density lipoprotein (LDL) is atherogenic. More recent epidemiological data have shown that a low level of high-density lipoprotein (HDL) is also associated with excessive CAD.[1] Hypertriglyceridemia, though not proven to be an independent risk factor for CAD, contributes indirectly to premature CAD because high triglyceride levels are usually associated with low levels of HDL cholesterol (HLD_{ch}). Extreme hypertriglyceridemia (greater than 1,000 mg/dL) can cause attacks of acute pancreatitis.

In the past, many workers in this field have hesitated to recommend aggressive treatment of blood lipid abnormalities because there were no proven benefits of lowering blood cholesterol or raising HDL levels. This deficiency has been remedied now by four clinical studies which have demonstrated that lowering cholesterol and/or raising HDL_{ch} levels reduces the incidence of coronary events (Table 1). The serious consequences of these events dictate aggressive treatment of abnormal plasma lipids and lipoproteins.

The Coronary Primary Prevention Trial (CPPT) of the Lipid Research Clinics,[2] published in 1984, was the first study to prove that lowering levels of LDL cholesterol (LDL_{ch}) decreased the incidence of coronary events. This study enrolled 3,806 men aged 35 to 59 years with cholesterol levels over 265 mg/dL and no evidence of heart disease at entry. Men were assigned randomly to either diet plus placebo or diet plus cholestyramine and were followed in a double-blind fashion for 7 to 10 years. An average 8% reduction of cholesterol in the drug-treated group was associated with a 19% decrease in the number of coronary events. Those who took the full dose of the drug throughout the study had a 25% fall in their cholesterol level and a 49% decrease in coronary events. These results suggested that a 2% fall in coronary events was associated with each 1% reduction in cholesterol in middle-aged men with modestly elevated cholesterol levels.[3] The reduction in coronary events would probably be smaller in those whose initial

TABLE 1.
Studies Showing a Beneficial Effect of Drug Treatment on Coronary Events

Study	Drug Treatment	Results
Coronary Primary Prevention Trial (CPPT)[2,3]	Cholestyramine	A 2% reduction in coronary events for each 1% decrease in cholesterol in middle-aged men with initial cholesterol over 265 mg/dL
Cholesterol-Lowering Atherosclerosis Study (CLAS)[4]	Colestipol + nicotinic acid	Slowed progression of narrowing in coronary arteries and bypass grafts in middle-aged men
Coronary Heart Project[5]	Nicotinic acid	An 11% reduction in overall mortality 9 years after taking the drug for a 6-year period
Helsinki Heart Study[6]	Gemfibrozil	A 34% reduction in coronary events in middle-aged men with non-HDL cholesterol > 200 mg/dL

cholesterol is less than 265 mg/dL. Often overlooked is the finding that subjects in the CPPT with HDLch levels of less than 40 mg/dL had no decrease in their incidence of coronary events despite reductions in cholesterol levels.[7]

The Cholesterol-Lowering Atherosclerosis Study (CLAS) included 162 men aged 40 to 59 years who had previous coronary bypass surgery.[4] Repeat coronary angiography was used to show that lowering cholesterol (average of 26%) and raising HDL_{ch} (average of 37%) by diet plus two drugs (colestipol and nicotinic acid) slowed the progression of narrowing in coronary arteries and bypass grafts. The authors also concluded that the marked reduction achieved in cholesterol levels (mean LDL_{ch} lowered below 100 mg/dL) produced some regression of coronary artery lesions, but the data supporting this interpretation are not convincing.

The Helsinki Heart Study[6] randomized 4,081 men, aged 40 to 55 years, with no prior CAD and a non-HDL_{ch} above 200 mg/dL to take either a placebo or gemfibrozil in a double-blind manner. The study showed an overall decrease of 34% in coronary events over a 5-year period of treatment with gemfibrozil. Although the most impressive effect of this drug on serum lipids was a 45% fall in plasma triglyceride levels, careful analysis of the data indicates that the reduction in coronary events resulted from a rise in HDL_{ch} of about 10% and a fall of similar magnitude in LDL_{ch}. Although no difference in coronary events was observed between the placebo and drug-treated groups during the first 2 years, the magnitude of the decline in events in the gemfibrozil group increased progressively over the final 3 years of the study. This finding suggests that a longer period of treatment would provide even greater benefits. Patients with Fredrickson's type II hypercholesterolemia had the greatest reduction in coronary events; benefits also were observed in patients with type IV hypercholesterolemia, but not in those with type II.

None of these trials found that lowering cholesterol reduced overall mortality, but such a result could hardly be expected due to the relatively small number of subjects enrolled in the studies and the short period of follow-up. However, in a 15-year follow-up of the Coronary Heart Project, the overall mortality decreased by 11% in a group of men treated earlier for 6 years with nicotinic acid.[5]

The reduction in coronary events in the CPPT can be attributed to the decrease in LDL_{ch}, since HDL_{ch} rose only a few percent. Because the medications used in the other studies not only raised HDL_{ch} but also lowered LDL_{ch}, none of these studies provides unequivocal evidence that an increase in HDL_{ch} reduces the incidence of coronary events.

Since all of these trials were carried out in middle-aged men, there is no direct evidence that lowering LDL_{ch} or raising HDL_{ch} will decrease coronary events in women or younger individuals. However, it seems reasonable to assume that women would benefit also, albeit possibly less dramatically, from a lowered cholesterol level. One might expect that reducing cholesterol levels in younger individuals could be especially beneficial because they have fewer established lesions and a longer period of potential treatment to slow the development of atherosclerosis.

Detection and Treatment Guidelines

Guidelines for the detection and treatment of high blood cholesterol levels in adults have been formulated by the Adult Treatment Guidelines Panel of the National Cholesterol Education Program sponsored by the National Institutes of Health.[8] These guidelines recommend that all adults have their cholesterol level determined at least every 5 years. A fasting measurement is not necessary, because recent food intake has little impact on the cholesterol level. Recommendations on ideal cholesterol levels were based largely on the relationship between serum cholesterol and deaths from CAD as reported in the Multiple Risk Factor Intervention Trial (MRFIT) study,[9] which was based on data obtained from a very large cohort of men between the ages of 35 and 57 years (Fig 1). As shown in Table 2, the panel selected a cholesterol below 200 mg/dL as desirable in adults. A cholesterol above 240 mg/dL is considered high, while values between 200 and 239 mg/dL are borderline. Those with desirable levels should have their cholesterol remeasured after 5 years. Patients with a high cholesterol need an overnight fasting lipid profile (cholesterol, triglycerides, and HDL_{ch}) to determine whether they have an elevated LDL_{ch}. Decisions regarding people with a borderline cholesterol depend on the presence or absence of other risk factors (Table 3). Those at high risk (confirmed CAD or positive for two risk factors) require a fasting lipid profile. A complete fasting lipid profile also should be done on all patients with established CAD, a family history of premature CAD, or unexplained pancreatitis to search for an abnormal HDL_{ch} in the former two cases and high triglycerides in the latter. Low-risk patients with borderline cholesterol levels are informed about proper dietary habits and have their cholesterol measured again after a year. My only disagreement with these recommendations concerns individuals between the ages of 20 and 30 years with borderline cholesterol levels. In my opinion, these people should have a fasting lipid profile regardless of their risk status.

All decisions for treatment are based on the LDL_{ch} level, because some patients may have a borderline or even high cholesterol as the result of elevated levels of HDL_{ch}. The LDL_{ch} can be estimated accurately, as long as the triglycerides are less than 500 mg/dL, by subtracting from the total cholesterol the HDL_{ch} and the triglycerides divided by six. LDL_{ch} values are considered desirable below 130 mg/dL, borderline between 130 and 159 mg/dL, and high above 160 mg/dL (Table 4).

The inclusion of overall risk status in the decision-making process for the management of hypercholesterolemia is one important advance made by the guidelines. Physicians should recognize that efforts to prevent CAD are

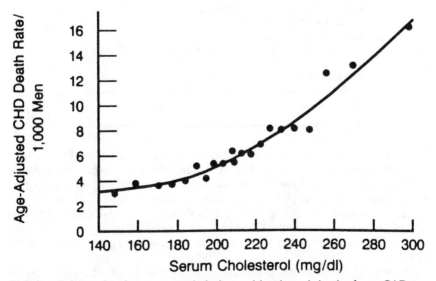

FIG 1. Relationship between total cholesterol levels and deaths from CAD in a cohort of 361,662 men aged 35 to 57 years in the MRFIT.[9] Note the steep increase in the slope for CAD death rate when cholesterol exceeds 200 mg/dL.

TABLE 2.
Classification and Actions Based on Screening Total Cholesterol

Cholesterol (mg/dL)	Classification	Risk Status	Action
< 200	Desirable		Repeat every 5 years
200–239	Borderline	Low	Give diet information and recheck annually
		High	Fasting lipid profile
> 240	High		Fasting lipid profile

TABLE 3.
Risk Factors for Coronary Artery Disease (CAD)

Male sex
CAD in a parent or sibling before the age of 55 years
Cigarette smoking
Uncontrolled hypertension
High-density lipoprotein (HDL) cholesterol < 35 mg/dL
Diabetes
Severe obesity (> 30% overweight)
Definite cerebrovascular or peripheral vascular disease

shortsighted if they focus only on a reduction of cholesterol levels in hypercholesterolemic patients. In fact, it is at least as important to convince patients to stop smoking and to initiate measures to control hypertension as it is to lower cholesterol levels in such patients.[10] Note that the higher frequency of heart disease in men places them at high risk when only one other risk factor is present. All diabetics are considered to be at high risk because the incidence of CAD in diabetic women is as great as in diabetic men.

An unresolved problem in the use of the guidelines is the variability of cholesterol determinations from one laboratory to another. The cholesterol and LDL_{ch} cut-points in the guidelines are based on measurements made with the methods of the Lipid Research Clinics (LRC) laboratories . Since other laboratory methods may give significantly different results, it is necessary to know how the values from other laboratories compare with those obtained using LRL methods. Now available and widely used are a number of desktop instruments for rapid cholesterol measurements on blood obtained by a finger stick. These machines generally give acceptably accurate determinations, provided the user is properly trained and careful in utilizing the instrument and obtaining the blood sample.

Before beginning possible lifelong treatment for hypercholesterolemia, adequate initial values must be obtained to be certain that treatment is needed and to judge its effectiveness. Usually recommended are at least two, and preferably three, baseline lipid profiles separated by about a week. Additional laboratory tests often are needed to identify secondary causes of hyper-cholesterolemia such as hypothyroidism, chronic renal disease, etc. Cholesterol elevations also may be caused by beta blockers or thiazide diuretics, drugs commonly used to treat patients with CAD or hypertension. Estrogens, corticosteroids, and retinoids can cause extreme hypertriglyceridemia.

One of the most difficult questions is whether to treat cholesterol elevations in the elderly. The need to address the issue is magnified by the greater frequency of borderline or high cholesterol levels in the elderly and by the extensive media coverage of cholesterol that has encouraged large numbers of people to participate in mass screening programs.

On the one hand, because angiographic studies have shown that lowering LDL_{ch} and raising HDL_{ch} slow the progression of CAD, it is difficult to decide when a patient is too old to benefit from lowered cholesterol. On the other hand, present evidence suggests that good levels of HDL_{ch} are more important than bad levels of LDL_{ch} in the elderly, and none of the intervention trials included subjects over the age of 60 years. Furthermore, does the

TABLE 4.
Classification and Actions Based on Low-Density Lipoprotein (LDL) Cholesterol

LDL_{ch} (mg/dL)	Classification	Risk Status	Action
< 130	Desirable		Repeat every 5 years
130–159	Borderline	Low	Give diet information and recheck annually
		High	Initiate diet
> 160	High	Low	Initiate diet
		High	Drug treatment if
> 190		High or low	elevation persists after 6-month trial of diet

relatively limited remaining lifespan of the elderly justify severe dietary restrictions or the costs and possible side effects of medications?

There is no easy answer to this question, but it is not sensible to set an arbitrary cutoff age for treatment. Decisions depend on the specific medical situation and the attitudes of each individual patient. I do not hesitate to give dietary instructions for lowering cholesterol levels to people of any age when they are especially concerned about a high cholesterol level. Decisions regarding the use of aggressive dietary measures or medications are more difficult. It is reasonable to use drugs in patients with recent coronary bypass surgery in an effort to prevent occlusion of the newly implanted vessels. In other patients, the presence or absence of other risk factors and the patient's general health status and degree of concern about high cholesterol all influence the decision to use drugs.

The guidelines of the National Cholesterol Education Program do not recommend the use of ratios of LDL_{ch} or total cholesterol to HDL_{ch} in making decisions on treatment. Since a high LDL and a low HDL are independent risk factors for CAD, each should be considered separately in making management choices. A high HDL_{ch} may give a "good" ratio of HDL_{ch} to LDL_{ch} and mask a significant elevation in LDL. Elevated levels of LDL_{ch} should be treated, even in patients with a high HDL. The best support for this position is the CPPT finding that patients with high levels of HDL_{ch} had the greatest reduction in coronary events when their cholesterol was reduced.

Aggressive treatment of hypercholesterolemia also implies the need to identify other family members with cholesterol problems. Approximately one half of the first-degree relatives of hypercholesterolemic patients also will have elevated cholesterol levels. Therefore, screening cholesterol measurements should be done in all children, siblings, and parents of hypercholesterolemic patients.

Dietary Treatment

Dietary measures are always the first step in the management of patients with any type of hyperlipidemia. The guidelines recommend dietary treatment when the LDL_{ch} exceeds 160 mg/dL for low-risk patients or 130 mg/dL for high-risk patients (Table 4). The initial, step 1 diet limits total fat to 30% of calories, saturated fat to less than 10% of calories, and cholesterol intake to 300 mg daily. If cholesterol levels remain too high after 3 months on this diet, the guidelines recommend a more restricted diet. This step 2 diet reduces saturated fat to less than 7% of total calories and cholesterol to 200 mg a day. Instructions for the step 1 diet are given by physicians or members of their staff; consultation with an experienced dietician is recommended at the onset of the step 2 diet.

Weight loss will often, but not always, lower cholesterol levels and should be incorporated into the dietary measures for obese patients. Weight loss in the obese may provide the additional benefit of raising the HDL_{ch}. An increased intake of water-soluble fibers, such as those found in oat bran, most beans, and the pectins of fruits and vegetables, also may help to lower cholesterol levels. It is often difficult to eat enough food rich in soluble fiber to have a major impact on blood cholesterol. Another option is the use of products such as Metamucil, which contain the water-soluble fiber of the psyllium seed. In one study, subjects who took a teaspoonful of Metamucil three times a day had a 12% reduction in their total and LDL cholesterol.[11] Fish oil capsules have been tried for a variety of ailments, but large doses of fish oil do not lower cholesterol or raise HDL_{ch}. However, fish oil capsules may be effective in treating some patients with hypertriglyceridemia.

Drug Treatment

Drug treatment generally is not considered until the patient has failed to reach acceptable cholesterol levels after a 3-month trial on the step 2 diet. Medications may be started earlier in patients with extreme cholesterol elevations when a maximal response to diet (25% to 30% fall in cholesterol) cannot lower cholesterol to a desirable range. The guidelines recommend that drugs should be used when the LDL_{ch} exceeds 160 mg/dL in high-risk patients or 190 mg/dL in low-risk patients (see Table 4).

The drugs of first choice to lower cholesterol are the bile acid sequestrants, cholestyramine or colestipol, and nicotinic acid. These medications are effective in lowering LDL_{ch}, have a long record of safety, and have been shown to reduce the number of coronary events in intervention trials. Their utility may be limited by the gastrointestinal side effects of the bile acid sequestrants or by the development of nausea and epigastric pain or abnormalities in liver enzymes with the use of nicotinic acid. Lovastatin, an inhibitor of cholesterol synthesis, is considered a drug of second choice because of limited experience with possible long-term complications and the lack of evidence for a reduction in coronary events. Probucol has the disadvantage of lowering both the LDL and HDL cholesterol to a similar degree. However, recent studies have shown that this drug inhibits the oxidation of the polyunsaturated fats in LDL and, thus, may prevent its uptake by macrophages in blood vessel walls. Based on the results of the Helsinki Heart Study, gemfibrozil is a good choice for patients with moderate cholesterol elevations, particularly when they have elevated triglycerides or a low HDL_{ch} also.

Drug combinations often are effective when a single medication does not lower cholesterol levels adequately. Because each of the drug classes mentioned above works by a different mechanism, the combination of two or even three drugs usually gives at least additive effects.[12] The best two-drug combinations are a bile acid sequestrant plus either nicotinic acid or lovastatin.

Triglycerides and HDL

A National Institutes of Health (NIH) Consensus Conference[13] recommended the following: triglycerides below 250 mg/dL do not require treatment; triglycerides above 500 mg/dL must be treated to avoid attacks of pancreatitis; decisions on the treatment of triglycerides between 250 and 500 mg/dL depend on the patient's cardiovascular risk status and HDL_{ch} level.

The most important measure in the treatment of hypertriglyceridemia is weight reduction to ideal body weight (usually based on a patient's own weight on reaching full maturity). Alcohol intake must be strictly limited in patients with elevated triglycerides. Other dietary restrictions are similar to the step 1 diet for the reduction of cholesterol. Patients with extreme hypertriglyceridemia (>1,000 mg/dL) may require more severe restriction of total fat intake. Nicotinic acid and gemfibrozil are the drugs of choice to treat hypertriglyceridemia. The bile acid sequestrants tend to increase triglycerides and are not a good choice in patients with elevated triglyceride levels.

It is difficult to raise HDL levels, but the effort is encouraged since available evidence suggests a 2% to 4% fall in the incidence of coronary events for every 1% increase in HDL_{ch}. Measures to raise HDL_{ch} include cessation of cigarette smoking, exercise, and weight loss in obese patients. Moderate alcohol use raises HDL_{ch}, but physicians should not encourage patients to increase their alcohol intake in an effort to raise their HDL. Instead, patients may be reassured that their present moderate alcohol consumption is not harmful to their cardiovascular status and may even be beneficial. Anabolic steroids cause marked reductions in HDL_{ch}; progestational agents, thiazides, and some beta blockers may also lower HDL_{ch}. Despite their capacity to raise HDL levels, neither nicotinic acid nor gemfibrozil is an approved treatment to raise HDL_{ch} except in patients with either hypercholesterolemia or hypertriglyceridemia.

References

1. Gordon T, Castelli WP, Hjortland MC, et al: High density lipoprotein as a protective factor against coronary heart disease: The Framingham Study. *Am J Med* 1977; 62:707–714. *These results from the Framingham Study showed that in both men and women aged 49 to 82 years a low HDL cholesterol was the most potent lipid risk factor for each manifestation of coronary heart disease (CHD). LDL cholesterol had a weaker association with CHD.*
2. Lipid Research Clinics Program: The Lipid Research Clinics Primary Prevention Trial Results: I. Reduction in incidence of coronary heart disease. *JAMA* 1984; 251:351–364. *This study in 3,806 asymptomatic middle-aged men with primary hypercholesterolemia was the first to show a significant*

*decrease in definite CHD death and/or myocardial infarction associated
with cholesterol reduction by diet plus cholestyramine treatment when
compared with a control group on placebo plus diet.*

3. Lipid Research Clinics Program: The Lipid Research Clinics Primary Prevention Trial Results: II. The relationship of reduction in incidence of coronary
   heart disease to cholesterol lowering. *JAMA* 1984; 251:365–374. *In men
   sustaining an average fall of 25% in total cholesterol while taking a full
   dose of cholestyramine (24 gm/day), the incidence of CHD was reduced by
   50% when compared with men taking a placebo.*

4. Blankenhorn DH, Nessim SA, Johnson ER, et al: Beneficial effects of
   combined cholestipol-niacin therapy on coronary atherosclerosis and coronary venous bypass grafts. *JAMA* 1987; 257:3233–3240. *Treatment of
   men aged 40 to 59 years with diet, colestipol, and niacin, which reduced
   LDL cholesterol by 43% and raised HDL cholesterol by 37%, was
   associated with angiographic evidence of slowed progression of coronary
   atherosclerosis in native vessels and a decrease in new lesions in bypass
   grafts.*

5. Canner PL, Berge KG, Wenger NK, et al: Fifteen year mortality in Coronary
   Drug Project patients: Long-term benefit with niacin. *J Am Coll Cardiol*
   1986; 8:1245–1255. *When followed up an average of 9 years after
   completion of the Coronary Drug Project, men who had earlier taken 3 gm
   niacin daily for a mean of 6.2 years had a mortality from all causes that was
   11% lower than that of the placebo group.*

6. Frick MH, Elo O, Haapa K, et al: Helsinki Heart Study: Primary prevention trial
   with gemfibrozil in middleaged men wtih dyslipidemia. *N Engl J Med* 1987;
   317:1237–1245. *When compared with placebo, gemfibrozil raised HDL
   cholesterol by 9% and lowered LDL cholesterol by 10% and triglycerides
   by 43% over a 5-year period; these changes were associated with a 34%
   reduction in CHD events.*

7. Gordon DJ, Knoke J, Probsfield JL, et al: High density lipoprotein cholesterol
   and coronary heart disease in hypercholesterolemic men: The Lipid Research
   Clinic Primary Prevention Trial. *Circulation* 1986; 74:1217–1225. *Lowering of LDL cholesterol levels with cholestyramine did not reduce the
   incidence of CHD events in subjects with HDL cholesterol levels less than
   40 mg/dL; maximal impact of cholestyramine treatment was observed in
   those with HDL cholesterol greater than 50 mg/dL.*

8. Report of the National Cholesterol Education Program Expert Panel on
   Detection, Evaluation and Treatment of High Blood Cholesterol in Adults.
   Arch Intern Med 1988; 148:36–69. *This report provides detailed recommendations on the use of cholesterol, LDL cholesterol, and other risk
   factors in making decisions on the dietary and drug treatment of hypercholesterolemia.*

9. Martin JJ, Hulley SB, Browner WS, et al: Serum cholesterol, blood pressure,
   and mortality: Implications from a cohort of 361,662 men. *Lancet* 1986;
   2:933–936. *Data from this huge cohort of men from MRFIT, showing the
   relationship between serum cholesterol and the incidence of death from
   CHD, formed the basis for the National Cholesterol Education Program to
   establish recommendations for when to intervene with diet or medications
   to lower cholesterol levels.*

10. Anderson JW, Zettwoch N, Feldman T, et al: Cholesterol-lowering effects of

psyllium hydrophillic mucilloid for hypercholesterolemic men. *Arch Intern Med* 1988; 148:292–296. *Treatment of 13 men with 1 tsp of psyllium mucilloid (Metamucil) three times daily for 8 weeks reduced their mean total cholesterol by 11% and LDL cholesterol by 17% when compared with a placebo-treated group.*

11. Kannel WB, Neaton JD, Wentworth D, et al: Overall and coronary heart disease mortality rates in relation to major risk factors in 325,348 men screened for MRFIT. *Am Heart J* 1986; 112:825–836. *This report shows the influence of cholesterol, blood pressure, and cigarette smoking on CHD deaths and all-cause mortality rates in 35 to 57 year–old men screened for MRFIT.*

12. Malloy MJ, Kane JP, Kunitake ST, et al: Complementarity of colestipol, niacin and lovastatin in treatment of severe familial hypercholesterolemia. *Ann Intern Med* 1987; 107:616–623. *Colestipol, niacin, and lovastatin were mutually complementary in lowering cholesterol levels; the combination of the three medications plus diet lowered serum cholesterol to levels similar to those associated with regression of atheromas in animals.*

13. National Institutes of Health Consensus Conference on the Treatment of Hypertriglyceridemia. *JAMA* 1984; 251:1196–1200. *The Consensus Conference concluded that individuals with triglyceride levels less than 250 mg/dL require no changes in life style; those with levels between 250 and 500 mg/dL require evaluation of family history, other risk factors, and the presence of dangerous genetic forms of hyperlipidemia before making decisions on treatment; and those levels greater than 500 mg/dL require treatment by diet and, if necessary, by drugs because of the risk of pancreatitis.*

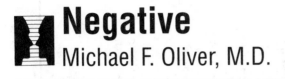

Negative
Michael F. Oliver, M.D.

Policy Statement

A debate on this question depends on the definition of hypercholesterol-emia and the interpretation of "aggressively." I shall assume from the outset that the question concerns the primary prevention of coronary heart disease (CHD) and not the treatment of hypercholesterolemia after the onset of clinical features of CHD.

If hypercholesterolemia is defined as serum concentrations above 250 mg/dL (approximately 6.5 mmol/L), then I have no argument about the need for aggressive treatment in order to reduce the risk of CHD, particularly if there are associated risk factors such as cigarette smoking, hypertension, and a family history of premature CHD. However, I do not consider that the evidence of likely benefit is strong enough to justify the aggressive treatment of serum cholesterol concentrations below about 250 mg/dL unless high-density lipoproteins (HDL) are lower than 40 mg/dL.

If "aggressively" is interpreted as the *mandatory* use of drugs, then I am only willing to endorse a policy which includes their use when serum cholesterol concentrations are rather high, say 280 mg/dL. In other words, much can be achieved by the less aggressive approach of rigorous attention to dietary intervention, although the weakness in the practice of this approach is the lack of compliance of many individuals to dietary change.

Modifications to Policy Statement

This policy statement is based largely on the results of the five major long-term controlled clinical trials of the primary prevention of CHD. These are the Los Angeles Veterans Administration[1] and the Helsinki Mental Hospital[2] dietary studies, the World Health Organization (WHO) Clofibrate Trial,[3] the Lipid Research Clinics Cholestyramine Trial,[4] and the Helsinki Heart Trial using gemfibrozil.[5] The latter four studies conducted in men with hyper-cholesterolemia above 250 mg/dL. I shall not trouble the reader with the details of the design and conduct of these, since I think for the purpose of this debate a superficial summary is all that is needed (Table 5). The results are consistent in showing a reduction in CHD events (fatal and nonfatal combined). The benefit is greater for nonfatal myocardial infarcts, although not significant in all trials, than for fatal events.

No primary prevention trials of the effectiveness of treating hyper-

Table 5.
Summary of Main Results of Cholesterol-Lowering Primary Prevention Trials

Trial	Preventive Regime	Numbers at Entry	Plasma Cholesterol	Nonfatal Infarction	Fatal Coronary Heart Disease	Total Coronary Heart Disease Events	Noncardiovascular Mortality
Los Angeles Veteran's Administration	Diet: P/S = 1.5	846	-13%	-32% n.s.	-18% n.s.	-23% n.s.	+12%*
Helsinki Mental Hospital	Diet: P/S > 1.5	922	-15%	-81%‡	-51% n.s.	-67%*	+21% n.s.
World Health Organization	Clofibrate	15,745	-9%	-26%*	+6% n.s.	-20%*	+32%‡
Lipid Research Clinic — Coronary Primary Prevention Trial	Cholestyramine	3,806	-13%	-19% n.s.	-24% n.s.	-19%*	+33% n.s.
Helsinki Heart	Gemfibrozil	4,081	-7%	-36% n.s.	-26% n.s.	-34%†	+21% n.s.

* $P < .05$
† $P < .02$
‡ $P < .01$

cholesterolemia have been conducted in women. It should not be assumed that their response will be identical or even similar. My *first modification,* therefore, is that the policies to be applied for the treatment of hyper-cholesterolemia should differ by gender. There is strong epidemiological evidence that the risk of developing CHD is of a lesser order of magnitude in women with hypercholesterolemia than in men. The 30-year follow-up of the Framingham Study[6] showed a significant association between choles-terol levels and CHD in men, after adjusting for blood pressure, smoking, relative weight, and diabetes, but not for women. Analysis of the relationship between cholesterol and CHD mortality in 19 countries[7] shows a significant correlation for men (r = .68), but not for women (r = .24). Low-density lipoproteins (LDL) are not an independent risk factor for CHD after controlling for age, blood pressure, smoking, high-density lipoprotein (HDL) cholesterol, and estrogen usage.[8] The difference in risk for CHD between the genders is likely to be related, at least in part, to the relatively high HDL cholesterol present in most women. The Framingham data have led to the conclusion that "the protective HDL cholesterol influence on CHD risk is about twice as strong as the atherogenic LDL effect."[9] The case for aggressive treatment of hypercholesterolemia in women is weaker than that for men and its effectiveness has yet to be demonstrated.

The *second modification* to my opening policy statement relates to HDL cholesterol. I consider that hypercholesterolemia in a man needs less vigorous treatment when the serum concentrations of HDL is in the region of 50 mg/dL or above, but more aggressive treatment when the HDL is less than approximately 40 mg/dL. It is not a bad rule-of-thumb approach to regard the ratio of total cholesterol to HDL as being definitely abnormal above 6 and to adopt an aggressive approach above this arbitrary threshold. A related point is that HDL levels should be part of any screening of the population (see later) and should be included in a second blood analysis when hypercholesterolemia is suspected.

The *third modification* to my initial policy statement involves age. It should be taken into account when considering any aggressive policy. The three drug trials cited[3-5] were conducted in men between the ages of 30 and 59 years; thus, the results, both good and bad, should relate to men of this age group only and should not be extrapolated to other ages until clinical trials have shown benefit. The association between total serum cholesterol and overall CHD mortality decreases with age and is not significant over the age of 50 years.[6] Those surviving over approximately 60 years with high cholesterol levels without CHD need not be concerned.

The Consensus Conference Statement

The most relevant recommendations of the Consensus Statement,[10] which I endorse fully, are that "individuals with high-risk blood cholesterol levels (values above the 90th percentile) be treated intensively by dietary means under the guidance of a physician...; if response to diet is inadequate, appropriate drugs should be added" and "adults with moderate-risk blood cholesterol levels (values between the 75th and 90th percentiles) be treated intensively by dietary means, especially if additional risk factors are present. Only a small proportion should require drug treatment."

But I contest and object to the unqualified statement that reduction of blood cholesterol *will* reduce the rate of coronary heart disease. Not "may," but "will." This promise has been promulgated extensively by health educators and is at the center of the National Cholesterol Education Program[11] and much media publicity. I have criticized the methods through which the consensus statement was reached elsewhere.[12] I also have indicated how very complicated are the problems of CHD prevention, and that reduction of hypercholesterolemia is not the panacea so many are being led to believe.[13] Others[14-16] similarly have tried to give perspective to this issue, and Palumbo[14] rightly emphasizes that arbitrary limits of serum cholesterol should not determine management and that clinical judgment should be the hallmark for optimum medical care. I also have drawn attention to the fact that total mortality was not reduced in any of the five key trials[17] (see Table 5).

One of the reasons that a debate such as this one is mounted at all is the extent to which it is justifiable for credible investigators and physicians to circumvent the precise facts and extend them into wishful thinking. Such projection and distortion of evidence is common in politics, although this does not make it acceptable. It is only permissible in clinical medicine if there is a very strong likelihood that most of the population will benefit greatly from intervention and at the same time will be at no risk from a change in lifestyle — reduction of obesity or fluoridation of water are examples. Unfortunately, this cannot yet be said for lowering serum cholesterol concentrations below the levels of those actually studied in formal clinical trials in men, in women, in the young, and probably also in the old. The American public should be told this more honestly and be alerted also to the very powerful pharmaceutical interests which favor a less exact interpretation.

The extension of advice beyond the facts is also one of my criticisms of the Lipid Research Clinic–Cholestyramine Primary Prevention Trial (LRC-CPPT)[4] proposal for a "broader interpretation" of the rather marginal reduction (see a relevant critique of the conduct and analysis of this trial[18]) in CHD events consequent upon giving cholestyramine to men between the ages of 35 and 64 years with marked initial hypercholesterolemia. The authors recommend that advice to reduce hypercholesterolemia should be extended to women, to younger and older ages, and to dietary change. The existing evidence to support these recommendations either does not exist, as is the case with women, or is very frail, as is true of diet.

Rationale of Aggressive Treatment of Hypercholesterolemia

The animal experimental evidence and human epidemiological and pathological evidence relating hypercholesterolemia to atherosclerosis, and particularly to coronary atherosclerosis, is impressive and incontrovertible. It would be unnecessarily repetitive and lengthy to list all the evidence supporting this conclusion, but it is also inappropriate not to refer to some of the key studies. Thus, the animal evidence is particularly impressive ranging from the early feeding experiments of Anitschkow[19] in rabbits through to the classical studies of induction and regression of aortic and coronary atherosclerosis in primates.[20-22] All of these studies and others have indicated that the feeding of excessive dietary cholesterol or excessive dietary saturated fat is associated with the development of cholesterol-rich atheromatous lesions, and that these can be severe enough to cause considerable arterial occlusion. They are, however, in the main remarkably free from any associated thrombosis. Regression studies, following the withdrawal of cholesterol-rich diets in animals and using cholesterol-lowering drugs in patients after coronary artery bypass surgery,[23] have reinforced the importance of hypercholesterolemia as a precursor of and as a potential therapeutic target for coronary atherosclerosis. They give credence to an aggressive approach.

Having stated this, the evidence relating hypercholesterolemia to coronary *heart* disease as distinct from coronary atherosclerosis or coronary *artery* disease is much less impressive. Many researchers fail to distinguish between these entities and there are frequent references in the literature to coronary artery disease as a generic description of angina and myocardial infarction and of coronary or ischemic heart disease as an indicator of coronary artery disease. There is no one-to-one relationship between these two. Coronary artery disease or atherosclerosis is mostly an asymptomatic condition which in its milder forms is compatible with survival into old age.[24] Coronary heart disease, on the other hand, is a descriptive term which should be confined to the clinical syndromes of angina pectoris (of different degrees), myocardial infarction, some forms of cardiac failure, and many, but not all, cases of sudden cardiac death. Those who expect or assume that there will be a huge reduction in the incidence of CHD by reducing serum cholesterol (and there are many claims and calculations made from simulation models that so-and-so many million lives will be saved) cannot have studied the complex pathogenesis of the clinical syndromes defined as CHD or understood the weakness of the relationship of cholesterol to each of these, particularly the mechanisms leading to death. Were clinical CHD to have a single or even a homogeneous etiology, and were this to be raised serum or LDL cholesterol or low HDL cholesterol, then the issue being debated would be very easy to answer in the affirmative. But the pathogenesis of clinical CHD and also of coronary artery disease (in view of the non–lipid-related activities of mono-cytes, macrophages, endothelium, and platelets) is too heterogeneous and complex for the aggressive treatment of hypercholesterolemia to produce a large benefit or to eliminate the disease, as some claim.

Everyone agrees that there are three classical risk factors identified with an increased risk of CHD: cigarette smoking, hypercholesterolemia, and hypertension. But these risk factors together explain no more than one half of the variance of CHD.[25] By definition, then, any one of these three risk factors will be responsible for only a minority of the incidence of CHD. It should not be surprising, therefore, that the epidemiological evidence relating hypercholesterolemia to CHD is less impressive than the animal experimental or pathological evidence referred to, briefly, earlier. Neverthe-less, there is a strong consistency from all the major epidemiological studies of a marked increase in the relative risk of CHD with increasing serum cholesterol concentrations. For example, the MRFIT data indicate that the risk of developing one of the clinical syndromes of CHD for men with a serum cholesterol in the top quintile of the distribution is 7 to 2.4 times (decreasing with age) that of those whose serum cholesterol is in the lowest quintile.[26] The same trend is true, inversely, for the relationship between the HDL cholesterol and CHD.[27] These within-population studies are amply sup-ported by between-population studies showing that communities with low serum cholesterol concentrations have appreciably less CHD than those with high serum cholesterol concentrations.[28]

Arguments Against Overaggressive Treatment

In formulating a policy for the aggressive treatment of hypercholesterol-emia, it is not only the increased relative risk of developing CHD with increasing serum cholesterol concentrations that needs to be taken into account but also the magnitude of the actual or absolute risk as a result of having a serum cholesterol concentration at a given level.

This forms the basis of my *first argument* against overaggressive treat-ment. The Pooling Project,[29] which includes Framingham data, has shown very clearly that the majority of men with serum cholesterol concentrations in the top quintile of the distribution do not develop CHD in the foreseeable future. Thus, 85% of those in the top quintile of cholesterol distribution in Framingham did not develop CHD over a 20-year follow-up period. It can be calculated from the Pooling Project that no more than one third of those men in the top quintile of serum cholesterol distribution will develop CHD over a period of 30 years. While this is a high proportion, it follows that two thirds will be treated unnecessarily, and potentially harmfully, if aggressive treatment includes drugs which have a degree of toxicity. Unfortunately, the specificity of lipoprotein and apoprotein measurements as predictors of CHD is too low to permit much improvement in the discrimination of those who will or will not develop CHD.

My *second argument* against overaggressive treatment of hypercholesterolemia is the curvilinear relationship between serum cholesterol concentrations and CHD mortality as defined by the MRFIT data.[30] This huge study of 361,000 middle-aged men is the largest set of data we have and are likely to have, and there is no doubt that the relationship between serum cholesterol concentrations and CHD mortality at 6 years is curvilinear and not linear. Opinions are put forth to suggest that this curvilinearity has been exaggerated. One of these is that, had two or three serum cholesterol estimations been made, there would have been a degree of regression toward the mean and therefore both ends of the curve would be less exaggerated. Another is that semilogarithmic transformation of the data will eliminate the curvilinearity. However, I know of no sound argument for such transformation of the data. Both of these opinions merely state the obvious.

Another view, which derives from the LRC-CPPT, is that it is relevant to apply to all cholesterol levels the calculated predicted linear reduction of CHD according to the degree of reduction of serum cholesterol (2% less CHD for every 1 mg/dL less of serum cholesterol). This calculation has been based on extrapolation to the central data of this study from a subgroup with a bigger response to cholestyramine. Such extrapolation is not justified, since the statistical design of the study was such that subgroups with more or less cholesterol response were not included initially and the total numbers in the LRC study are such that significant changes in CHD incidence cannot be demonstrated for a given subgroup. Thus, the assumed linearity between reduction of cholesterol and reduction of CHD is not based on fact. Further, to apply this calculation to population expectation is a *reductio ad absurdum*[14] as it implies that by reducing cholesterol levels by 50% CHD would be eliminated!

My *third argument* against overaggressive treatment is the unexplained increase in noncardiovascular mortality in each of the five key primary prevention trials (see Table 5). The evidence of the effectiveness of lowering cholesterol relates mostly to the reduction of nonfatal myocardial infarction and this is impressive, but analysis of the results of all primary and secondary prevention drug trials shows a significant 17% excess of noncardiovascular deaths in those treated with cholesterol-lowering drugs[31] and a nonsignificant excess of 11% in noncardiovascular deaths for those treated with cholesterol-lowering diets.[32] It has been argued that the majority component of the adverse response to drugs is contributed by the WHO Clofibrate Trial[3] and, since it may be a phenomenon of one trial, it can be dismissed. However, the consistency and the lack of reduction of total mortality in all of the five major trials must be taken seriously and caution is needed.[17] The possibility that a reduction in cellular cholesterol in some individuals may produce an adverse biological response should not be ignored. There is always a danger of being too influenced to look for good results at the expense of not being alert to adverse results; the LRC-CPPT findings in relation to cancer are an example.[4] While there were 57 cases of cancer in the cholestyramine-treated group and 57 in the placebo group, it is within the gastrointestinal tract that one would look for adverse effects in relation to the usage of nonabsorbable anion exchange of resin, and there were 21 incident cases (11 deaths) of gastrointestinal cancer in the cholestyramine-treated group as compared with 8 cases (1 death) in the placebo group. The difference was not significant, but surely should not be dismissed.

In contrast to these three arguments against the overaggressive treatment of hypercholesterolemia there is one in its favor. This relates to post–coronary artery bypass patients, in whom everything possible should be done to maintain graft patency, and control of hypercholesterolemia has been shown to aid this.[23] With this exception, I shall not address the question of whether aggressive treatment of hypercholesterolemia is of value in the secondary prevention of CHD. This is a separate and complex issue, particularly since prognosis is determined principally by left ventricular function and damage and not by hypercholesterolemia.

Screening — National or Opportunistic

The National Cholesterol Education Program[11] has produced glossy brochures entitled "Remember to ask for your cholesterol number," backed up by multiple support articles and programs through the media. A statement is made that "future efforts… will focus on providing health care professionals and the public with updated information and guidance so that they can make more effective decisions regarding the detection and treatment of high blood cholesterol." These initiatives are, in my opinion, misleading and mistaken. They are misleading because the inference is that knowledge of one's cholesterol level is sufficient to determine whether action should or should not be taken. They are mistaken because they place the onus on the individual and not on the physician.

There are two reasons for my criticism of this effort. The first is that a given "cholesterol number," particularly from a single determination, provides insufficient information for action or inaction. Many of us already will be aware of examples of misinterpretation of a particular serum cholesterol concentration. In my view, the interpretation should be carried out by a physician (although some health professionals may have learned enough to make responsible decisions) and not by the public itself. There are many examples of anxious but entirely healthy individuals referring themselves to offices and hospitals because of serum cholesterol concentrations of 200 to 220 mg/dL, a range in which I consider intervention to be not needed, unless perhaps there is a very unusually low HDL cholesterol as well. Not only does

---

TABLE 6.
Unreliability of Cholesterol Estimations

Laboratory Weaknesses
    Error between laboratories ($\approx$ 5%) and within laboratories ($\approx$ 3%)
    Quick methods versus laboratory analyses
    Quality controls not used uniformly
Methods of Venipuncture
    Sitting vs. lying—lower when sitting
    Venous congestion—increases
Other Influences
    Seasonal (lowest in autumn, highest in spring)
    Menstrual cycle (low at ovulation, high in post-luteal phase)
    Post-menopausal rise
Conclusion
    Two are minimum
    Regression to mean, therefore three are more reliable

---

the knowledge of serum cholesterol create unnecessary anxiety or even false security (in view of the other factors leading to CHD), but the subsequent referrals are time-consuming and costly. Admittedly, it is difficult to avoid identifying ranges of serum cholesterol where action of different degrees is indicated, but over-rigid interpretation of arbitrary numbers should be recognized and combatted with wise and experienced advice.

The second reason why I am opposed to the advice that all Americans should know their cholesterol level is the unreliability of cholesterol estimations. This is discussed rather infrequently and, certainly, the average member of the public has little or no idea that a single estimation of serum cholesterol by a rapid method, giving a result of 200 mg/dL might in fact be 190 mg/dL, 210 mg/dL, or worse according to the circumstances of the venipuncture, the time of the year, or the time of the menstrual cycle, for example (Table 6).

It might be supposed, then, that I am opposed to screening. My view[33] is that this is best conducted on an opportunistic basis when the opportunity presents, and in conjunction with physicians who know how to interpret the results and who know the weaknesses of a single estimation of serum cholesterol and not through uneconomic national screening campaigns. I am concerned by the intrusion of pharmaceutical companies into this field with their widespread offers of free estimation of serum cholesterol concentration, coupled with a brochure about their particular drug.

It is true, however, that there will be a proportion of individuals with hypercholesterolemia who will be missed by a policy of opportunistic screening; an important question is how big is this proportion. It certainly can be minimized by focusing the public's attention on the risks within a family when premature vascular disease has occurred, by alerting them to the significance of corneal arcus and xanthomata, and especially by ensuring that physicians actually do screen for serum cholesterol concentrations whenever an individual presents to them. The latter is difficult and does not occur as frequently as it should. For example, many patients are admitted to the hospital with surgical conditions and serum cholesterol is not measured.

Intravascular Thrombosis

It may seem surprising to introduce thrombosis into a critique of policies for the treatment of hypercholesterolemia. However, one of the reasons for the rather weak relationship between serum cholesterol concentrations and the development of clinical CHD (as distinct from the acquisition of coronary atherosclerosis) is that intravascular thrombosis is often the critical influence converting asymptomatic coronary artery disease to CHD, and its occurrence or onset is independent of a given level of serum cholesterol. It is only recently that thrombogenic indices of significance have been identified as precursors of clinical CHD. The dominance of the cholesterol hypothesis undoubtedly has had an adverse effect on clinical studies of the relationship between thrombogenesis and fibrinolysis and CHD. However, it now has been shown clearly that fibrinogen and Factor VIIc have an equal or even more powerful predictive power for CHD than serum cholesterol,[34,35] and inhibition of some of the mechanisms associated with fibrinolysis (particularly tissue plasminogen–activated inhibitor) is correlated significantly with CHD.[36] I take the view that the prevention or reduction of a thrombogenic tendency in middle-aged adults may have a yield as great or greater than that of lowering hypercholesterolemia. Factors influencing the "thrombosis equation," and also LP(a), are at last a focus of intense research and one of very considerable potential.

Justifiable Action

There are four essential considerations regarding the aggressive treatment of hypercholesterolemia. These are the likely benefit to the community and the individual, the cost financially and in terms of lifestyle, the risks and potential adverse effects, and the priority that should be given by nations with a restricted health budget and other important health needs.

Based on the view that there is a true curvilinear relationship between serum cholesterol and CHD, it is obvious that more individuals will be benefitted by the reduction of cholesterol levels when their serum cholesterol concentrations are in the top few deciles compared with the bottom few deciles. This is illustrated in Figure 2 and is a strong argument for the high-risk strategy. I indicated at the outset that I am strongly in favor of aggressive treatment when plasma concentrations are about 250 mg/dL or above and, by inference, that I am much less enthusiastic for aggressive action below these levels because the benefit is manifestly less.

The costs, both financial and psychological, must be brought into the equation. I am all for the adoption of a prudent diet by most or all of those individuals whose serum cholesterol concentrations lie between 200 and 250 mg/dL. The sort of prudent diet that I recommend is one in which total fat calories are not much above 30% of total calories and in which saturated fat calories make up no more than 10% to 12%. This is a practical diet and not a punitive one. I am unconvinced, however, that the evidence for lowering dietary cholesterol from an average of, say, 500 to 600 mg/day to 250 to 300 mg/day is that compelling or that it is likely to contribute much to the reduction of the total incidence of CHD. I am completely opposed to the use of expensive drugs for those whose serum cholesterol concentrations are below 250 mg/dL or thereabouts. I do not even make an exception for individuals with multiple risk factors, since I think that most of these people can and should be guided in a sensible life style and even they do not need recourse to expensive drugs. Drugs may be indicated for those with higher levels, but it is often forgotten that drugs used to lower serum cholesterol concentrations must be taken for life. This may be a tough sentence, financially and psychologically, on a man 40 years old, for example. There

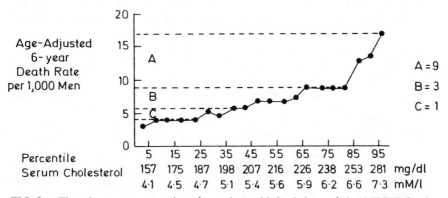

FIG 2. The above curve is taken from the published data of the MRFIT Study (361,662 men). Example *A* indicates the number of deaths per 1,000 men which might be saved if serum cholesterol were to be reduced throughout the 6 years from about 280 mg/dL to 250 mg/dL; example *B* indicates that there might be 3 fewer deaths with reduction from a level of 250 mg/dL to 200 mg/dL; and example *C* indicates that there might be 1 death less with reduction from 200 mg/dL to 160 mg/dL.

is increasing evidence, and it is not in the least surprising, that compliance to drug regimens falls within a year or two of starting the drugs. The question of financial expense is particularly important with the availability of HMGCoA reductase inhibitors, and consideration of the best alternative, such as combined treatment with an anion exchange resin and a fibrate, may be acceptable to some. Too little attention has been given to the psychological dependence on drug treatment for a condition which the majority of healthy individuals did not know they had until they were screened for one reason or another. It is one thing to take drugs for symptomatic disease but quite another to take them for an asymptomatic risk. The anxiety produced by the knowledge of this risk is justified when the risk is great, but not when it is only marginally increased; the same is true of the dependency on drugs.

The risks of treating hypercholesterolemia aggressively are probably less than the risks of leaving really high cholesterol levels untreated, but there is a point in the continuing relationship between serum cholesterol and coronary heart disease where the risks of using drugs on an indefinite basis may outweigh the risks of leaving cholesterol concentrations untreated.[37] It also is far from clear that lowering serum cholesterol to very low levels (overaggressive treatment) is biologically desirable or safe (see above). Very strict monitoring of the long-term clinical safety of drugs which lower cholesterol is a priority, although it is largely ignored because of the intrinsic difficulties.

The final consideration in terms of justifiable action is whether the aggressive reduction of hypercholesterolemia should be a priority in terms of health care and in relation to other health issues presenting to government health departments. To some extent these questions are political ones and, certainly, it is a brave doctor (and an unwise one) who would advocate that aggressive treatment of hypercholesterolemia should be the number one priority for a nation. The argument advanced for this is that CHD is the principal cause of mortality. However, most CHD deaths occur over the age of 65 years and hypercholesterolemia is a weak risk factor at that age. In my view, there is strong justification for adopting a policy for the aggressive treatment of hypercholesterolemia (particularly really high concentrations) in young and middle-aged men, and this is probably an economic investment. However, it is not cheap. One estimate of the cost-benefit situation has been calculated to be $56,100 per life-year saved for a cohort of 40-year-old men with cholesterol levels of 315 mg/dL treated with lifelong cholestyramine.[38] The costs for intervention rise steeply with increasing age and lower cholesterol levels. These estimates relate only to the cost of drug treatment. I doubt if it should be given priority over all other health questions, however. I am quite sure that the benefits of aggressive treatment of hypercholesterolemia currently are being exaggerated. I am also concerned that many doctors and people are being made to feel guilty if raised cholesterol levels are not treated aggressively, and that this guilt is largely a result of excesses and extravangancies of a relatively few vociferous self-styled health educators.

Conclusion

I have tried to give some perspective concerning the treatment of hypercholesterolemia by indicating, first, that I support such a policy for those with serum cholesterol concentrations above levels of about 250 mg/dL and for those with total cholesterol/HDL ratios above about 6. Moderation in life-style and diet, neither of which needs to be particularly aggressive, is to be commended for those with serum cholesterol concentrations between about 210 and 250 mg/dL.

I am opposed to overaggressive treatment for several reasons and believe that almost all men and women with levels below about 210 mg/dL should be reassured. The chief reason is that serum cholesterol concentrations relate to asymptomatic coronary *artery* disease rather than to symptomatic coronary *heart* disease, and that 90% of those with cholesterol levels below 200 to 210 mg/dL will not develop CHD over the next 20 years. The argument that CHD is the most common cause of death in those with low serum cholesterol levels is not, in view of the heterogeneous pathogenesis of CHD and lack of reduction in total mortality, a compelling argument for lowering everyone's serum cholesterol into their boots!

References

1. Dayton S, Pearce ML, Hashimoto S, et al: A controlled clinical trial of a diet high in unsaturated fat in preventing complications of atherosclerosis. *Circulation* 1969; 40 (suppl II):1–62. *This is the first clinical trial to show a significant reduction in CHD events using a diet with a P/S radio of > 1.5. There was also a significant increase in noncardiovascular mortality, particularly cancer.*
2. Turpeinen O, Karvonen MJ, Pekkarinen M, et al: Dietary prevention of coronary heart disease: The Finnish Mental Hospital Study. *Int J Epidemiol* 1979; 8:99–118. *This is a rather complicated clinical trial using a high polyunsaturated/saturated ratio in a changing population in two mental hospitals. There was a significant reduction in CHD events and no change in total mortality.*
3. World Health Organization: A co-operative trial in the primary prevention of ischaemic heart disease using clofibrate. *Br Heart J* 1978; 40:1069–1118. *The first drug trial of the effectiveness of lowering raised cholesterol in healthy men is reported. This showed a significant reduction in nonfatal myocardial infarction, no change in cardiac events, and a significant increase in noncardiovascular mortality.*
4. The Lipid Research Clinics Coronary Primary Prevention Trial results. 1. Reduction in incidence of coronary heart disease. *JAMA* 1984; 251:351–374. *This showed a marginally significant (P = .04 using a one-sided test) reduction of total CHD events and this could be related to a degree of reduction of serum cholesterol. There was no change in total mortality.*

Cholestyramine was used and there were more oral-gastrointestinal cancers.

5. Frick MH, Elo O, Haapa K, et al: Helsinki Heart Study: Primary Prevention Trial with gemfibrozil in middle-aged men with dyslipidemia. *N Engl J Med* 1987; 317:1237–1245. *This is a controlled trial using a fibrate with a significant reduction of CHD events but no change in total mortality. Gemfibrozil produced a profound reduction in triglyceride concentration and a rise in HDL cholesterol.*

6. Anderson KM, Castelli WP, Levy D: Cholesterol and mortality: 30 years of follow-up from the Framingham Study. *JAMA* 1987; 257:2176–2180. *Life tables are presented showing the relationship of serum cholesterol by quartile to prognosis in men and women. The relationship between raised serum cholesterol and CHD prognosis disappears in men after 55 years and is not significant in women.*

7. Simons LA: Interrelations of lipids and lipoproteins with coronary artery disease mortality in 19 countries. *Am J Cardiol* 1986; 57:5G–10G. *While there is a strong correlation between serum cholesterol and LDL cholesterol and CHD in men, none exists for women. There is also a strong negative relationship for HDL in men but not in women.*

8. Bush TL, Barrett-Connor E, Cowan LD, et al: Cardiovascular mortality and noncontraceptive use of estrogen in women: Results from the Lipid Research Clinics' program follow-up study. *Circulation* 1987; 75:1102–1109. *Lack of a relationship between LDL as an independent factor and CHD in women is documented.*

9. Kannel WB: Metabolic risk factors for coronary heart disease in women: Perspective from the Framingham study. *Am Heart J* 1987; 114:413–419. *LDL is only weakly related to CHD in women; the inverse relationship with HDL is stronger.*

10. Consensus Conference: Lowering blood cholesterol to prevent heart disease. *JAMA* 1985; 253:2080–2086. *This is an assembly of evidence indicating that the reduction of cholesterol particularly from high levels, may reduce CHD incidence.*

11. National Heart, Lung and Blood Institute: Report of the National Cholesterol Education Program: Expert Panel on Detection, Evaluation and Treatment of High Blood Cholesterol levels in adults. *Arch Intern Med* 1988; 148:36–69. *Recommendations to the medical profession and the public as to how high blood cholesterol might be reduced are given.*

12. Oliver MF: Consensus or nonsensus conference on coronary heart disease. *Lancet* 1985; 1:1087–1089. *This is a critique of the structure and procedure of consensus conferences.*

13. Oliver MF: Prevention of coronary heart disease — propaganda, promises, problems and prospects. *Circulation* 1986; 73:1–9. *This paper provides a critical examination of current dogma concerning the prevention of CHD and a plea to consider other approaches as well as reduction of serum cholesterol.*

14. Palumbo PJ: National Cholesterol Education Program: Does the Emperor have any clothes? *Mayo Clin Proc* 1988; 63:88–90. *This is an editorial criticizing the consensus and other reports suggesting that reduction of cholesterol is all that is necessary to reduce CHD.*

15. Becker MH: The cholesterol saga: Whither health promotion? *Ann Intern Med* 1987; 106:623–626. *As above.*
16. Fihn SD: A prudent approach to control of cholesterol levels. *JAMA* 1987; 258:2416–2418. *A conservative and well balanced point of view is given.*
17. Oliver MF: Reducing cholesterol does not reduce mortality. *JACC* 1988; 12:814–817. *This is an editorial reviewing the evidence that total mortality is not reduced by lowering cholesterol and that noncardiovascular mortality is often increased in the trials.*
18. Kronmal RA: Commentary on the published results of the Lipid Research Clinics Coronary Primary Prevention Trial. *JAMA* 1985; 253:2091–2093. *This is a survey criticizing the design, conduct, and reporting of the Lipid Research Clinic Trial.*
19. Anitschkow N: Experimental arteriosclerosis in animals, in Cowdry EV (ed): *Arteriosclerosis*, New York, Macmillan Publishing Co Inc, 1933, pp 271–322. *This is the first experimental evidence that feeding a diet rich in cholesterol can lead to arteriosclerosis in rabbits.*
20. Armstrong ML, Warner ED, Connor WE: Regression of coronary atheromatosis in rhesus monkeys. *Circ Res* 1970; 27:59–67. *This is a demonstration that the discontinuation of a high-cholesterol, high-fat diet in primates is associated with the regression of atheromatous lesions.*
21. Wissler RW, Vesselinovitch D: Regression of atherosclerosis in experimental animals and man. *Med Conc Cardiovasc Dis* 1977; 46:27–32. *As above.*
22. Clarkson TB, Lehner NDM, Wagner WD, et al: A study of atherosclerosis regression in Macaca mulatta. *Exp Mol Pathol* 1979; 30:360–385. *As above; but also taking into consideration the effects of stress on atherosclerosis progression and regression.*
23 Blankenhorn DH, Nessim SA, Johnson RL, et al: Beneficial effects of combined colestipol-niacin therapy on coronary atherosclerosis and coronary venous bypass grafts. *JAMA* 1987; 257:3233–3240. *Evidence that colestipol-niacin reduces the extent of progression in coronary venous bypass grafts but has no effect on the frequency of thrombosis is given.*
24. McGill HC: *The Geographic Pathology of Atherosclerosis.* Baltimore, The Williams & Wilkins Co, 1968. *The frequency and benign nature of atherosclerosis in old age are documented.*
25. Wilson PWF, Castelli WP, Kannel WB: Coronary risk prediction in adults (The Framingham Heart Study). *Am J Cardiol* 1987; 59:91G–94G. *The classical risk factors of smoking, cholesterol, and blood pressure account for no more than one half of the cause of CHD, even when multiplicative.*
26. Stamler J, Wentworth D, Neaton JD: Is the relationship between serum cholesterol and risk of premature death from coronary heart disease continuous and graded? Findings in 356,222 primary screenees of the Multiple Risk Factor Intervention Trial (MRFIT). *JAMA* 1986; 256:2823–2828. *An analysis of the relationship between serum cholesterol and coronary heart disease mortality is provided.*
27. Miller GJ, Miller NE: Plasma-high-density-lipoprotein concentration and development of ischemic heart disease. *Lancet* 1975; 1:16–20. *This is a review showing a strong inverse relationship between plasma HDL and CHD experimentally, clinically, and epidemiologically.*
28. Epstein FH: Nutrition, atherosclerosis and coronary heart disease: Evidence

from epidemiological observations. *Atherosclerosis Rev* 1979; 5:149–182. *Low-cholesterol populations have low CHD rates.*

29. Pooling Project Research Group: Relationship of blood pressure, serum cholesterol, smoking habit, relative weight and ECG abnormalities to incidence of major coronary events. Final Report of the Pooling Project. *J Chron Dis* 1978; 31:201–306. *This is an assessment of the relative risks of developing CHD according to the presence of risk factors.*

30. Martin MJ, Hulley SB, Browner WS, et al: Serum cholesterol, blood pressure and mortality: Implications for a cohort of 361,662 men. *Lancet* 1986; 2:933–936. *A clear demonstration of a curvilinear relationship between serum cholesterol and CHD mortality is given.*

31. Yusuf S, Cutler J: Single factor trials: Drug studies, in Olsson AG (ed): *Atherosclerosis. Biology and Clinical Science.* Edinburgh, Churchill Livingstone, 1987, pp 393–397. *This report provides aggregated evidence from all drug trials of cholesterol lowering of a reduction in nonfatal myocardial infarction but an increase in noncardiovascular deaths.*

32. Yusuf S, Furberg CD: Single factor trials: Control through life-style changes, in Olsson AG (ed): *Atherosclerosis. Biology and Clinical Science.* Edinburgh, Churchill Livingstone, 1987, pp 389–391. *Aggregated evidence of the effect of cholesterol lowering by diet is reported. Unimpressive results.*

33. Oliver MR, Ashley-Miller M, Wood D: *Screening for Risk of Coronary Heart Disease.* Chichester, England, John Wiley & Sons, 1985. *This is a survey of the pros and cons, and the economics, of screening for risk factors for coronary heart disease.*

34. Meade TW, Mellows S, Brozovic M, et al: Haemostatic function and IHD: Principal results of the Northwick Park Heart Study. *Lancet* 1986; 2:533–537. *This study reports evidence that raised fibrinogen and raised factor VIIc are strong predictors of subsequent CHD and that this prediction is independent of serum lipid levels.*

35. Stone MC, Thorp JM: Plasma fibrinogen — a major coronary risk factor. *J Roy Coll Gen Pract* 1985; 35:565–569. *As above.*

36. Hamsten A, Wiman B, DeFaire U, et al: Increased plasma levels of a rapid inhibitor of tissue plasminogen activator in young survivors of myocardial infarction. *N Engl J Med* 1985; 313:1557–1563. *This report offers evidence of impaired fibrinolysis in patients with myocardial infarction — a new predictor of CHD.*

37. Oliver MF: Risks of correcting the risks of coronary disease and stroke with drugs. *N Engl J Med* 1982; 306:297–298. *This is an editorial indicating that the long-term and widespread use of drugs is not without harm.*

38. Oster, G, Epstein AM: Cost-effectiveness of antihyperlipidemic therapy in the prevention of coronary heart disease: The case of cholestyramine. *JAMA* 1987; 258:2381–2387. *An appraisal of the economics of using drugs to prevent CHD is given.*

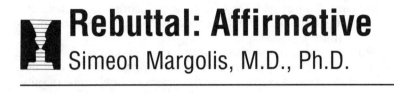

Rebuttal: Affirmative
Simeon Margolis, M.D., Ph.D.

Dr. Oliver and I agree on most of the fundamental issues related to the aggressive treatment of hypercholesterolemia. We agree that the "evidence relating hypercholesterolemia to atherosclerosis and particularly coronary atherosclerosis is impressive and incontrovertible." We agree that intervention trials have shown that lowering cholesterol levels does reduce the incidence of coronary events, nonfatal more than fatal. Although Dr. Oliver strongly and sensibly argues that there is no one-to-one relationship between coronary atherosclerosis and coronary heart disease (CHD), he cites ample evidence for a very strong correlation between plasma cholesterol levels and CHD.

Selection of Patients for Treatment

We both believe that hypercholesterolemic men between the ages of 30 and 59 years should be placed on a diet, and that the use of drugs should be limited to those patients whose more severe hypercholesterolemia persists despite dietary efforts. Dr. Oliver defines these two groups by their total cholesterol level: above 250 mg/dL as hypercholesterolemia and above 280 mg/dL as severe hypercholesterolemia. I prefer the recommendations made by the National Cholesterol Education Program (NCEP) which use the level of LDL cholesterol (LDL_{ch}) rather than the total cholesterol as a basis for therapeutic decisions.[1] Use of the LDL_{ch} allows the identification of patients who need no treatment because their high cholesterol is due to a high HDL cholesterol (HDL_{ch}) as well as those whose total cholesterol is not impressively elevated but who have a high LDL_{ch} associated with a low HDL_{ch}. I would go even further than Dr. Oliver or the NCEP guidelines in obtaining HDL_{ch} determinations. I believe this measurement should be carried out in any individual with a strong family history of premature coronary artery disease (CAD) or any of the other major risk factors for CAD. On the other hand, I do not agree with Dr. Oliver that management decisions should be based on the ratio of cholesterol or LDL_{ch} to HDL_{ch}. Both a high LDL and a low HDL contribute independently to the development of CAD. The risk of a significantly elevated LDL_{ch} persists even if the HDL_{ch} is high and therefore the ratio is relatively low. In fact, the Lipid Research Clinics Coronary Primary Prevention Trial[2] showed that the incidence of coronary events was reduced when cholesterol was lowered in subjects with an HDL_{ch} above 40 mg/dL, but not in those with lower levels of HDL_{ch}. Based on these findings, I also cannot agree with Dr. Oliver's conclusions that a low HDL_{ch} should be a requisite for the treatment of moderate hypercholesterolemia or an indication for more aggressive treatment.

I agree with Dr. Oliver that hypercholesterolemia should not be treated overaggressively, which I interpret to mean by the inappropriate use of drugs. However, I do think it makes sense to use the presence or absence of other risk factors in choosing the cholesterol or LDL_{ch} level necessary for initiating treatment.

One major area in which I disagree with Dr. Oliver relates to his strong objections to generalizing from the results of past intervention trials in making decisions on the treatment of women and people younger or older than those included in the trials. Strictly speaking, his arguments are indisputable; we have no data on the impact of lowering cholesterol on coronary events in women or in those younger than 30 years or older than 59 years. On the other hand, the extraordinary costs of intervention trials, especially in women and younger subjects, make it extremely unlikely that such data ever will be available. From what we know about the biology of atherosclerosis, it certainly seems reasonable to assume that controlling hypercholesterolemia in young people will slow their development of CAD. Similarly, it is hard to believe that hypercholesterolemia is not harmful in women, though probably less so than in men. We should consider some alteration in the present cut-points for making decisions on drug treatment in women but should not ignore hypercholesterolemia in them altogether.

More difficult are decisions in men and women older than 60 years. The findings in the Cholesterol-Lowering Atherosclerosis Study (CLAS) study[3] that a reduction in cholesterol slowed the progression of coronary artery lesions make it difficult to deny the possible benefits of treating hyper-cholesterolemia in older patients. These decisions should be based on the clinical judgment of the physician regarding the overall health, risk status, and desires of the patient. There seems to be no risk in putting elderly patients on a prudent diet; in the midst of the cholesterol frenzy in this country, many elderly patients are eager for (will even demand) some treatment of their elevated cholesterol and will be grateful for an improvement. When choles-terol levels are extremely high, I believe it is reasonable to use drugs gingerly in elderly patients who do not respond to diet and are especially apprehensive about their cholesterol values.

Dr. Oliver and I recommend the same dietary approach to the manage-ment of hypercholesterolemia. However, he states that he is not convinced that restricting the intake of cholesterol is likely to contribute much to the reduction of CHD. Moderate restriction of dietary cholesterol will not lower plasma cholesterol levels by much in most individuals. On the other hand, 30% to 50% of dietary cholesterol is absorbed and must be transported through the bloodstream and eventually eliminated from the body. Evidence in both animals and humans indicates that high-cholesterol diets lead to the formation of cholesterol-rich lipoproteins that are extremely atherogenic.[4]

"Overselling" the Importance of Hypercholesterolemia

I agree with Dr. Oliver that the treatment of hypercholesterolemia should not be the number one health priority. In fact, the treatment of hyper-cholesterolemia ranks third on my priority list among the major risk factors for coronary disease, far behind cigarette smoking and below hypertension, both of which produce major ill effects other than CHD. I also agree that the relationship between CAD risk and cholesterol levels is curvilinear rather than linear. And clearly the conclusion that every 1% fall in cholesterol levels is associated with a 2% reduction in coronary events holds true only for those individuals with higher levels of cholesterol (and possibly only for men). For these reasons, I try to address all risk factors in management and to dissuade overeager adult patients from the inconvenience of rigid diets and the dangers of drugs when their cholesterol is less than 200 mg/dL. Patients and physicians alike should understand that a reduction in cholesterol, whatever its starting level, *may* (rather than *will*) decrease the likelihood of CHD.

Dr. Oliver points out that many physicians do not screen for cholesterol despite the presence of a strong family history or other risk factors for CAD. At the same time, he objects to the strategy of the NCEP in urging every individual to ask about his or her cholesterol number. I believe this strategy makes good sense. The goal is not to place the onus of decisions on the patient but rather, by educating the public, to raise the level of physician consciousness about cholesterol in general and especially in the patients who ask about their number. This approach has caused excessive concern about cholesterol in the general public and considerable, often unnecessary, anxiety in many individuals who are the victims of inaccurate laboratory tests or who do not understand their implications. In the long run, however, the furor will quiet and with luck we will be left with physicians who are more alert to cholesterol and other risk factors for CAD.

Dangers of Lowering Cholesterol

I do not agree with Dr. Oliver's concern that lowering plasma cholesterol levels may produce an adverse effect by reducing cellular cholesterol. There is no evidence for ill effects in normocholesterolemic people in the Western world or in those with extremely low cholesterol levels in underdeveloped countries. The notion that a low cholesterol is causally related to an increased risk of cancer, especially of the colon, has not withstood the test of further studies. One recent study concluded that the association between a low serum cholesterol level and cancer is due at least partly to a lowering of cholesterol levels by the presence of preclinical cancer.[5] Another study found a positive association between the serum cholesterol level and both rectal and colon cancer.[6]

There is no doubt that the methods used to lower cholesterol can cause adverse effects: economic, psychological, and physical. Physicians must be aware of these costs and not undertake lightly the aggressive treatment of hypercholesterolemia which must be continued for many years. Dietary treatment appears to have no harmful physical effects, but patients should be cautioned to avoid excessive dietary regimens that have not been proven safe by long use in some population (for example, diets with an extremely high intake of polyunsaturated fats). Physicians need to be especially aware of the immediate side effects and possible long-range complications of all medications. As indicated by Dr. Oliver, the optimum medical care of each patient depends upon clinical judgment in weighing the possible benefits against the adverse effects of aggressive treatment of hypercholesterolemia.

"Beyond Cholesterol"

Dr. Oliver emphasizes the critical importance of intravascular thrombosis in converting asymptomatic CAD to CHD, and the need for intensive research on the role of thrombogenesis and fibrinolysis in the development of CHD. I agree completely, and would only add the importance of expanded efforts to understand the detailed mechanisms whereby LDL and HDL, respectively, enhance and lessen atherogenesis. An excellent recent review illustrates the value of such studies by examining the way that oxidation of polyunsaturated fatty acids in LDL may accelerate its uptake by macrophages in the arterial wall.[7]

References

1. Report of the National Cholesterol Education Program Expert Panel on Detection, Evaluation and Treatment of High Blood Cholesterol in Adults. *Arch Intern Med* 1988; 148:36–69.
2. Gordon DJ, Knoke J, Probstfield JL, et al: High density lipoprotein cholesterol and coronary heart disease in hypercholesterolemic men: The Lipid Research Clinics Primary Prevention Trial. *Circulation* 1986, 74:1217–1225.
3. Blankenhorn DH, Nessim SA, Johnson ER, et al: Beneficial effects of combined colestipol-niacin therapy on coronary atherosclerosis and coronary venous bypass grafts. *JAMA* 1987; 257:3233–3240.
4. Mahley RW, Innerarity TL, Bersot TP, et al: Alterations in human high density lipoproteins induced by diets high in cholesterol with or without a plasma cholesterol elevation. *Lancet* 1978; 2:807.
5. Sherman RW, Wentworth DN, Cutler JA, et al: Serum cholesterol levels and cancer mortality in 361,662 men screened for the Multiple Risk Factor Intervention Trial. *JAMA* 1987; 257:943–948.

6. Tornberg SA, Holm L-E, Carstensen JM, et al: Risks of cancer of the colon and rectum in relation to serum cholesterol and beta-lipoprotein. *N Engl J Med* 1986; 315:1629–1633.
7. Steinberg D, Parthasarathy S, Carew TE, et al: Beyond cholesterol: Modifications of low-density lipoprotein that increase its atherogenicity. *N Engl J Med* 1989; 320:915–924.

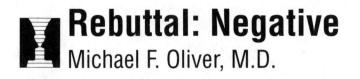

Rebuttal: Negative
Michael F. Oliver, M.D.

When I agreed to participate in this "Debate in Medicine," I expected that there would be a greater difference of opinion concerning the treatment of hypercholesterolemia. In the event, there has been no question of an excessively enthusiastic protagonist or a nihilistic antagonist confronting each other. In other words, I agree with many of Dr. Margolis' views (as must be evident from my text) and such differences as exist probably relate to those between our two cultures, with the American attitude having high expectations and the European being traditionally more cautious.

Agreements

We both have already addressed the influence of gender, age, and HDL cholesterol concentrations in determining a policy for screening and treating hypercholesterolemia. We both have discussed the inferences which should be drawn from the primary prevention trials, although with slightly different emphasis. We also have considered the unreliability of a single estimation of serum cholesterol or LDL cholesterol as an index for action and the difficulties which result as a consequence of selecting any arbitrary cutoff point. We are clearly in agreement that dietary measures always should be the first step in the management of patients with any type of hyperlipidemia, and that drugs generally should not be considered until a real effort has been made to adhere rigorously to the recommended diet.

Alternative Views

There are four issues arising from Dr. Margolis' statement that I think are worth expanding with alternative interpretations.

First, the statement by the Adult Treatment Guidelines Panel of the National Cholesterol Education Program (NCEP) sponsored by the National Institutes of Health recommends that "all adults have their cholesterol level determined at least every 5 years." I consider that the recommendation is not soundly based and is insufficiently precise, although I have no strong difference of opinion with Dr. Margolis regarding this recommendation. The failure of the National Cholesterol Education Program to make different recommendations for the two genders is one major fault or serious oversight. I have indicated already the lack of a relationship between serum cholesterol concentrations in women and their subsequent prognosis, the lack of a relationship internationally between cholesterol and coronary heart disease (CHD) mortality, and the lack of a major clinical trial indicating a reduction in nonfatal myocardial infarction conducted in women. Another weakness of the NCEP recommendation is that it is not age-related; both Dr. Margolis and I have considerable doubts as to the value of estimating serum cholesterol over the age of, say, about 60 years. Additionally , I know of no strong reasons why estimations of serum cholesterol should be conducted every 5 years. The increase in serum cholesterol concentrations in men under 50 years old is probably in the region of about 10% every 10 years and, if this is agreed to be an accurate assessment, the increased risk of CHD in those with serum cholesterol concentrations below about 220 mg/100 mL is minimal indeed. However, I do support a policy of estimating serum cholesterol every 10 years in those with concentrations around and above about 220 mg/100 mL.

Second, Dr. Margolis refers to a cholesterol-lowering atherosclerosis study[1] (CLAS) and rightly concludes that there are no convincing data to support the authors' interpretation that a marked reduction of serum cholesterol levels produces some regression of coronary artery lesions. It is unconvincing not only because of the relatively small size of the trial, but also because the incidence of thrombotic occlusion (as distinct from the extent of atheromatous lesions) was unchanged. It is of little consequence clinically if a treatment which causes regression of coronary atherosclerotic lesions (and this trial did not clearly show that) leaves the extent of thrombotic occlusion unchanged because, clearly, the supply of blood to a potentially ischemic myocardium is unlikely to be improved greatly. It will be important to study carefully the results of the ongoing atheroma-regression trials (several of which are using HMGCoA reductase inhibitors) in order to see whether the expected regression in coronary atheroma is associated with less thrombotic occlusion. It is conceivable that it may not be, because "healing" changes which take place in the subendothelial and smooth muscle tissue in coronary arteries may be associated with increased platelet-fibrin repair activity and hence the formation of microthrombi may occur which from time to time may lead to an occlusive thrombus at the point where regression is taking place. We should keep our minds open about this.

Third, Dr. Margolis refers to the 15-year follow-up of the Coronary Drug Project in which it has been suggested that a decrease in overall mortality by 11% may relate to the reduction of serum cholesterol which was achieved when the men were treated with nicotinic acid for a 6-year period 9 or more years before their death.[2] The reason for relating the reduction in death to cholesterol reduction many years earlier appears to be the marginal improvement in incidence in those receiving nicotinic acid at the end of the 6-year period of treatment. However, there are other interpretations. Nicotinic acid has a profound effect in lowering serum triglycerides, largely as a consequence of decreasing very-low-density lipoprotein (VLDL) production, but also due to the inhibition of lipoprotein lipase activity. Nicotinic acid also has been established for many years as a vasodilator and has been used in many countries for the treatment of peripheral vascular disease. This vasodilator effect is not different from that which may be obtained from long-acting nitrate treatment and is likely to reduce left ventricular work which, in the presence of coronary artery disease, all previous myocardial infarction might postpone the onset of myocardial ischemia and infarction. Also, the vasodilator effect might actually improve myocardial flow; it is worth noting that nicotinic acid was one of two drugs used in the CLAS study already discussed. Thus, to attribute the minor change in mortality to cholesterol lowering many years earlier is only one interpretation.

Fourth, both Dr. Margolis and I have referred to the relevance and importance of raised serum triglycerides. In the World Health Organization (WHO) Clofibrate Trial and the Helsinki Heart Study using gemfibrozil, there was a relatively greater reduction in serum triglycerides compared with serum cholesterol, and both of these trials showed a significant reduction in nonfatal myocardial infarction. When combined with the reciprocal rise in HDL, these changes may be at least as important as a reduction in cholesterol. Recently, an "open" Swedish Primary Prevention Trial[3] has indicated that CHD mortality was reduced with nicotinic acid treatment (see earlier). In this trial, the reduction in CHD was related to the decrease in serum triglycerides and not to changes in cholesterol. A reduction of hypertriglyceridemia may lead to a reduction of the risk of intravascular thrombosis. This possibility needs intensive study in view of the strongly positive correlation between serum triglycerides and one of the major indices of thrombogenesis, Factor VIIc,[4] and one of the major indices of fibrinolysis, tissue plasminogen activator inhibitor (tPAI).[5] Since intravascular thrombosis may be the most important "trigger" converting clinically occult coronary artery disease to clinically manifest coronary heart disease, modification or even aggressive treatment of hypertriglyceridemia in some individuals may be even more important than aggressive treatment of hypercholesterolemia.

References

1. Blankenhorn DH, Nessim SA, Johnson ER, et al: Beneficial effects of combined colestipol-niacin therapy on coronary atherosclerosis and coronary venous bypass grafts. *JAMA* 1987; 257:3233–3240.
2. Canner PL, Berge KG, Wenger NK, et al: Fifteen year mortality in Coronary Drug Project patients: Long-term benefit with niacin. *J Am Coll Cardiol* 1986; 8:1245–1255.
3. Carlson LA, Rosenhamer G: Reduction of mortality in the Stockholm Ischaemic Heart Disease Secondary Prevention Study by combined treatment with clofibrate and nicotinic acid. *Acta Med Scand* 1988; 223:405–418.

4. Mitropoulos KA: Hypercoagulability and Factor VII in hypertriglyceridemia. *Semin Thromb Hemost* 1988; 14:246–252.
5. Hamsten A, Wiman B, DeFaire U, et al: Increased plasma levels of a rapid inhibitor of tissue plasminogen activator in young survivors of myocardial infarction. *N Engl J Med* 1985; 313:1557–1563.

Editor's Comments
H. Verdain Barnes, M.D.

The "Cholesterol Era" is here especially in the United States. Our national emphasis on cholesterol has been, is currently being, and will continue to be substantially underwritten by the federal government, i.e., the taxpayer. Is it justified? If so, how can we identify those individuals at greatest risk, and how should we manage their care? These important issues are debated enthusiastically by two major contributors to this field, Drs. Simeon Margolis from the United States and Michael F. Oliver from Scotland.

Is a national health priority to reduce cholesterol justified by current data? Here, our debators have substantive agreements and disagreements. They agree that data from a variety of studies clearly support a strong association between hypercholesterolemia and atherosclerosis including the coronary arteries. Their conclusion based on the findings of several major intervention trials is that there is a decrease in the incidence of nonfatal coronary events in those subjects whose cholesterol was lowered. However, both note that available data do not answer the question for populations other than males 30 to 60 years old. On the other hand, they disagree as to the degree to which this male data can be extrapolated to females of all ages and to males outside the age range targeted in the intervention trials. For practical purposes, Dr. Margolis strongly favors extrapolation and Dr. Oliver does not. Based on their position statements and rebuttals, neither believes that lowering cholesterol merits being the number one national health priority. Dr. Margolis, for example, ranks hypercholesterolemia third behind hypertension and smoking as the major risk factors for coronary artery disease. In this editor's view, the data substantiating the association between hypercholesterolemia and atherosclerosis are clear for "middle-aged" males. However, in my view, a cause and effect relationship has not been unequivocally established. Philosophically, I find Dr. Margolis' arguments for extrapolating the male data to females and younger males persuasive, but would hasten to add that from a purely scientific perspective Dr. Oliver is correct. As practitioners, we rarely have an absolute scientific base from which to derive our medical decisions. In our current setting, I am not convinced that with increasing patient awareness and sophistication, a hypercholesterolemic female or young male can be educated adequately to allay their concerns. Thus, to do nothing because of our lack of specific age-group or gender data seems impractical if not impossible in the United States. For patients over the age of 60 years, the issue appears to fall in a similar category, but this editor would prefer to see additional data on atherosclerosis regression by lowering cholesterol before embarking on aggressive pharmacological therapy in this age group.

Who is at substantial risk? Here, our debators support different views which highlight the relatively arbitrary features of our current information. The "cutoff" values for major hypercholesterolemia proposed by both have supporters in the literature. Few, if any, would argue that total cholesterol values above 280 mg/dL on two or three determinations should not be treated aggressively. Both debators emphasize that practitioners must be knowledgeable about and convinced that their laboratory's values are accurate. This is not an easy task in my experience, albeit a critical one. This editor agrees with Dr. Margolis that the various ratios proposed for making clinical management decisions are to a degree suspect and that the use of LDL_{ch} and HDL_{ch} levels along with total cholesterol currently provides the clinician with the most useful and reliable information upon which to base management decisions.

Both debators agree that a "prudent diet" is the preferred first-line therapy. If one defines "aggressive therapy" as a stringent diet and/or pharmacological therapy, both debators advocate a more conservative approach. Dr. Oliver, however, is more conservative than Dr. Margolis. They agree that the available methods for lowering cholesterol can result in adverse psychological, physical, and economic problems, but Dr. Margolis does not believe there is sufficient reason to be concerned about potential adverse effects due to a concomitant lowering of intracellular cholesterol with pharmacological therapy. Most importantly, I believe, our debators agree that cholesterol levels alone are not sufficient and that sound clinical judgment based on a complete history and physical examination plus a knowledge of the possible advantages and disadvantages of second-line (pharmacological) therapy are essential for optimal patient management. This editor fully agrees.

Finally, our debators call for accelerated research on intravascular thrombosis (thrombogenesis and fibrinolysis) as it relates to the development of coronary heart disease in the asymptomatic patient with coronary atherosclerosis. This editor enthusiastically endorses our debators' focus on this critical area which may result in greater sensitivity and specificity in evaluation and therapy.

What should we tell our patients who have been prodded into a "cholesterol frenzy"? In my view, we should tell them that the data available are incomplete, the problem is multifactorial, the standards for "aggressive intervention" are not absolute, a "prudent diet" as defined in these position statements is desirable for most if not all, and pharmacological therapy is not a panacea and should be reserved for patients whose cholesterol remains high following a full effort using diet alone. As always, however, management should be tailored to the individual patient's needs, using all of the parameters available to us for making a sound clinical decision.

Should Asymptomatic Cigarette Smokers Have Annual Chest X-Rays After Age 55 Years?

Chapter Editor: Richard H. Winterbauer, M.D.

Affirmative: Myron R. Melamed, M.D.
Attending Pathologist, Memorial Sloan-Kettering Cancer Center, and Professor of Pathology, Cornell University Medical College, New York, New York

Betty J. Flehinger, Ph.D.
Manager, Statistics, Department of Mathematical Sciences, International Business Machines (IBM) Thomas J Watson Research Center, Yorktown Heights, New York

Negative: Robert S. Fontana, M.D.
Professor of Medicine, Mayo Medical School, Rochester, Minnesota

Editor's Introduction

The debate to follow explores a dilemma common to all physicians practicing internal medicine. Mr. Smith, age 55 years, with a 70 packs/year history of smoking, has just completed his physical examination. He feels well and has no respiratory symptoms save for the ubiquitous morning cough of the smoker. The physical examination is normal. Should a screening chest x-ray be done? The American Cancer Society says no. However, in each clinician's personal experience are examples of patients with stage I bronchogenic carcinoma discovered by screening chest x-ray and successfully operated upon. This debate addresses the role of the annual chest x-ray as a screening test for bronchogenic carcinoma. Both debaters were major investigators in the National Cancer Institute's Lung Cancer Detection Study and have arrived at opposing viewpoints in the interpretation of results from this landmark study.

Richard H. Winterbauer, M.D.

Affirmative

Myron R. Melamed, M.D.
Betty J. Flehinger, Ph.D.

Lung cancer is the most common cause of death from cancer in the United States today, among women as well as men. Approximately 90% of those who develop the disease will die of it, most in less than 3 years. In 1987 there were an estimated 139,000 deaths from lung cancer in the United States.[1] The long-term solution eventually will have to be prevention of this disease, and the most important preventive measure is the elimination of cigarette smoking. For the present and foreseeable future however, we must be concerned with the care of patients who have and will develop lung cancer. The only curative treatment presently available is surgery and, with rare exceptions, cure is possible only for those patients with cancers confined to the lung and regional lymph nodes who have tumors amenable to complete resection. Few patients with these early-stage lung cancers are symptomatic. Diagnosis generally hinges on the discovery of a radiological abnormality in an "incidental" chest x-ray taken during the course of hospitalization for another reason or as part of a routine "check-up."

In 1974 we undertook a 10-year study of the possible value of regular, periodic screening examinations to detect lung cancer in an early, asymptomatic, and potentially curable stage. The study was carried out with the support of the National Cancer Institute (NCI) at three institutions: the Memorial Sloan-Kettering Cancer Center in New York (MSKCC), the Johns Hopkins Medical Institutions in Baltimore, and the Mayo Clinic in Rochester, Minnesota. Approximately 10,000 men were recruited into the study at each institution. They were all cigarette smokers over the age of 45 years considered to be at high risk of lung cancer but without known evidence of the disease at the time of enrollment.[2] Interestingly, 223 of the total 31,360 participants at all three institutions were found to have lung cancer on their initial examination — a prevalence rate of slightly over 7 per 1,000,[3] equaling or exceeding the rate of detection, for example, in screening for carcinoma in situ of the uterine cervix by Papanicolaou smears. In the MSKCC study, one sixth of all deaths were due to lung cancer (the total mortality from lung cancer at the end of 7 years equaled 1.7% of the population compared with 8.6% for all other causes of death combined).

There are only two screening tests available for the detection of early or asymptomatic lung cancer: the chest x-ray and sputum cytology. The MSKCC, Hopkins, and Mayo studies were designed primarily to evaluate sputum cytology, so evidence with respect to the value of the chest x-ray is indirect, accounting for differences in opinion regarding its worth. It should be noted also that differences in design between the studies were intended to provide complementary information. At MSKCC and Hopkins the men were volunteers, recruited from the general population of large urban communities; at Mayo they were recruited from a patient population coming for reasons unrelated to possible lung cancer. At MSKCC and Hopkins they were randomly assigned into two approximately equal groups, one receiving dual screening with sputum cytology every 4 months as well as an annual posteroanterior (PA) and lateral chest x-ray, the other receiving only the annual chest x-ray. At Mayo, all men received the dual screening initially, and then were randomized into an intensive screen group which was instructed and reminded to obtain a chest x-ray and submit a sputum cytology at intervals of 4 months after returning home, and a control group simply advised at the initial examination to obtain an annual chest x-ray.[4] Follow-up was excellent at all three institutions. At MSKCC, 99.4% of the men enrolled in the program were followed for 5 to 7 years during the period of active screening, and for 2 years post-screening.

Data from these studies have now been reported in a series of publications.[3-9] We have concluded that, while sputum cytology supplementing the chest x-ray can detect as many as 23% more cancers than can x-rays alone on the initial examination, these additional cancers can be identified on later chest x-rays while still resectable and curable. Thus, sputum cytology does not lower the death rate from lung cancer (Fig 1) and does not benefit the individual who adheres to a conscientious program of annual chest x-rays (Table 1). It may be useful to screen a population that cannot be followed easily. However, we are concerned here with the value of screening for lung cancer by means of annual chest x-rays.

We consider the following to be established by our own study (MSKCC)[6,8,9] and by those at Hopkins[5] and Mayo,[7] and it is the basis for our recommendations regarding screening for lung cancer:

1. Forty percent of all lung cancers can be detected at an early stage, i.e., stage I of the American Joint Committee on Cancer Staging (AJC stage I); they are localized to the lung with or without peribronchial or hilar lymph node involvement.

2. Seventy percent to 80% of the patients who have AJC stage I lung cancer treated surgically do not die of that disease (Fig 2).

3. Overall, the 5-year survival of all patients who developed lung cancer while enrolled in the screening program was 35%, contrasted with 13% for the United States as a whole.

4. The proportion of early (stage I) lung cancers dropped from 41% to 20% during the 2 years following cessation of screening, and survival decreased from 47% at 4 years for lung cancer diagnosed during the screening period to 20% at 4 years for lung cancer diagnosed in the post-screening period (Table 2, Fig 3).[9] Patients with lung cancer diagnosed in the post-screening period were comparable both by stage and survival to patients whose lung cancer developed undetected by us during the screening period (interval cases) (Table 3).

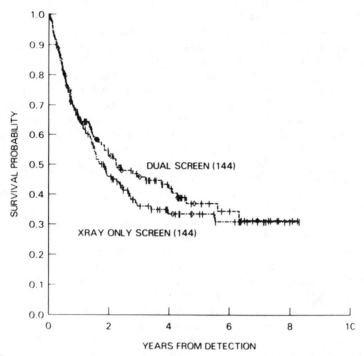

FIG 1.
Survival from lung cancer of men who were in the dual screening group (annual chest x-ray and sputum cytology every 4 months) compared with those in the single screening group (annual chest x-ray only). While sputum cytology detected radiologically occult, very early lung cancers which were successfully resected and cured, x-rays detected those same cancers later, although still early enough to be resected and cured. (From Melamed MR, Flehinger BJ, Zaman MB, et al: *Chest* 1984; 86:44–53. Used by permission.)

5. The interval and post-screening cases of cancer detected by "incidental" or "routine" chest x-rays, while still asymptomatic (other), had essentially the same survival as those diagnosed by screening, while survival among cases diagnosed because of symptoms (symptomatic) was comparable to the reported survival of lung cancer in the general population of the United States, i.e., 13%. (Fig 4).

6. Nearly one half of all lung cancers in the MSKCC study were adenocarcinomas, which is consistent with reports from other institutions suggesting that adenocarcinoma is becoming the predominant type of lung cancer. Unlike squamous carcinoma, adenocarcinoma of the lung tends to be peripheral in origin and can be detected in chest x-rays while still very small.

The argument may be made that the increased survival of patients with lung cancer in this study compared with the general population can be explained by lead time, length bias, and overdiagnosis bias. Phrased another way, the stage I lung cancers detected by screening are presumed to be a special type of slow-growing cancer that might never progress to symptomatic disease, dissemination, and death. They grow so slowly that unscreened individuals remain unaware of their cancer and eventually die of other causes. No evidence is yet available to affirm or deny this possibility. However, with this reservation in mind, we undertook to build a mathematical model of the development and progression of lung cancer in a high-risk population to whom we offered screening by annual chest x-ray.[10] The data from our 10-year screening program were used to estimate the parameters of this model. It was found that the mean duration of early-stage adenocarcinoma and large-cell undifferentiated carcinoma of the lung is at least 4 years, that the probability of detecting it in an early stage on any given examination is less than 20%, and that the cure probability is 50% at most. Based on these figures, the decrease in lung cancer mortality from annual screening and prompt surgical treatment starting at age 45 years might be as much as 18%.[11]

Table 1.
Lung Cancer Stage — Dual Screen vs. X-ray Only,* All Cases Detected[†]

Stage	Dual Screen	X-ray Only
Stage I	59	58
Stage II	7	11
Stage III	78	75
Total	144	144

*Dual Screen = annual chest x-ray and sputum cytology every 4 months; X-ray Only = Annual PA and lateral chest x-ray.

[†]The 288 lung cancer cases proven by the end of the screening period do not include 5 cases proven in the post-screening period as a result of prior suspicious screening examinations (compare with Table 2).

[‡]Adapted from Flehinger BJ, Melamed MR, Heelan RT, et al: Accuracy of chest film screening by technologists in the New York Early Lung Cancer Detection Program. *AJR* 1978; 131:593–597. Used by permission.

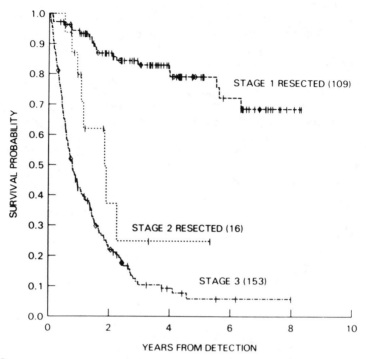

FIG 2.
Survival from lung cancer by stage. Three deaths from lung cancer after 5 years in the stage I resected group were due to new primary lung cancers. (From Melamed MR, Flehinger BJ, Zaman MB, et al: *Chest* 1984; 86:44–53. Used by permission.)

Whether one considers a potential salvage rate of up to 18% insufficient to justify the cost of an annual chest x-ray is perhaps a matter of philosophy, perhaps a matter of relative values. It is very possible that the health care planner with legislated budget restrictions may have a different opinion than the individual at high risk who is concerned about his personal health. From a national perspective, assuming 135,000 deaths per year from lung cancer in the United States and excluding the 17% that are small-cell carcinomas that cannot be salvaged by surgery, a reduction of even 10% would result in more than 10,000 lives saved annually. This is comparable to all the deaths from uterine cancer, cancer of the urinary bladder, or brain tumors.[1]

Ideally, one would like a direct evaluation of the chest x-ray as a means of screening for lung cancer. There have been attempts to do so, most recently in the Mayo lung study which compared approximately 4,500 patients who were screened by chest x-ray and cytology every 4 months with a like number who were recommended (but not reminded) to have annual chest x-rays.

While the results of that study showed more lung cancers detected in the intensively screened population, they failed to show a significant difference in lung cancer deaths due to the screening. The Mayo study does *not* prove that there is no difference, however. Let us assume that the death rate from lung cancer in a population of mature smokers is 3 per 1,000 per year. In order to design a controlled trial to detect a 20% reduction in that mortality, we would require that 60,000 smokers be monitored for 5 years, with 30,000 of them randomly allocated to a group receiving annual chest x-rays and 30,000 to a control group forbidden to have any routine chest x-rays. Alternatively, one could study 30,000 smokers for 10 years. If the goal were to detect 10% reduction in lung cancer mortality, it would require the study of 200,000 smokers for 5 years or 100,000 for 10 years.

Clearly, the Mayo lung study did not have a sufficiently large population for such an evaluation. Furthermore, the control population of once-screened Mayo Clinic patients who were not reminded to obtain chest x-rays is hardly comparable to a control group known not to have had x-rays. Even if it were feasible to recruit and hold the enormous number of subjects required in a long-term screening study, one might question the ethics as well as the practicality of denying chest x-rays to one half the participants of a study of many years' duration. Thus, it is not realistic to expect a direct evaluation of the possible benefits of chest x-ray screening for lung cancer. The approach we have taken is indirect, but gives a close approximation and places outer bounds on estimates derived from a mathematical model to which we can fit data from the NCI and other lung cancer studies.

Table 2.
Lung Cancer Stage — Memorial Sloan-Kettering Cancer Center (MSKCC) Screening Program*

Stage	Detected by Screening	Interval[†] Cases	Post-screening	Total
Stage I	100 (53%)	20 (20%)	12 (20%)	132
Stage II	15	3	5	23
Stage III	75	80	44	199
Total	190	103	61	354

*From Flehinger BJ, Melamed MR, Heelan RT, et al: Accuracy of chest film screening by technologists in the New York Early Lung Cancer Detection Program. *AJR* 1978; 131:593–597. Used by permission.
[†]Interval Cases = cases diagnosed during the screening period but not as a result of the screening examination.

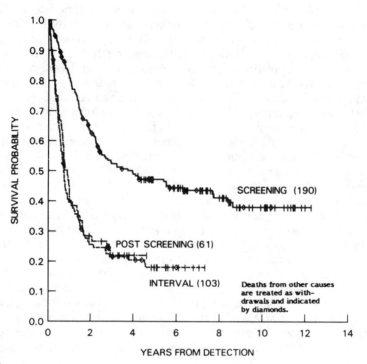

FIG 3.
Survival from lung cancer detected by screening compared to interval and post-screening cases. (From Melamed MR, Flehinger BJ: *Schweiz Med Wochenschr* 1987; 117:1457–1463. Used by permission.)

The amount of radiation sustained from an annual chest x-ray is negligible, particularly for the older age group of individuals who are most at risk of lung cancer. The argument against chest x-ray screening is essentially one of cost-effectiveness. Lung cancer incidence is strongly age-related, increasing sharply at 50 to 55 years (Fig 5), and the cost of case finding could be reduced by recommending that screening begin at age 50 or 55 years. Also, single anatomic site screening studies can be disproportionately expensive. A considerable part of the cost of the three NCI lung screening studies, for example, was in recruiting, holding, and following the men who enrolled. The detailed data collection and analysis necessary for this study also would not be required for screening per se. Even the cost of double-reading films, which may be necessary to achieve maximum sensitivity in detecting radiological abnormalities, could be minimized by using specially trained radiological technologists for the preliminary examination.[12] The costs of administration, maintenance of the physical plant, record-keeping, and correspondence with participants, their families, and their physicians could be minimized by including the screening chest x-ray as part of the physical examination carried out in a comprehensive health care facility. In fact, the added cost of a screening chest x-ray is relatively small for the middle-aged cigarette smoker who seeks medical evaluation from his physician in an office, hospital, or other medical facility. In this setting, even if there is only a 40% chance of detecting and resecting an early lung cancer (i.e., stage I), it seems irresponsible to deny that chance to the patient who requests and expects a complete medical evaluation from his physician. Would an informed patient at risk of lung cancer consent to a physical examination that excludes the chest x-ray? How, in good conscience, can the physician assure his middle-aged male patient who is known to be a cigarette smoker that he is in good health if he does not have a chest x-ray?

The MSKCC, Hopkins, and Mayo studies did not prove that the chest x-ray was an effective detection technique for lung cancer, but they were not designed to do so. Conversely, they did not prove that the chest x-ray is ineffective, and the shift to earlier stage at diagnosis, increased operability, and increased survival all suggest that it is of value. Until there is good evidence that treatment is ineffective, or until treatment becomes so very effective that cure no longer depends on detection at an early stage, the medical profession in our view is obliged to make every effort possible to identify and treat lung cancer at an early and potentially curable stage. At present, the most effective detection technique is the annual chest x-ray, particularly in the case of adenocarcinomas of the lung (which are now the most common type of lung cancer). The chest x-ray is a simple examination that is relatively inexpensive and harmless. Our best efforts to quantify the

Table 3.
Method of Detection of Interval and Post-screen Cases of Lung Cancer According to Stage of Disease*

	Interval Cases		Post-screen Cases	
Stage	**Asymptomatic[†]**	**Symptomatic**	**Asymptomatic[†]**	**Symptomatic**
Stage I	12	7	10	2
Stage II, III	5	81	14	35

[†]Chest x-rays of asymptomatic individuals were taken as part of a routine physical examination or on hospitalization for unrelated illness.

*Adapted from Flehinger BJ, Melamed MR, Heelan RT, et al: Accuracy of chest film screening by technologists in the New York Early Lung Cancer Detection Program. *AJR* 1978; 131:593–597. Used by permission.

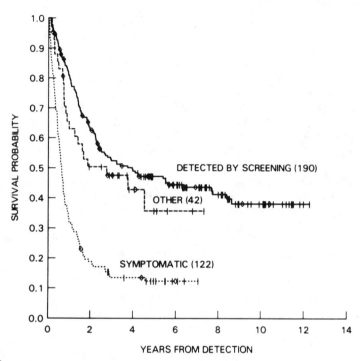

FIG 4.
Survival of lung cancer according to method of detection. The survival of patients
with asymptomatic lung cancer detected by chest x-rays taken as part of a routine
physical examination or incidental to hospitalization for unrelated illness (other) is
essentially the same as for men with lung cancer detected by screening. Survival of
patients with symptomatic lung cancer was comparable to overall survival from lung
cancer in the United States. (From Melamed MR, Flehinger BJ: *Schweiz Med
Wochenschr* 1987; 117:1457–1463. Used by permission.)

effect of screening with the chest x-ray by mathematical modeling indicate
that up to 18% of lung cancer deaths can be prevented by present techniques
of early detection and treatment. If we are to improve survival from lung
cancer it will be by building on this base and improving detection and
treatment of early cases of lung cancer, not by a fatalistic acceptance of
failure. Who among us truly believes that we should seek no cases, be content
to treat no cases, and can cure no cases of early lung cancer?

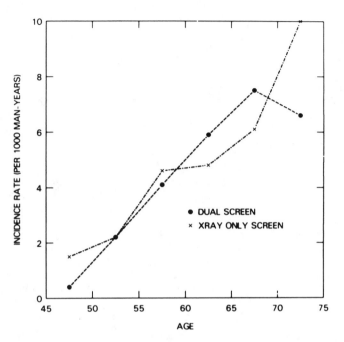

FIG 5.
Incidence of lung cancer by age. (From Melamed MR, Flehinger BJ, Zaman MB, et al: *Chest* 1984; 86:44–53. Used by permission.)

References

1. American Cancer Society, *Cancer Facts and Figures.* 1988. *This interesting report provides data on the estimated frequency of various cancers in the United States.*
2. National Cancer Institute Cooperative Early Lung Cancer Group: *Manual of Procedures,* 2nd ed. Revised April 1979, NIH Publication No 79-1972. *A detailed description of the procedures used in the Cooperative Early Lung Cancer Detection Study is provided.*
3. Early lung cancer detection: Summary and conclusions. *Am Rev Respir Dis* 1984; 130:565–570. *A summary of the combined prevalence data which compares findings in the three collaborating studies of early lung cancer is given.*
4. Berlin NI, Buncher CR, Fontana RS, et al: The National Cancer Institute Cooperative Early Lung Cancer Detection Program. Results of the initial screen (prevalence). Early lung cancer detection: Introduction. *Am Rev Respir*

Dis 1984; 130:545–549. *This manuscript provides an introduction and description of the early lung cancer detection program.*

5. Frost JK, Ball WC Jr, Levin ML, et al: Early lung cancer detection: Results of the initial (prevalence) radiologic and cytologic screening in the Johns Hopkins study. *Am Rev Respir Dis* 1984; 130:549–554. *The results of prevalence data from one of the three institutions involved in the early lung cancer detection program are reported.*

6. Flehinger BJ, Melamed MR, Zaman MB, et al: Early lung cancer detection: Results of the initial (prevalence) radiologic and cytologic screening in the Memorial Sloan-Kettering study. *Am Rev Respir Dis* 1984; 130:555–560. *This paper gives the results of prevalence data from one of the three institutions involved in the early lung cancer detection program.*

7. Fontana RS, Sanderson DR, Taylor WF, et al: Early lung cancer detection: Results of the initial (prevalence) radiologic and cytologic screening in the Mayo clinic study. *Am Rev Respir Dis* 1984; 130:561–565. *The results of prevalence data from one of the three institutions involved in the early lung cancer detection program are reported.*

8. Melamed MR, Flehinger BJ, Zaman MB, et al: Screening for early lung cancer. *Chest* 1984; 86:44–53. *Incidence data from the Memorial Sloan-Kettering Cancer Center Early Lung Cancer Detection Program are given.*

9. Melamed MR, Flehinger BJ: Detection of lung cancer: Highlights of the Memorial Sloan-Kettering Study in New York City. *Schweiz Med Wochenschr* 1987; 117:1457–1463. *A comparison of lung cancer occurrence during the screening period and for 2 years after screening terminated in the Memorial Sloan-Kettering Cancer Center Early Lung Cancer Detection Program is documented.*

10. Flehinger BJ, Kimmel M: The natural history of lung cancer in a periodically screened population. *Biometrics* 1987; 43:127–144. *This report provides a mathematical model of the development and progression of lung cancer in a periodically screened population based on data from the early lung cancer detection program.*

11. Flehinger BJ, Kimmel M, Melamed MR: Natural history of adenocarcinoma — large cell carcinoma of the lung: Conclusions from screening programs in New York and Baltimore. *J Natl Cancer Inst* 1988; 80:337–344. *This study documents the observations that adenocarcinoma and large-cell carcinoma of the lung have a preclinical period of development estimated to be at least 4 years and perhaps as long as 10 years.*

12. Flehinger BJ, Melamed MR, Heelan RT, et al: Accuracy of chest film screening by technologists in the New York Early Lung Cancer Detection Program. *AJR* 1978; 131:593–597. *Specially trained senior radiological technologists are capable of screening routine chest x-rays and identifying subjects with abnormalities that can be evaluated by the radiologist later.*

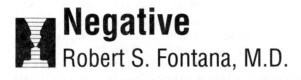

Negative
Robert S. Fontana, M.D.

The question I was asked to address in this debate is whether "all asymptomatic smokers over 55 years of age should receive an annual chest x-ray." I am assuming that the question refers to asymptomatic smokers in the United States and other technologically developed countries where excellent radiological facilities and qualified personnel are available. I am also assuming that the reason for obtaining the chest x-ray is to try to detect presymptomatic lung cancer. Thus, I have narrowed the question to the search for lung cancer in an asymptomatic population at increased risk for developing the disease. I presume this is the primary intent of the debate.

To me, the key words in the question are "all" and "asymptomatic." No reference has been made to traditional clinical practice in which the patient seeks the physician's aid and the physician uses his or her best judgment to try to help the patient. Rather, the protagonists in this debate favor the application of yearly chest roentgenography to an asymptomatic, high-risk population numbering in the millions. This is large-scale screening for lung cancer which has not necessarily been sought by the smokers and for which there is the implicit promise of benefit, including treatment of proven efficacy.[1]

The optimal approach to an evaluation of roentgenographic screening for asymptomatic lung cancer is the randomized controlled trial. Mortality from lung cancer is the preferred and always applicable endpoint for measuring the results of such screening.[2] Other methods formerly used to evaluate lung cancer screening, including assessment of survival, distribution of cancers by stage, and numbers of cancers detected, are subject to various biases. Among these biases are lead-time bias (the time by which screen-detected cancer is discovered earlier than symptom-diagnosed cancer), length bias (the over-representation in an asymptomatic population of more slowly growing cancers with longer presymptomatic phases), and selection bias (the over-representation among volunteers for screening of persons who tend to be more affluent and health conscious). As a consequence, these previous methods of evaluating screening for lung cancer are no longer considered appropriate.[2]

There has never been a randomized controlled trial of yearly screening for presymptomatic lung cancer alone using full-size chest x-rays compared with no screening at all. However, in 1964 the Kaiser Foundation Research Institute began conducting a randomized trial of multiphasic health screening that included chest roentgenography.[3] Approximately 5,000 members of the Kaiser Health Plan, aged 35 to 54 years old, were assigned at random to a study group that was urged to undergo multiphasic screening once each year. A comparable number of members were randomly assigned to a control group that was not encouraged to be screened, although members could obtain screening on their own initiative. About 60% of the study group and 20% of the control group had the multiphasic check-up each year. After 11 years of follow-up there was no significant difference in lung cancer mortality between the study group (25 lung cancer deaths) and the control group (26 lung cancer deaths). It has been stated that there is a 20% chance that the Kaiser trial would have missed a true impact of 50% decrease in lung cancer mortality.[4]

From 1960 through 1968 the Mass Radiography Service of North West London conducted a controlled (but not randomized) study of screening for lung cancer by means of chest photofluorograms.[5] A test group of 29,723 men 40 years of age and older, drawn mainly from industrial establishments, was offered chest x-rays every 6 months for 3 years. A control group of 25,311 men of similar age and smoking habits, drawn from other industries within the same area, was offered chest x-rays at the beginning and end of the study. There were 101 lung cancers discovered in the test group, compared with 76 in the control group. In the test group, 44% of the lung cancers were resectable, and the 5-year lung cancer survival rate was 15%. In the control group these percentages were 29% and 6%, respectively. Lead-time bias must be considered in interpreting these results, but even without adjusting for lead time there was no significant difference in lung cancer mortality in the two groups (0.7 lung cancer deaths per 1,000 person-years in the test group and 0.8 in the control group).

Two other well-known studies of roentgenographic screening for lung cancer should be mentioned. Both were uncontrolled studies. The Philadelphia Pulmonary Neoplasm Research Project, which began in 1951 and ended in 1965, offered chest photofluorograms every 6 months to 6,136 male volunteers aged 45 years or more.[6] The 5-year survival rate for newly detected cases of lung cancer was only 8%, about the same as the national rate for unscreened persons at the time this investigation took place.

The South London Cancer Study (1959–1963) offered chest photofluorography every 6 months for 3.5 years to 67,400 male volunteers, aged 45 years and older.[4] The overall 4-year survival rate for 234 lung cancer cases discovered during and between screenings was 18%, compared with an expected 9% estimated from regional historical data. Results were influenced by lead-time and selection biases.

The dismal results observed in the forgoing studies led to the opinion that annual (or semi-annual) chest photofluorograms (or x-rays) would not alter the poor prognosis for lung cancer. It was stated that the prognosis was determined largely by the biological nature of the disease.[6] Nevertheless, it was recognized that symptomatic lung cancer was usually fatal, and the notion persisted that the detection of presymptomatic (potentially localized and resectable) lung cancer was advantageous.

There have been only two reliable tests for detecting early-stage, presymptomatic lung cancer, namely the chest x-ray and the cytologic examination of sputum. The x-ray is most useful for detecting early-stage peripheral tumors, while sputum cytology specifically detects early-stage centrally located, intrabronchial squamous cancers.[7]

During the 1960s there were three important technological advances that encouraged renewed efforts to screen for asymptomatic lung cancer. First, there were refinements in roentgenographic technology, including the routine use of full-size (36 × 43 cm) chest x-rays (photofluorography produced too much radiation), the introduction of new film-screen combinations plus large capacity x-ray generators yielding high kilovoltage, and improvements in film processing. Second, techniques for inducing the production of sputum were devised, and better methods of preserving and processing sputum were developed which enabled the collection of multiple-day sputum specimens. Third, the flexible fiberoptic bronchoscope was introduced, greatly expanding the range of endoscopic visibility.[7]

Spurred by these developments and the relentless rise in the incidence and mortality rates of lung cancer, the National Cancer Institute (NCI) sponsored three randomized controlled trials of screening for asymptomatic lung cancer in the United States.[8] These trials, for which the endpoint was mortality from lung cancer, began in 1971. They were conducted at the Johns Hopkins Medical Institutions, the Memorial Sloan-Kettering Cancer Center, and the Mayo Clinic. Each trial involved about 10,000 men who were at high risk for lung cancer (age 45 years or older with a history of chronic heavy cigarette smoking).

In the Mayo trial, all subjects were offered an initial (prevalence) screening that included a chest x-ray and a sputum cytology test. Subjects whose initial screens were considered satisfactory and negative for lung cancer were randomly assigned either to a study group, which was offered chest x-rays and sputum cytology tests every 4 months for a period of 6 years, or to a control group, which was not systematically rescreened but which was advised to receive the two testing procedures annually. In the Hopkins and Memorial trials, subjects assigned to the study group were offered annual chest x-rays plus sputum cytology every 4 months. Control subjects were offered annual chest x-rays only.

The prevalence screening at Mayo and the initial roentgenographic and cytologic screening of the study groups at Hopkins and Memorial yielded 160 cases of lung cancer (combined prevalence rate 7.6 per 1,000).[8] Nearly 60% of these prevalence cancers were early-stage (International stages 0, I, II) and resectable. At Hopkins and Memorial the 5-year survival rate (calculated by the Kaplan-Meier method) of the prevalence cases exceeded 50%, while at Mayo it approached 40%. There were 63 prevalence cases of lung cancer detected in the control populations at Hopkins and Memorial that were screened by chest x-rays only (6.2 per 1,000 screened).[8] About 45% of these cases were early-stage and resectable, and approximately 35% survived lung cancer for 5 years. While these prevalence data were encouraging, the influence of lead-time bias, length-biased sampling, and selection bias must be kept in mind. Moreover, prevalence data do not allow estimations of lung cancer mortality rates. It was specifically for the purpose of obtaining information on mortality from lung cancer that the three NCI-sponsored randomized trials of periodic rescreening for lung cancer (incidence rescreening) were undertaken.[8]

These trials are now complete. Both the study group and the control group in each trial were followed closely for nearly 40,000 person-years. Significant results of the trials have been recorded in Table 4.[7,9,10] In all three trials, less that 13% of lung cancers in the study groups were detected by cytology alone. In the Hopkins and Memorial trials, which assessed the addition of sputum cytology every 4 months to annual chest roentgenography, no significant reduction in lung cancer mortality could be attributed to cytology.[2] In the Mayo trial, which compared sputum cytology and chest roentgenography every 4 months to a recommendation that the two tests be obtained yearly, there was substantially increased detection of early-stage, more resectable lung cancers, and improved survivorship within the study group compared with the control group. However, there was no significant difference in lung cancer mortality between the two groups.[7]

In all of the trials, stage distribution of the screen-detected cancers was favorably shifted toward earlier-stage, resectable disease, but this appears to be attributable to lead time.[7,9,10] There were no differences in either mortality from lung cancer or the number of advanced-stage lung cancers (International Staging System stages III and IV) between the two study groups in any of the trials, and these were the crucial issues.[7,9,10]

One critic of the NCI trials has commented:

> It is difficult to avoid two conclusions: (1) preclinical lung cancer is not a suitable condition for which to screen, either because the disease is too advanced at the time it is detectable by current screening modalities, or because current therapies have no better outcome if applied at an earlier than at a later phase of disease; and (2) sputum cytology and chest x-ray film are not sensitive enough to detect the biological precursors of clinical cancer. Most simply stated, the rate of biological progression of most lung cancer appears to be too rapid to be amenable to screening by existing modalities.[11]

These are strong statements, but concerned reservations about the effectiveness of current management of lung cancer, including surgical treatment, have been expressed by others.[12]

After reviewing preliminary data from the NCI trials and the earlier lung cancer screening programs already cited, the American Cancer Society has changed its policy and no longer recommends any tests for the early detection of lung cancer.[4] In addition, the group that prepared the section on screening and detection of cancer for the NCI monograph "Cancer Control Objectives for the Nation: 1985–2000" has concluded:

TABLE 4.
Staging (International System*), 5-Year Survival Rates, and Mortality Rates From Lung Cancer: Incidence Lung Cancers in Hopkins, Memorial, and Mayo Randomized Controlled Trials

Institution	Screening Tests	Lung Cancers, Total Cases (detected by) (cytology only)	Stages 0, I, II (early-stage)	Stages III, IV (advanced-stage)	5-Year Survival Rate, % (Kaplan-Meier)	Lung Cancer Mortality Rate (per 1,000/year)
Johns Hopkins[9]	4-month cytology Yearly x-ray	194 (22)	83	111	28	3.4
	Yearly x-ray only	202	93	109	18	3.8
Memorial[10]	4-month cytology Yearly x-ray	143 (18)	58	85	37	2.7
	Yearly x-ray only	154	68	86	33	2.7
Mayo[7]	4-month cytology & x-ray	206 (18)	99	107	33	3.2
	None scheduled	160	51	109	<15	3.0

*From Mountain CF: *Chest* 1986; 89:225S–233S.

Several clinical studies conducted in the 1960s and the 1970s, involving chest x-rays, sputum cytology, and questionnaires delivered in various combinations and frequencies, did not indicate that lung cancer screening significantly affects mortality from that disease. Also, three recent randomized controlled trials, involving chest x-rays and sputum cytology given as often as every 4 months, have not shown that lung cancer screening has an effect on mortality. Although some individual practitioners and researchers have expressed dissent, virtually every organization that has reviewed the available data has concluded that lung cancer screening with these techniques is not effective.[13]

One is reminded of the words of the well-known, contemporary American philosopher, Yogi Berra: "It's like déjà vu all over again."

Since the previously stated policies and conclusions were published, another randomized, controlled trial of screening for lung cancer by chest roentgenography and sputum cytology has been reported from Czechoslovakia.[14] While the results of this trial are a bit difficult to evaluate, they do seem to lend support to the findings of the three NCI-sponsored randomized trials. In particular, the tabulated causes of death list 19 lung cancer deaths in the study population (N = 3,172) which was screened semi-annually for 3 years, compared with 13 lung cancer deaths in the control population (N = 3,174) which was screened only at the beginning and at the end of the trial. There also appeared to be more advanced-stage lung cancers encountered in the study group (19) than in the control group (17).

In the NCI-sponsored randomized trials, many more lung cancers were detected by chest x-ray than by sputum cytology. Furthermore, a number of early-stage, resectable lung cancers were discovered by nonstudy chest x-rays obtained for various reasons during medical encounters that occurred between scheduled screening of study subjects in all three trials, as well as in the control population at Mayo.[7,9,10]

As noted previously, the randomized controlled trial is the optimal method of evaluating the effectiveness of screening.[2] However, problems may arise in evaluating a procedure, such as chest roentgenography, that is already common in medical practice. Study and control populations are then susceptible to "contamination" by procedures performed for indications other than screening. While contamination itself can be evaluated, it can complicate things. It may be worthwhile to consider alternative approaches to screening.[2] Case-control studies have been proposed recently, and one such study of screening for lung cancer has been reported from the German Democratic Republic.[15] The results suggested that the risk of dying from lung cancer was not significantly less for persons screened by 70-mm chest films within 2 years preceding a diagnosis of lung cancer than it was for unscreened individuals. However, the results of this study must be viewed with caution because of the rather small sample size.

Available evidence simply does not support an unqualified recommendation that "all asymptomatic smokers over 55 years of age should receive an annual chest x-ray." The best recommendation any physician (or any other concerned individual) can give any smoker today is the strongest possible encouragement to quit. Help in quitting also should be offered. The primary prevention of lung cancer is the watchword today and, thankfully, that word is now being heard, heeded, and implemented.

References

1. Sackett DL, Holland WW: Controversy in the detection of disease. *Lancet* 1975; 2:357–359. *This report provides a commentary on the important distinction between population screening (for diseases for which early diagnosis and treatment have been proven beneficial) and case finding (among patients who have sought medical attention without promise of benefit).*

2. Prorok PC, Miller AB: Screening for cancer: I-General principles on evaluation of screening for cancer and screening for lung, bladder and oral cancer. UICC Technical Report Series. Geneva, International Union Against Cancer, 1984. *An excellent summary of the principles of screening for cancer. Discussions of the Memorial and Mayo lung cancer screening programs are included, and there is a thoughtful critique of screening for lung cancer (pages 136–142).*

3. Dales EG, Friedman GD, Collen MF: Evaluating periodic multiphasic health checkups: A controlled trial. *J Chronic Dis* 1979; 32:385–404. *This is a somewhat complicated report of the results of a randomized, controlled trial of screening for various diseases. Data on lung cancer are included.*

4. Eddy DM: Guidelines for the cancer-related checkup: Recommendations and rationale. *CA* 1980; 30:194–240. *This is the controversial 1980 report announcing the American Cancer Society's new policies toward periodic testing for cancer, especially cancers of the lung, colon and rectum, cervix, and breast.*

5. Brett GZ: Earlier diagnosis and survival in lung cancer. *Br Med J* 1969; 4:260–262. *This was a nonrandomized, controlled trial of screening for lung cancer, with data on lung cancer detectability, resectability, survivorship, and mortality that were quite similar to the Mayo screening data.*

6. Weiss W, Boucot KR, Seidman H: The Philadelphia Pulmonary Neoplasm Research Project. *Clin Chest Med* 1982; 3:243–256. *This is a long-term, retrospective look at the first study specifically designed to screen for lung cancer. Neither randomized nor controlled, it utilized semi-annual chest photofluorography.*

7. Fontana RS: Screening for lung cancer: Recent experience in the United States, in Hansen HH (ed): *Lung Cancer: Basic and Clinical Aspects.* Boston, Martinus Nijhoff, 1986, pp 91–111. *This is a review of and comparison of results from the three NCI-sponsored randomized, controlled trials of screening for lung cancer, with emphasis on the Mayo trial.*

8. Flehinger BJ: The National Cancer Institute cooperative early lung cancer detection program. Summary and conclusions. *Am Rev Respir Dis* 1984; 130:565–570. *This concise summary presents the salient results of the initial (prevalence) screening for lung cancer from the three NCI-sponsored randomized trials.*

9. Johns Hopkins Medical Institutions, Baltimore, Md: *Final Report, Lung Cancer Control Detection and Therapy, Phase II, NCI-PHS Contract No N01-CN-4537*. Bethesda, Md, National Cancer Institute, 1984. *As the title indicates, this detailed report summarizes data collected by the Johns Hopkins lung cancer screening program through 1984. Also offered are interpretations of these data.*

10. National Lung Program, Memorial Sloan-Kettering Cancer Center, New York City: *Final Report and Data Summary*. Bethesda, Md, National Cancer Institute. *This is a summary, without commentary, of the results of the Memorial Sloan-Kettering lung cancer screening program, including data accrued through 1984.*

11. Hulka BS: Screening for cancer: Lessons learned. *J Occup Med* 1986; 28:687–691. *The author presents her views on the general principles of screening for cancer, as well as the pros and cons of site-specific screening for cancers of the cervix, breast, and lung.*

12. Ball WC: The effect of surgical treatment on the natural history of lung cancer (editorial). *Am Rev Respir Dis* 1983; 127:1. *This one-page, extremely provocative editorial questions the effectiveness of early diagnosis and surgical treatment for lung cancer. Required reading!*

13. Greenwald P, Sondik EJ (eds): *National Cancer Institute Monograph. Cancer Control Objectives for the Nation: 1985–2000*. Washington, DC, US Government Printing Office, 1986. NIH Publication No 86–2880, number 2. *As its foreword states, this monograph, with objectives for the year 2000, is an "analysis and synthesis of current knowledge about the prevention and control of cancer through life-style factors, screening and treatment."*

14. Kubik A, Polak J: Lung cancer detection: Results of a randomized prospective study in Czechoslovakia. *Cancer* 1986; 57:2427–2437. *This randomized, controlled trial of cytologic and photofluorographic screening for lung cancer yielded results comparable to those of Brett's study (reference 5) and the Mayo screening program.*

15. Ebling K, Nischan P: Screening for lung cancer — a case-control study. *Int J Cancer* 1987; 40:141–144. *This case-control study, designed to evaluate biennial chest photofluorography, showed no trend in relative risk of lung cancer death with respect to frequency of testing or interval since the last test.*

Rebuttal: Affirmative

Myron R. Melamed, M.D.
Betty J. Flehinger, Ph.D.

Dr. Fontana makes several important points, with which we agree. It is essential, of course, that excellent radiological facilities and qualified personnel be available to carry out the recommended annual chest x-rays. Equally essential is ready access and prompt referral to a modern hospital with the facilities and personnel to investigate any radiologically suspicious lesions and to carry out the necessary thoracic surgery. Thus, the argument for annual chest x-ray screening does indeed apply specifically to the United States and other technologically advanced countries.

By the same token, we dismiss the results of studies in which photofluorograms were used for screening,[1-7] since full-size, high-quality films are necessary to detect the very early carcinomas with the best cure rates, as is implicitly acknowledged in Dr. Fontana's call for excellent radiological facilities. If one needs further confirmation, it is only necessary to compare the 6% and 15% 5-year lung cancer survival of the North West London study,[1,2] the 8% overall 5-year survival for lung cancer in the Philadelphia Pulmonary Neoplasm Research Project,[3,4] and the overall 4-year survival rate of 18% for the South London Cancer Study[6] with the overall 5-year survival of 35% of the Memorial Sloan-Kettering study. Of course, improvements in surgical treatment, anesthesia and pre- and postoperative care also play an important role.

Even with high-quality, full-size x-rays, however, the present predicted upper boundary for long-term reduction in mortality is 18%, based on our mathematical model using data from the Memorial Sloan-Kettering study.[8,9] Long-term mortality reduction of this order of magnitude is very likely to be missed in the data presently available from short-term screening programs or studies of relatively small populations, as in the Kaiser Foundation Research Institute study.[10] Since it is not feasible and perhaps not possible to undertake a sufficiently long-term randomized study of the large population required to establish (or refute) a 10% to 20% mortality reduction, our best estimate of "truth" lies in mathematical modeling.

Dr. Fontana has defined early-stage lung cancer as stages 0, I and II. We do not accept stage II lung cancer as "early," since the 5-year survival rate following resection is only 50%.[11] We restrict "early" lung cancer to stage I cases (includes stage 0), and they account for 47% of all prevalence cases (detected by cytology and x-ray) at the three institutions in the National Cancer Institute (NCI) study. The survival of these prevalence cases following resection is 80% at 5 years and 75% at 10 years.[11]

As noted by Dr. Fontana, 24 of 63 prevalence cases of lung cancer (38%)

detected by chest x-rays in the control populations at Hopkins and Memorial were early-stage (i.e., stage I). Survival of the resected stage I lung cancers at these two institutions was about 85% at 5 years; the 35% 5-year survival he reports applies to the entire control population and includes stage II and III cases.[11] These data only emphasize the importance of early detection in achieving long survival. Stage I lung cancer constituted 120 of the 293 cases of lung cancer that developed during the entire period of screening in the Memorial Sloan-Kettering Cancer Center (MSKCC) study (41%) (i.e., prevalence and incidence). Survival of all resected stage I lung cancers (prevalence and incidence) was 65% at 10 years in the MSKCC study.[12] Dr. Fontana is also correct, of course, that there was no difference in lung cancer mortality between the study and control groups. Thus, we concluded that cytology added nothing to the annual chest x-ray, as we have discussed already. Since both the study and control groups at Hopkins and MSKCC had annual chest x-rays, there could not possibly be differences in mortality or number of advanced-stage cancers attributable to the chest x-rays. However, a striking shift to advanced-stage disease was noted at MSKCC during the 2 years following cessation of screening; stage I/stage II–III = 120/173 (2:3) during screening, and 12/49 (1:4) after cessation of screening.

In summary, the Mayo, Hopkins, and MSKCC studies were designed to assess sputum cytology as a screening technique and have done so effectively. They were not designed to and cannot directly answer whether chest x-ray screening is of value. A mathematical model using data collected in the MSKCC and Hopkins studies indicates that a reduction in death from lung cancer due to annual x-ray screening is not greater than 18%. A decrease in mortality of this order cannot be confirmed directly with any existing screening data, and would require an unrealistically large, long-term study for proof. Yet a decrease in lung cancer mortality of even 10% would result in nearly 15,000 lives saved annually. In the absence of hard statistical proof of efficacy, we believe the softer evidence of earlier detection and longer survival, supported by mathematical modeling estimates of a modest decrease in mortality, justify our recommendation for annual chest x-rays of high-risk cigarette smokers.

References

1. Brett GZ: Bronchial carcinoma in men detected by selective and unselective miniature radiography. A review of 228 cases. *Tubercle* 1959; 40:192–195.
2. Brett GZ: Earlier diagnosis and survival in lung cancer. *Br Med J* 1969; 4:260–262.
3. Bucot KR, Cooper DA, Weiss W: The Philadelphia Pulmonary Neoplasm Research Project: An interim report. *Ann Intern Med* 1961; 54:363–377
4. Weiss W, Boucot KR, Seidman H: The Philadelphia Pulmonary Neoplasms Research Project. *Clin Chest Med* 1982; 3:243–256.

5. Kubik A, Polak J: Lung cancer detection. Results of a randomized prospective study in Czechoslovakia. *Cancer* 1986; 57:2427–2437.
6. Nash FA, Morgan JM, Tomkins JG: South London Lung Cancer Study. *Br Med J* 1968; 2:715–721.
7. Ebeling K, Nischan P: Screening for lung cancer — results from a case-control study. *Int J Cancer* 1987; 40:141–144.
8. Flehinger BJ, Kimmel M: The natural history of lung cancer in a periodically screened population. *Biometrics* 1987; 43:127–144.
9. Flehinger BJ, Kimmel M, Melamed MR: Natural history of adenocarcinoma - large cell carcinoma of the lung: Conclusions from screening programs in New York and Baltimore. *J Natl Cancer Inst* 1988; 80:337–344.
10. Dales EG, Friedman GD, Collen MF: Evaluating periodic multiphasic health checkups: A controlled trial. *J Chronic Dis* 1979; 32:385–404.
11. Early lung cancer detection: Summary and conclusions. *Am Rev Respir Dis* 1984; 130:565–570.
12. Melamed MR, Flehinger BJ: Detection of lung cancer; highlights of the Memorial Sloan-Kettering (MSKCC) study in New York City. *Schweiz Med Wochenschr* 1987; 117:1457–1463.

Rebuttal: Negative
Robert S. Fontana, M.D.

The proposition I was asked to debate is whether "all asymptomatic smokers over 55 years of age should receive an annual chest x-ray." So phrased, the proposition mandates yearly chest x-rays for all mature, asymptomatic smokers, male and female, regardless of the circumstances. To me, this is screening. Drs. Melamed and Flehinger agree. In their initial argument they state, "we are concerned here with the value of screening by means of annual chest x-rays."

In this debate it is not the mature, asymptomatic smoker who is seeking a chest x-ray each and every year. No, it is we health providers who are telling him (or her) to have one each and every year. Since we are initiating the action by recommending annual screening, we should be able to demonstrate tangible benefits for these asymptomatic smokers.

The only acceptable proof of the effectiveness of any screening procedure is a reduction in mortality from the disease for which screening is being conducted. Unless the death rate from lung cancer is reduced, the routine annual chest x-ray wil have accomplished very little. It may result in some alleviation of discomfort, or it may even enable surgical treatment to be utilized instead of radiation therapy or chemotherapy, but unless it results in a reduction in mortality from lung cancer, it will have failed to achieve its main objective.

As I stated in my initial argument, increased lung cancer detection, a shift to an earlier stage at diagnosis, or improved lung cancer survival rates are not valid alternatives as proofs of the effectiveness of screening. On the contrary, such findings are to be expected as a consequence of the various screening biases described in both initial arguments. Such findings were encountered in all three of the National Cancer Institute (NCI)-sponsored randomized, controlled trials of screening for early lung cancer. Yet in each of these trials there was no significant difference in lung cancer mortality between the study (more intensively screened) group and the control group.

The protagonists' arguments in this debate are eloquent but empty. Drs. Melamed and Flehinger have based their case on observations of improved lung cancer survival rates and downstaging of tumors; on misconceptions concerning the aim, design, and results of the Mayo screening program; and on overly zealous conclusions derived from a mathematical model.[1,2] They have reiterated an appeal that all mature smokers should receive annual chest x-rays because they believe that this is the prudent thing to do.[3] They have ignored their charge in our debate, namely, advocacy of mandated, large-scale screening for lung cancer by means of annual chest x-rays. Instead, they have chosen to praise the virtues of case finding in the individual "middle-aged smoker who seeks medical evaluation from his (or her) physician." This is laudable, for such patient-initiated consultations require that we physicians exercise our best judgment, but to me *this is not large-scale screening.*

I sincerely believe that Drs. Melamed and Flehinger have failed to substantiate their position in the debate, and their arguments require no further rebuttal. Nevertheless, I will challenge each of the "paper tigers" they have created. However, before proceeding further I should address the matter of the differences that exist in the tabulated data from our two initial arguments.

Drs. Melamed and Flehinger have utilized an older lung cancer staging system formulated by the American Joint Committee on Cancer (AJCC).[4] This has been superseded by a new International Staging System, which I have employed.[5] Stages I and II of the AJCC staging system now have been replaced by stages 0, I, and II of the International system, while AJCC stage III has been subdivided into stages III and IV in the new system. These differences are minor and should not confuse the reader. The most important point to remember is that International stages 0, I, and II (AJCC stages I and II) are more likely to be resectable, whereas International stages III and IV (AJCC stage III) are usually unresectable.

More substantial tabular differences also exist. Drs. Melamed and Flehinger have explained some of these in their footnotes. Their Table 2 is identical to a table published in the journal *Chest* in 1984.[3] Tables 1 and 3 are similar to tables published more than 3 years later in *Surgical Clinics of North America.*[6] The differing dates of publication account for the differences in total cases tabulated. In Tables 1 and 2, data from the initial screening for lung cancer (prevalence screening) have been combined with data from subsequent periodic rescreenings (incidence screening).

For reasons already elaborated in my initial argument, I have elected to tabulate only incidence screening data. Prevalence data are more likely to be affected by screening biases. In addition, prevalence data alone do not permit calculations of lung cancer mortality rates. Incidence data do, since they represent the results of rescreening at regular intervals over a prolonged period. In order to obtain maximum comparability, I have tabulated only the incidence data appearing in the final reports of the three NCI-sponsored randomized trials of screening for early lung cancer. These reports include all data accrued prior to Jan 1, 1985.

But enough of classification and tabulation; it is time to expose the protagonists' paper tigers. Drs. Melamed and Flehinger have stated that all three of the NCI-sponsored lung cancer screening programs "were designed primarily to evaluate cytology," but this is not so. The aim of the Mayo screening program was to evaluate both the chest x-ray and sputum cytology.

Elsewhere in their initial argument Drs. Melamed and Flehinger call attention to the limitations of the Mayo study. They write, "while the results of that study showed more lung cancers detected in the intensively screened population, they failed to show a significant difference in lung cancer deaths due to the screening. The Mayo study does not prove that there is no difference, however." Then, assuming "the death rate from lung cancer in a population of mature smokers is 3 per 1,000 per year," they proceed to demonstrate why it would be enormously unwieldy, and probably unethical, to attempt a randomized trial of yearly radiological screening that would be capable of detecting a 10% to 20% reduction in lung cancer mortality.

Of course the Mayo study had its limitations, but it was still reasonably robust. Using the lung cancer death rate of 3 per 1,000 per year observed in the Mayo control population (and a one-tailed $\alpha = .05$ test), the probability of detecting a true reduction in lung cancer mortality in the group screened every 4 months was 90% for detecting a 35% reduction and 80% for detecting a 30% reduction. Furthermore, in this debate I am not obliged to prove that there is not a reduction in lung cancer mortality. It is up to my opponents to prove that there is one if they wish to justify annual screening chest x-rays as a (potentially subsidized?) health policy for all mature, asymptomatic smokers. This they have not done.

The six points used by my opponents as "the basis for our recommendations regarding screening for lung cancer" all can be explained, as they themselves admit, "by lead time, length bias, and overdiagnosis bias." I agree with this explanation, but they would rather not. Instead, they do their utmost to substitute the increased lung cancer resectability and survivorship that they did observe in the Memorial study for the decrease in lung cancer mortality that they did not observe. The same pattern was observed in the Mayo study. In that study, there were 94 resected lung cancers and a 5-year lung cancer survival rate of 33% in the group screened every 4 months. In the control group, there were 51 resected lung cancers and a 5-year lung cancer survival rate of less that 15%. Notwithstanding these substantial differences in resectability and survivorship, there was no significant difference in lung cancer mortality between the two groups.

A close observer of the NCI-sponsored lung cancer screening programs has written, "The opinion based on survival studies that the annual chest x-ray film does result in an improved mortality is one which I feel can be challenged by the Mayo study. ..." The writer concludes, "It seems to me inconceivable that annual chest x-ray films will be proven, in a much larger study, to be beneficial when chest x-ray films every 4 months showed no benefit compared with a validly selected and studied control group."[7]

Failing to demonstrate any real reduction in lung cancer mortality in their, or anyone else's, lung cancer screening program, Drs. Melamed and Flehinger resort to a mathematical model of screening for lung cancer by annual chest x-rays. The model was originally constructed and published by Drs. Flehinger and Marek Kimmel.[1] It was based on data from the Memorial Sloan-Kettering study, and it referred only to adenocarcinomas in self-selected New York City male volunteers, all of whom were smokers aged 45 to 80 years. The model assumed perfect compliance with screening in the study group and no testing of the control group. It also assumed that all lung cancers detected by screening would be treated promptly. The estimated impact on mortality from adenocarcinoma of the lung in these male smokers ranged from a 0% to an 18% reduction. The publication concluded, "It is clear that currently available screening techniques will not solve the problem of lung cancer mortality in smokers."

Subsequently, the mathematical model appeared in another publication.[2] This time, adenocarcinoma was linked with large-cell carcinoma, and the model was applied not only to the Memorial data, but also to data from the identically designed lung cancer screening study conducted at the Johns Hopkins Medical Institutions. This publication concluded, "From the Sloan-Kettering data, one might conclude that ALCA (adenocarcinoma-large cell carcinoma) mortality reduction associated with screening and surgical treatment could be as great as 18%, while the Hopkins study leads to the conclusion that 5% is an upper bound." It should be remembered that adenocarcinoma and large-cell carcinoma together account for only 50% of all lung cancers. However, in this debate the mathematical model has been applied to all lung cancers. The protagonists have stated, "Based on these figures, the decrease in lung cancer mortality from annual screening and prompt surgical treatment starting at age 45 years might be as much as 18%." The model appears to have gained bias with the passage of time.

The final, emotional paragraph of the argument by Drs. Melamed and Flehinger brazenly recommends that all mature, asymptomatic smokers receive chest x-rays annually until there is proof of *ineffectiveness!* There is one last hurrah for the vainglories of downstaged tumors, increased lung cancer resectability and survival rates, and magnified mathematical models. The protagonists plead that since they can offer nothing better, we should accept what they do offer. And what is that? Regrettably, because I also wish it were otherwise, it is not proof that "all asymptomatic smokers over 55 years of age should receive an annual chest x-ray."

References

1. Flehinger BJ, Kimmel M: The natural history of lung cancer in a periodically screened population. *Biometrics* 1987; 43:127–144.
2. Flehinger BJ, Kimmel M, Melamed MR: Natural history of adenocarcinoma - large cell carcinoma of the lung: Conclusions from screening programs in New York and Baltimore. *J Natl Cancer Inst* 1988; 80:337–344.
3. Melamed MR, Flehinger BJ, Zaman MB, et al: Screening for lung cancer: Results of the Memorial Sloan-Kettering study in New York. *Chest* 1984; 86:44–53.
4. American Joint Committee on Cancer: *Manual for Staging for Cancer.* Philadelphia, Lippincott, 1983.
5. Mountain CF: A new international staging system for lung cancer. *Chest* 1986; 89:225S–233S.

6. Melamed MR, Flehinger BJ, Zaman MB: Impact of early detection on the clinical course of lung cancer. *Surg Clin North Am* 1987; 67:909–924.
7. Miller AB: Synthesis of papers on biological monitoring, case studies in screening, and social and economic issues. *J Occup Med* 1986; 28:782–788.

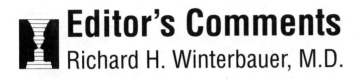

Editor's Comments
Richard H. Winterbauer, M.D.

Lung cancer remains the most common cause of death from cancer in both men and women in the United States, with an estimated 140,000 deaths annually. The American Cancer Society in 1980 concluded that screening chest roentgenograms did not reduce the mortality from lung cancer and recommended against their use. The recommendation struck at the heart of a deeply ingrained American practice pattern which had been sustained in major part by physicians' personal experience in recognizing small, asymptomatic, curable lung cancers through screening chest x-rays. Such stage I bronchogenic carcinomas have a 70% to 75% 5-year survival with surgery.

The major study responsible for shaping the American Cancer Society's recommendation was the National Cancer Institute (NCI) Lung Cancer Detection Study of 1974 through 1984 conducted at the Mayo Clinic in Rochester, the Memorial Sloan-Kettering Cancer Center (MSKCC) in New York, and the Johns Hopkins Medical Institutions in Baltimore. Interestingly, this debate is between two senior investigators in the NCI Lung Cancer Detection Study who arrived at opposite conclusions regarding the value of screening chest roentgenography. Each of the three participating institutions recruited 10,000 male cigarette smokers over the age of 45 years. The patients at MSKCC and Johns Hopkins were recruited from the general population, while those at the Mayo Clinic were selected from patient groups seeking medical attention unrelated to lung cancer. The MSKCC and Johns Hopkins populations were randomized either to screening with both sputum cytology every 4 months and an annual posteroanterior (PA) and lateral chest x-ray or with an annual chest x-ray alone. At the Mayo Clinic, all men received dual screening initially and then were randomized to either chest x-ray and sputum cytology every 4 months or to a control group advised at the initial examination to obtain annual chest x-rays, with no efforts made to ensure compliance with this recommendation. Nine percent to 12% of the lung cancers recognized at all three institutions had a positive cytology with a negative chest x-ray, but there was no reduction in mortality in this radiographically negative group. It was concluded that carcinomas recognized by cytology alone can be identified on later chest x-rays while still resectable and, thus, sputum cytology does not lower the death rate from lung cancer compared to groups receiving annual chest x-rays. All patients from each institution had an annual chest x-ray recommended, with varying degrees of reinforcement and compliance. The point of Drs. Melamed and Flehinger that the study design does not allow a direct assessment of the value of screening chest x-rays on lung cancer mortality is well taken. However,

Drs. Melamed and Flehinger argue quite convincingly for the value of screening x-rays by citing the following results: (1) the 5-year survival of all patients who developed lung cancer while receiving chest x-ray screening was 35% contrasted with 13% for the United States as a whole; (2) in the 2 years following the cessation of screening, the proportion of stage I lung cancers dropped from 41% to 20%; and (3) in the years after the conclusion of the screening study, the 4-year survival dropped to 20% compared to 47% during the screening period.

It would appear that flaws in study design, such as the use of photofluorograms for screening, small sample size, screening young populations at low risk for lung cancer, and a variable frequency of annual chest x-rays in the control group, still leave screening chest x-rays for the detection of early lung cancer an unproven, yet not discredited, clinical practice. Careful definition of the group to be screened is exceedingly important. Smokers at the age of 50 years or greater seem a reasonable target group. Every 1% reduction in mortality would save approximately 1,000 lives annually.

Should Thyroid Hormone Be Used for the Diagnosis and Treatment of Patients With a Thyroid Nodule?

Chapter Editor: H. Verdain Barnes, M.D.

Affirmative: Manfred Blum, M.D.
Professor of Clinical Medicine and
Radiology, Director, Nuclear Endocrine
Laboratory, New York University Medical
Center, New York, New York

Don Zwickler, M.D.
Fellow in Endocrinology, Department of
Medicine, New York University Medical
Center, New York, New York

Negative: Ernest L. Mazzaferri, M.D.
Professor and Chairman, Department of
Internal Medicine, Ohio State University
College of Medicine, Columbus, Ohio

Editor's Introduction

As many as 7% of all U.S. adults have a clinically apparent thyroid nodule(s), making diagnosis and mangement of these entities relatively common problems for the practicing physician. This debate focuses on the issue of whether or not thyroid hormone is useful in the diagnosis and/or treatment of these patients. Our debators are internationally recognized authorities in thyroid disease. Dr. Ernest L. Mazzaferri is from Ohio State University and Drs. Manfred Blum and co-author Don Zwickler are from New York University Medical Center.

These debators agree that fine-needle aspiration biopsy (FNB) of the nodule is currently the diagnostic procedure which provides the greatest accuracy. They differ, however, as to whether thyroid hormone (TH) suppression is of value in diagnosis. Dr. Mazzaferri espouses the negative position, while Drs. Blum and Zwickler take the affirmative position in a setting where the FNB is equivocal. The latter authors detail their protocol for using TH. Next, they address the issue of whether TH should be used in the long-term management of a benign nodule in a euthyroid patient. They present cogent arguments on both sides of the issue from the perspectives of rationale, clinical effect, potential undesirable side effects, and therapy monitoring.

Can a definitive approach to these issues be derived from the current data? How should you manage your next patient? In this chapter, you will find provocative discussions which have useful clinical implications.

H. Verdain Barnes, M.D.

Affirmative
Manfred Blum, M.D.
Don Zwickler, M.D.

Some thyroidologists would have us believe that there is no role for thyroid hormone in the management of a patient with a thyroid nodule. Their concept is that fine-needle biopsy (FNB) is the only way to select a patient with thyroid cancer for surgery. Furthermore, many of these physicians contend that if cancer is not found in this way, the nodule is almost certainly benign and usually needs no treatment. The major reason for these changes in thinking have come from experiences with FNB that were validated in special centers. In addition, there are assertions from a few clinicians that the suppression of thyrotropin (TSH) with thyroid hormone is not effective in selecting cancers or shrinking benign nodules and there is increased awareness that excessive thyroid medication can have untoward effects. We believe that, while these concepts are useful, they go too far and may be counterproductive in many situations.

Clinical medicine is an imprecise discipline that stems from science, experience, and the professional desire to do the best that one can with incomplete information. At times, an apparent breakthrough like FNB or the recognition of a potentially serious adverse effect alters our thinking and patterns of professional behavior. *Primum non nocere,* we are taught. Recently we have been told that the administration of excessive thyroid hormone may cause osteoporosis, because sometimes osteoporosis is seen in patients who have prolonged and severe thyrotoxicosis. However, we do not know if osteoporosis follows the use of quantities of thyroid hormone that do not cause thyrotoxicosis but just barely suppress TSH into the low normal or minimally depressed level. Nor do we know the cost/benefit relationships of untreated enlarging goiters or thyroid nodules when compared with the unknown (if any) propensity to osteopenia from modulated amounts of thyroid hormone.

We do not challenge the consensus that properly performed, FNB is a safe, inexpensive, and accurate procedure for the diagnosis of cancer in a thyroid nodule. A positive diagnosis of cancer is almost completely reliable. There is no argument about procedure or protocol when cancer is found; surgery is indicated. However, most thyroid nodules are benign and FNB is not always as simple or as reliable as some authors report. We feel that FNB is often only one step in the diagnosis in a sizeable portion of the patients who are encountered by the average clinician. In addition, the long-term management of patients with benign nodular thyroid disease must be addressed.

In many patients, FNB is a simple procedure. However, there are limitations to FNB, including (1) difficulty in reliably puncturing a nodule that is smaller than 1.5 cm in diameter or deep in the neck; (2) a 10% to 20% error, especially when a nodule has undergone cystic and/or hemorrhagic degeneration (which is the case in almost all large nodules); (3) sampling error, especially when aspirating a nodule in a goiter; (4) a high number of nonspecific results; (5) uncertainty about management when the findings are "suspicious;" (6) suboptimal results when the procedure is performed by clinicians who are not experts; (7) results which often are inconclusive when interpreted by cytologists who are not specially trained; (8) controversies about cytologic classification and an inability to differentiate follicular adenoma and follicular carcinoma; and (9) the need to do something for a patient who cannot have an FNB or who refuses to have one. Thus, we feel that the ideal diagnostic goal of FNB is not practical in some circumstances and not always achievable, even in the best of hands. Furthermore, we believe that it is inappropriate, as has been suggested, to refer all patients who are perceived to have a dominant thyroid nodule to a special center for FNB. Consequently, we should not ignore whatever additional help is available to us.

We will address the subject of the "cold" thyroid nodule and submit that other approaches have been useful and can continue to contribute to the management of these patients. Fundamental to our concept is the realization that thyroid cancer is rare and usually of low virulence. There is no controversy if the diagnosis is made with a FNB. However, if cancer is not found or if cytology is ambiguous, malignancy still may be present and suppressive therapy can be effective in identifying thyroid tumors. Moreover, there is extensive opinion that patients with benign disease who do not need surgery can benefit from lifelong treatment with thyroid hormone.

Are Clinical Factors Useful in Diagnosing Malignancy?

It has been shown that an analysis of the history and physical examination can detect clinical thyroid malignancies. Blum and Rothschild employed clinical factors that suggested a high risk of malignancy to select 30 patients for surgery from 220 patients with a "cold" thyroid nodule.[1] Of these, 15 had cancers and 10 had adenomas. It does not seem prudent to ignore this kind of information. The criteria that suggest malignancy include male sex, youth, enlargement of the nodule without evidence of hemorrhage, history of exposure to ionizing radiation during youth, firmness to palpation, fixation to surrounding tissue, local adenopathy, and evidence of distant spread. Because of the significant false-negative rate of FNB, we do not see how one can avoid recommending surgery when these factors suggest a high risk of cancer, even when the cytology is benign. On the other hand, a positive FNB in patients with these criteria can be useful in leading to a preoperative surgical plan. In our judgment, the decision about the extent of the surgery should not be confused by a negative or inconclusive intraoperative frozen section when the FNB showed malignancy. The result of this pitfall is a second operation.

Defining Therapy With Thyroid Hormone

It is important to differentiate replacement and suppressive therapy with thyroid hormone. Replacement therapy uses the least amount of the medication that is required to return TSH to a physiological level. In distinction, suppressive therapy requires adequate thyroid hormone to lower TSH to undetectable levels when measured by a specific and highly sensitive assay such as the two-site, monoclonal antibody immunoradiometric method (IRMA). A more rigorous definition of suppression requires using that amount of thyroid hormone which blocks the responsiveness of TSH to an administration of thyrotropin-releasing hormone (TRH). It is also important to the concept of suppressive therapy to distinguish its use for a short time as a diagnostic trial to assess the shrinkage of a nodule from long-term treatment to inhibit thyroid tissue. An unresolved issue regarding suppressive therapy relates to the difference, if any, between the suppressive potential of L-thyroxine (T_4) and triiodothyronine (T_3).

Is There Any Role for a Diagnostic Trial of Suppressive Therapy in the Patient With a Thyroid Nodule?

The utility of a trial of suppressive therapy with thyroid hormone to diagnose a thyroid nodule is controversial.[2,3] Some investigators are opposed to it because an unequivocal difference in nodule size has not been shown between untreated controls and patients who are given euthyroid doses of T_4. In distinction, when given for only 3 months, supraphysiological quantities of T_3 have been shown to shrink nontumorous nodules.[1] Both T_4 and T_3 are generally conceded to reduce the size of euthyroid goiters which masquerade as thyroid nodules. In these cases, there is one clinically dominant portion of the goiter and the rest of it is not obvious; this is a common occurrence. Fortunately, one recent and comprehensive review has concluded that it makes no difference whether suppressive therapy or FNB is used to identify thyroid cancer with regard to overall diagnostic success, morbidity, or mortality.[4]

A summary of the clinical research with thyroid hormone during the last

100 years will be helpful to understand suppressive therapy. Some of the studies with adequate control groups can be found in very old data and there actually has been a relatively orderly sequence of events in the use of thyroid suppression through history. These steps have led to the clinical use of thyroid hormone in managing patients with diffuse goiter, nodular goiter, solitary nodule, and differentiated carcinoma. We will not discuss cancer therapy here.

As early as 1890, thyroid extract was found to be effective in decreasing the size of a goiter. Kocher characterized the effectiveness of therapy based on the type of goiter. Diffuse goiter responded better than nodular goiter and enlargement of short duration responded better than chronic swelling. Bruns suggested the concept that the remaining portion of a thyroidectomized gland would undergo compensatory hypertrophy due to deficiency of endogenous thyroid. Unfortunately, thyroid hormone was touted as a panacea, then all but abandoned as a medicinal agent when it became apparent that it was not a cure-all.

In 1953, Greer and Astwood reviewed the experience with thyroid medication of the prior 60 years and revived interest in its use.[5] They noted that the last decade of the 19th century marked a transition from the sole use of iodine as therapy for the suppression of goiter to the use of exogenous thyroid hormone which caused shrinkage of goiters in iodine-sufficient areas and in people who were apparently euthyroid. Fifty patients with goiter who had suppression therapy and 40 patients with goiter who had no therapy were examined. Superior partial and complete shrinkage was achieved in thyroid-treated patients when compared with controls. This observation held true for solitary nodules and goiters alike.

In the following years it was reported that 30% to 60% of goiters and nodules were reduced in size as a result of treatment although the studies are difficult to compare because the types of thyroid problems were not uniform, the criteria of size were imprecise, and the regimens varied. In 1953, it was noted astutely in one study that all but 1 of 36 patients had some reduction in goiter size. This patient had a follicular adenocarcinoma. In 1960, Astwood provided additional information.[6] It was recognized that thyroid suppression shrank hypothyroid goiters most effectively, and was less effective in shrinking diffuse euthyroid goiters, multinodular goiters, and solitary nodules, in that order. Glasford noted that, among 111 patients with nodular goiters undergoing suppressive therapy, 20% got smaller, 20% grew, and 60% showed no change.[7] He used 2 to 8 grains of desiccated thyroid extract for 3 to 6 months. Since 2 of 4 carcinomas shrank on suppressive therapy, he concluded that it was useless as a diagnostic modality. In contrast, Hill reported the value of suppressive therapy in selecting patients for surgery.[8] A threefold decrease in operations per year was accompanied by a similar increase in surgical yield in 167 patients with nodules.

Improved clinical selection of patients with thyroid cancer for surgery was reported by Blum and Rothschild.[1] In the first part of their protocol, they showed the value of clinical factors as discussed earlier. The second part of their study evaluated the diagnostic use of suppressive therapy. They defined shrinkage of a nodule as 50% reduction of its diameter as measured by perimetry and sonography. Sufficient T_3 (75 to 100 µg a day in divided doses) was used as the pharmaceutical agent to reduce circulating T_4 to low levels and to produce minimal thyrotoxicosis for 3 months. The identification of 5 cancers and 19 adenomas among 83 patients who consented to this form of diagnostic treatment was achieved. A diagnostic utility for thyroid suppression was emerging and the discovery of the reciprocal relationship between TSH and T_4 provided a physiological rationale for this therapy. However, a general concern with the diagnostic use of suppressive therapy was the observation that a few malignant nodules shrank during the treatment. It was unclear if the cancer shrank or if the surrounding thyroid gland responded to reducing TSH, until sonography provided an easily available answer to that question.

During recent years, although the focus of our attention has been largely on the solitary nodule, high-resolution sonography has shown that many nodules that appear to be solitary clinically actually are associated with minute, often multiple, nodules;[9,10] many are part of a multinodular goiter. Now, some investigators have not been able to find any value to suppressive therapy. Gharib et al. reported that suppression with T_4 is not effective in reducing the size of a thyroid nodule compared to placebo.[11] Thus, there still is no consensus regarding the value of suppressive therapy. Furthermore, the fear of overlooking carcinomas persists to this day, even in the era of FNB.

Many papers about FNB have revealed results that are impressive, but really not any more impressive than those obtained using T_3 as a diagnostic tool.[3] The apparent advantage of FNB is the rapidity with which most of the cancers can be identified. This rapidity is certainly desirable for both the patient and the physician, but probably is not of major clinical consequence considering the benign behavior and slow growth of thyroid carcinoma. In the cases where there is a false-negative result, the quick results are misleading. To minimize this concern, patients with a suspicious, inconclusive, or negative cytology are sometimes subjected to repeat FNB, with T_4 generally used in the interval between aspiration (which may be as long as a year or more). Although some thyroidologists report that they rely entirely on the results of FNB, others advise surgery when fluid reaccumulates in a complex nodule or when a solid nodule either fails to shrink or grows during suppressive therapy. The important issues would seem to be how and when suppression is used; there are situations in which thyroid hormone is useful and times when it may be dangerous.

A Suggested Way to Use Diagnostic Suppressive Therapy

Although FNB is the preferred way to diagnose malignancy in a thyroid nodule, sometimes aspiration cannot be done, is refused by the patient, or gives equivocal results. A management decision still has to be made for such patients. In these cases, we employ a 3-month course of T_3, using the criteria mentioned above. One reason for using T_3 rather than T_4 is the rapidity of its cessation of effect, which is a desirable attribute if adverse effects should occur. However, many physicians prefer to use a longer course of T_4. Shrinkage of a nodule on suppressive therapy is reassuring, while growth of a nodule when TSH is suppressed is suspicious of tumor unless proven otherwise by surgery. However, as mentioned, some clinicians have concluded that even benign nodules do not shrink on suppressive therapy and that the procedure is not useful.

It is important to note that in the study by Gharib et al., some of the nodules were "functioning" and not "cold." It is unclear whether any of the former were autonomous and therefore not expected to shrink on thyroid medication. Nevertheless, the reasons for the disparate conclusions are not clear. They may relate to such factors as selection bias, differing definitions of suppressive therapy, or the use of T_4 for many months (rather than T_3 for 3 months) as the drug regimen. The two drug regimens may have differences. For instance, it is difficult to avoid mild thyrotoxicosis in the process of extinguishing TSH when T_3 is the suppressive agent. Full suppression of TSH by mild thyrotoxicosis may be required for the desired effect during the diagnostic trial. However, when T_4 is employed, one keeps the patient euthyroid with greater certainty by monitoring T_4 as well as TSH. In distinction, it is easier to monitor a patient's compliance when T_3 is used rather than T_4. With T_3 administration, depressed levels of T_4 signify compliance, which can be verified frequently, inexpensively, and without risk. It is unclear if single daily administration of T_3 is as safe or effective as divided doses, but it is a more convenient regimen that will contribute to compliance.

Monitoring compliance is difficult when euthyroid-producing quantities of T_4 are used; T_4 remains normal both when the medication is used properly and when it is not. Theoretically, the TSH (IRMA) should be maintained at the lowest limit of the normal range without allowing it to become undetectable. How often TSH should be checked is unclear. In any event, the goal is hard to achieve, of unproven value, expensive to test, and probably not attainable for the 6 months or 1 year that is required for T_4 diagnostic suppression. The best way to test compliance with T_4 involves assessing blockade of the uptake of radioactive iodine by the thyroid gland via a procedure which is costly, inconvenient, poorly standardized and open to artifact, and which requires exposure to radiation. Indeed, the question of long-term, regular compliance may be one reason that it has been difficult to document shrinkage of a nodule on T_4 suppression. It is easier to get a patient's cooperation for 3 months than for 6 or 12 months.

Suggested Management When There Is Benign Cytology

In our opinion, patients who have a benign diagnosis on FNB should be given "cautious" suppressive therapy, which is different from a 3-month diagnostic trial. By that, we mean thyroid hormone should be administered in quantities sufficient just to suppress or keep TSH very low without free hyperthyroxinemia. We use T_4 for this purpose on the possibility that it may be safer than T_3 for chronic therapy. We engage in this protocol because of the evidence that whether or not T_4 suppression is associated with shrinkage of a nodule, it prevents the growth of thyroid tissue. Exceptions include enlargement that is caused by hemorrhage, non-TSH humoral growth factors, or inflammation, situations that usually are detectable. Otherwise, the presence or absence of growth during suppressive therapy signifies a benign or malignant tumor which should be treated accordingly. In distinction, it is our experience that if suppressive therapy is not employed, then most nodules (or goiters that appear to be nodules) grow over the years, impose the fear of malignancy, occasionally obstruct the thoracic inlet, and lead to avoidable surgery. On the other hand, shrinkage of a nodule on suppressive therapy after a FNB has failed to show malignant disease is reassuring, but is still no guarantee of benign disease. Therefore, most clinicians continue suppressive therapy and periodic reassessment.

There is no consensus concerning management when the FNB is negative but the nodule does not shrink on suppressive therapy. Some authorities advocate repeat FNB, long-term suppressive therapy, and observation if interval biopsies are consistent with benign pathology. Others recommend surgery if there is no shrinkage on adequate suppressive therapy after a specified time interval. At this juncture, the prudent appraoch would appear to be discussing the relative risks and advantages of observation or surgery with the patient and individualizing management according to the clinical situation and the patient's wishes.

Suppressive Therapy After Surgery for Benign Disease

Enlargement of the post-surgical thyroid remnant and a way to avoid it have been known for many years. Recent data have shown that after partial thyroidectomy the TSH will increase significantly to the high normal range for approximately 3 months, while the T_4 will decrease slightly and there will be an exaggerated response of TSH to TRH. Thereafter, the biochemical values will return to baseline. However, a euthyroid enlargement of the remnant ensues in several years unless too little tissue is left after surgery or the tissue is so diseased that any enlargement is accompanied by hypothyroidism. The historical, clinical, and chemical data provide a strong rationale for the prophylactic use of thyroid hormone postoperatively, unless there is a medical contraindication. One has the impression that prevention of regrowth is accomplished more easily and uniformly than is shrinkage of tissue that has grown and perhaps scarred after surgery. The actual long-term benefits and risks of this type of therapy have not been evaluated adequately, but one is persuaded to employ conservative judgment, especially when heart disease is present or advanced age approaches.

Concern About Using Suppressive Therapy

If chronic suppressive therapy is maintained, T_4 levels should not be permitted to rise significantly above normal because of the well-known untoward effects of thyrotoxicosis, which we shall not review. Although it has been shown recently that osteoporosis may occur as a result of prolonged and severe thyrotoxicosis, it is unclear whether it will occur as a consequence of a 3-month trial of T_3 or a minimal, chronic elevation of T_4. Nevertheless, it would be prudent to avoid very high levels of the thyroid hormones, especially when treating benign disease. However, we see nothing in the current literature that would lead us to deny our patients the probable benefits of carefully regulated suppressive therapy.

Cost-effectiveness

It has become necessary to address more than the management of a single patient. Rather, the cost-effectiveness of management in entire populations has become a focus of the attention of industry, labor unions, insurance companies, and the government. FNB is cost-effective when cancer is found. However, the economic impact of false-negative results, additional tests, diagnostic trials, and long-term suppressive therapy must be compared to the consequences of diverse situations. Among these are the "human" factors and occasional delayed recognition or emergence of cancer which may or may not have an adverse effect on the patient and could result in medicolegal implications for the physician. Furthermore, the impact of preventable surgery when a nodule or goiter becomes larger and the cardiovascular and osteoporotic risks of treatment need to be analyzed as well.

Conclusion

One may conclude that FNB is very useful in the diagnosis of the solitary "cold" thyroid nodule. Sometimes it may be the only procedure that is required, especially if the aspiration shows a thyroid malignancy which should lead to surgery. However, there are limitations to FNB. In many patients, careful analysis of the entire clinical picture is needed for a management decision. Suppressive therapy with thyroid hormone is diagnostically useful when there is a benign or equivocal cytology and particularly when there is a dominant nodule in a goiter. When employing this treatment, one should be cautious not to make the patient thyrotoxic. Because there are false-negative results with FNB, nodules that do not regress during long-term treatment with suppressive therapy should be biopsied again or possibly treated surgically, depending upon the physician's and the patient's philosophy and choice. There also is a prophylactic role for suppressive therapy after thyroid surgery.

References

1. Blum M, Rothschild M: Improved nonoperative diagnosis of the solitary "cold" thyroid nodule: Surgical selection based on risk factors and three months of suppression. *JAMA* 1980; 243:242–245. *After most of the cancers were selected by using clinical criteria and factors associated with a high risk of cancer, 3 months of thyroid suppression with triiodothyronine resulted in shrinkage of the non-neoplastic solitary thyroid nodules. The tumors (adenomas and carcinomas) did not shrink and were selected for surgery.*
2. Van Herle AJ: The thyroid nodule. *Ann Intern Med* 1982; 96:221–232. *The diagnostic accuracy and cost-effectiveness of various techniques in the evaluation of the thyroid nodule are examined, including fine-needle aspiration, ultrasonography, and thyroid scanning.*
3. Rojeski MT, Gharib H: Nodular thyroid disease. *N Engl J Med* 1985; 313:428–436. *This is an in-depth review of the evaluation and management of nodular thyroid disease utilizing sonography, thyroid hormone suppression, radionuclide imaging, and fine-needle aspiration. The authors believe fine-needle biopsy is the best diagnostic tool.*
4. Molitch ME, Beck JR, Dreisman M, et al: The cold thyroid nodule. An analysis of diagnostic and therapeutic options. *Endocr Rev* 1984; 5:185–197. *A decision analysis reveals that thyroid suppression is as useful a diagnostic and therapeutic tool in the management of the thyroid nodule as fine-needle biopsy or surgery.*
5. Greer MA, Astwood EB: Treatment of simple goiter with thyroid. *J Clin Endocrinol Metab* 1953; 1:1312–1331. *Suppressive therapy is successful in shrinking diffuse and nodular goiter during a 5-year period.*
6. Astwood EB, Cassidy CE, Aurbach GE: Treatment of goiter and thyroid nodules with thyroid. *JAMA* 1960; 174:459–464. *A retrospective study of*

the effectiveness of thyroid hormone suppression on goiter and thyroid nodules.

7. Glasford GH, Fowler EF, Cole WH: The treatment of nontoxic nodular goiter with desiccated thyroid: Results and evaluation. *Surgery* 1965; 58:621–625.

8. Hill LD, Beebe HG, Hipp R, et al: Thyroid suppression. *Arch Surg* 1974; 108:403–405. *Thyroid suppression is analyzed in terms of selecting patients for surgery.*

9. Blum M: The role of imaging in the management of thyroid nodules: A personal perspective. *Thyroid Today* 1986;9:1–7. *A discussion of the role of imaging in the management of thyroid nodules is presented.*

10. Blum M: Ultrasonography and computed tomography of the thyroid gland, in Ingbar SH, Braverman LE (eds): *Werner's The Thyroid,* 5th ed. New York, JB Lippincott, 1986, pp 576–591. *This is a comprehensive review of the utility of ultrasound and computed tomography (CT) imaging of the thyroid. Echography is useful as an adjunct to needle biopsy in the management of the cold thyroid nodule.*

11. Gharib H, James EM, Charboneau J: Suppressive therapy with levothyroxine for solitary thyroid nodules. *N Engl J Med* 1987; 317:70–75.

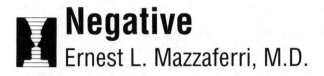

Negative
Ernest L. Mazzaferri, M.D.

Management of the isolated thyroid nodule is an important and controversial clinical problem. Over the past several decades thyroid hormone suppression has gained wide acceptance, both for diagnosis and for long-term management of thyroid nodules. Its goal is to suppress thyrotropin (TSH) production, based upon the notion that TSH initiates and/or promotes the growth of thyroid nodules, particularly benign nodules. The hypothesis is that neoplastic nodules treated with thyroid hormone will continue to grow, while benign nodules will shrink and may disappear. However, despite its wide application, this hypothesis continues to be unproven and suppressive therapy remains controversial.[1-5]

The aim of this paper is to examine the rationale and results of thyroid hormone suppression for both the diagnosis and long-term management of thyroid nodules. The current data do not support routine use of L-thyroxine in either situation, and I believe this practice is no longer justified.

The Prevalence of Thyroid Nodules and Thyroid Cancer

Thyroid nodules are important because they are so common. Anxiety about a nodule's malignant potential, the principal fear of both patient and physician, generally prompts a careful diagnostic evaluation of a large number of patients with nodules each year in this country. However, since thyroid cancer is relatively rare (only about 10,000 new cases are diagnosed each year in the United States), most nodules eventually prove benign. Once the nodule has been diagnosed as a benign lesion, thyroid hormone is often given because of concern about the nodule's continued growth, even though most tend to grow very slowly.

An estimated 4% to 7% of adults in the United States have thyroid nodules.[1,2] Each year, new nodules are detected in about 1 person per 1,000 in the United States. Their incidence increases linearly with age, and at least 5% to 7% of adults over the age of 50 years have palpable thyroid nodules.[1,2] They are three- to fourfold more common in women than men, and most are asymptomatic. Clinically solitary nodules, which have the greatest risk of harboring a malignancy, are about three times more frequent than multiple nodules. Prior head or neck x-ray therapy eventually leads to palpable thyroid abnormalities in about 20% to 30% of subjects so exposed during childhood.[1,2] Because they are so common, thyroid nodules contribute substantially to the cost of medical care, particularly for the elderly.

The diagnosis of thyroid nodules is difficult, because they are difficult to classify and their anticipated clinical behavior is nearly impossible to define. Thyroid nodules may be caused by thyroid cancer, metastatic cancer, primary thyroid lymphoma, benign adenoma, colloid nodule, thyroiditis, infection, developmental abnormalities, cysts, and other disorders. It is not surprising that a nodule's response to thyroid hormone suppression is unpredictable and nonspecific.

The selection of thyroid nodules for surgery is a difficult and controversial problem. When selected for surgery on clinical grounds, only 10% to 20% of thyroid nodules are cancers, an incidence that increases to 30% to 50% when there has been prior head or neck irradiation.[1-3] Most malignant tumors are papillary or follicular thyroid carcinomas which typically have slow growth rates not clinically distinguishable from those of benign lesions. The diagnostic problem is complicated further by the fact that both occult benign nodular disease and microscopic thyroid carcinoma (which rarely poses a threat to survival) occur with high frequency in carefully examined autopsy and surgical specimens.[1,2] These lesions may cause serious diagnostic and therapeutic dilemmas, since ultrasonography can identify solid lesions as small as 3 mm and cystic lesions as small as 1 mm.[1] In the population over the age of 50 years, about one half of the palpably normal glands have discrete nodules detected by high resolution ultrasonography, an incidence that parallels the frequency of benign nodules found at autopsy.[1] In addition, many thyroid glands previously exposed to ionizing irradiation show small defects by radionuclide scanning.[2] Sensitive diagnostic techniques that uncover such small lesions, but which do not sharply discriminate malignant from benign disease, can lead to an unnecessarily high number of thyroidectomies being recommended. Thyroid hormone suppression used for diagnostic purposes suffers from this problem.

The Rationale for Using Thyroid Hormone to Suppress Thyroid Nodules

The basic assumption that has led to the commonplace use of thyroid hormone in the management of thyroid nodules is that TSH is a potent thyroid growth factor. This assertion may be flawed. There is both in vitro and in vivo evidence suggesting that TSH is not a thyroid growth factor.

Westermark et al.[6] studied thyroid cells from normal human thyroid tissue and benign nodular goiter grown and maintained in tissue culture for 4 to 18 passages. Thyroid cells grown in the presence of TSH for 1 to 2 weeks had a slower growth rate and the culture dishes showed 24% to 36% lower cell numbers than did controls. The authors concluded that the primary action of TSH in vivo is not stimulation of growth. Other in vivo studies corroborate this notion.[3] Clinical studies support the idea that TSH is not the principal growth-promoting factor for thyroid nodules or nontoxic goiters.[6-9] The growth of residual thyroid tissue and the appearance of new nodules after subtotal thyroidectomy occurs despite thyroid hormone suppression therapy, and appears to be independent of TSH.[6-9]

Why Controversy Exists

Despite its use for a number of decades, controversy continues to exist regarding thyroid hormone suppression of thyroid nodules for several reasons. Older studies did not use fine-needle biopsy (FNB) to describe the nodule's pathology before long-term thyroid hormone suppression or sensitive diagnostic methods such as ultrasonography to assess nodule size during this therapy.[3] Modern laboratory tests such as sensitive TSH assays or free thyroid hormone measurements have been used only recently to accurately gauge the degree of suppression.[3] Many studies are flawed insofar as they are not prospective, placebo-controlled, double-blind, long-range studies. The form, dosage, and duration of thyroid hormone therapy have differed among studies, and there is little consensus regarding the definition of a positive response (i.e., "suppression") either for diagnosis or for long-term therapy. Few studies compare the cost of one approach over the other, and virtually none considers the potentially harmful long-term effects of chronic thyroid hormone suppression of benign thyroid nodules.

Evidence Against the Use of Thyroid Hormone for the Diagnosis of Thyroid Nodules

There is considerable evidence from published studies that thyroid hormone suppression is not as effective as newer diagnostic methods, particularly FNB, for the diagnosis of thyroid nodules. Substantial variability has been reported among different authors in the criteria for suppression and the response rates to thyroid hormone. However, combining the data gathered by Gharib et al.[3] and Molitch et al.[4] from 13 different series of patients comprising 912 individuals, the overall response rate to thyroid hormone has been 43%. Highly variable response rates, ranging from 9% to 69%, have been reported in these series.[3,4] The reason for this difference relates in part to the unique definitions of a positive response used by various authors. In contrast, an abundant literature in recent years substantiates the efficacy of FNB for the diagnosis of thyroid carcinoma.

In 1981, Ashcraft and van Herle[5] reported an exhaustive survey of the American and foreign literature on the evaluation of thyroid nodules. Their findings permit a unique comparison of thyroid hormone suppression and FNB for the diagnosis of thyroid nodules in a large number of patients. Table 1 is a summary of their review of ten series that reported the responses to thyroid suppressive therapy in 446 patients with solitary thyroid nodules. Of this group, 36.8% were considered to be "responders" and 63.2% "nonresponders" to thyroid hormone, according to the various definitions used by the different authors (see Table 1). The percentage of malignancy found in all surgically excised nodules evaluated by thyroid hormone suppression was 13.9%. This resulted in a false-negative rate* (malignant nodules responding to thyroid hormone suppression) of 8.7%, and a false-positive rate (benign nodules failing to respond) of 80.3% (Table 2). The sensitivity and specificity of thyroid hormone suppression in these studies was 91.3% and 19.7%, respectively.

The results of FNB for thyroid nodules were also reported by Ashcraft and van Herle[5] in the same review. Table 3 summarizes their findings in 28 series that reported the results of FNB in 10,872 patients with thyroid nodules in whom the procedure produced sufficient material for cytologic interpretation. Of the entire group, the cytology was considered to be benign in 84.3% and malignant or suspicious in 15.7% (see Table 3). Of the surgically excised nodules, 20.6% were malignant, compared with 13.9% for the group initially subject to thyroid hormone therapy (Table 4). False-negative tests occurred at about the same frequency with FNB and suppression (7.7% vs. 8.7%, respectively; see Tables 2 and 4). However, false-positive tests occurred with a fourfold lower frequency following FNB than with suppression (20% vs. 80.3% respectively; see Tables 2 and 4). The sensitivity and specificity of thyroid FNB was 92.3% and 80%, respectively, compared with 91.3% and 19.7% for thyroid hormone suppression. Thus, while the sensitivities of the two diagnostic methods are very similar, there are striking differences in their

---

* The definitions used in this text are as follows:

$$\text{False-negative rate} \ = \ \frac{\text{number of diseased patients with a negative test}}{\text{number of diseased patients}}$$

$$\text{False-positive rate} \ = \ \frac{\text{number of nondiseased patients with a positive test}}{\text{number of nondiseased patients}}$$

$$\text{Sensitivity (true positive)} \ = \ \frac{\text{number of diseased patients with positive test}}{\text{number of diseased patients}}$$

$$\text{Specificity (true negative)} \ = \ \frac{\text{number of nondiseased patients with negative test}}{\text{number of diseased patients}}$$

TABLE 1.
Response to Thyroid Hormone Suppressive Therapy in Patients With Solitary Thyroid Nodules in Ten Series Reviewed by Ashcraft and van Herle*

	All Patients	**Responders**	**Nonresponders**
Number (%) in group	446 (100)	164 (36.8)	282 (63.2)
Number (%) to surgery[†]	165 (40)	30 (18.3)	135 (47.9)
Number malignant	23	2	21
(%) operated[‡]	(13.9)	(6.7)	(15.6)
(%) in group[§]	(5.2)	(1.2)	(7.4)
Number benign			
Number (%) operated[¶]	142 (86.1)	28 (93.3)	114 (84.4)
Number (%) in group[‖]	423 (94.8)	162 (98.8)	261 (92.6)

* Data from Ashcraft MW, van Herle AJ: *Head Neck Surg* 1981; 216–227.
† Percentage of total patients in each column operated upon, but two series reviewed did not report the number of patients sent to surgery.
‡ Percentage of malignancy found in operated cases in each column, but several series did not report the number with malignancy.
§ Percentage of malignancy found in total cases in each column.
¶ Number and percentage of benign lesions found in operated cases in each column.
‖ Number and percentage of cases in each column not operated and presumed benign (total cases minus cases malignant at surgery).

TABLE 2.
Final Diagnosis*

	Malignant (13.9%)	**Benign (86.1%)**
Nonsuppressible	21 (91.3%)	114 (80.3%)
Suppressible	2 (8.7%)	28 (19.7%)
Total	23	142

*Cases from Table 1 that went to surgery. Sensitivity = 91.3% and specificity = 19.7%.

TABLE 3.
Results of Fine-Needle Aspiration Biopsy (FNB) of Thyroid Nodules in 28 Literature Series Reviewed by Ashcraft and van Herle*

	All[†]	Benign FNB	Suspicious/ Malignant FNB
Number (%) in group	10,872 (100)	9,161 (84.3)	1,711 (15.7)
Number (%) to surgery[‡]	3,639 (33.5)	2,368 (25.8)	1,271 (74.3)
Number malignant	750	58	692
(%) operated[§]	(20.6)	(2.4)	(54.4)
(%) in group[¶]	(6.9)	(0.6)	(40.4)
Number benign			
Number (%) operated[││]	2,889 (79.4)	2,310 (97.6)	579 (45.6)
Number (%) in group[**]	10,112 (93.1)	9,103 (99.4)	1,019 (59.6)

* Data from Ashcraft MW, van Herle AJ: *Head Neck Surg* 1981; 216–227.
† All patients in whom sufficient material was obtained by FNB for cytology.
‡ Percentage of patients operated upon in each column, but several series did not report the number of patients sent to surgery.
§ Percentage of malignancy in operated cases in column, but several series did not report the number of patients sent to surgery.
¶ Percentage of malignancy in total number of cases in column, including those not operated upon.
││Number and percentage of benign nodules in cases sent to surgery in column.
**Number and percentage of all benign cases (total cases minus malignant) in column, including those not operated upon.

TABLE 4.
Final Diagnosis*

	Malignant (20.6%)	Benign (79.4%)
Malignant/suspicious fine-needle biopsy	692 (92.3%)	579 (20.0%)
Benign fine-needle biopsy	58 (7.7%)	2,310 (80%)
Total	750	2,889

*Cases from Table 3. Sensitivity = 92.3% and specificity = 80%.

specificities, an observation which has important diagnostic and cost impli-cations.

Table 5 considers the posttest probabilities of cancer when thyroid hormone suppression or FNB is either positive or negative. The likelihood of a nodule being malignant before any testing is done (the pretest probability) is about 10%, an assumption made by Molitch et al.[4] in their careful decision

---

TABLE 5.
Posttest Probability of Disease With Positive and Negative Tests*

Probability of Disease if Test is Positive[†]

$$P = \frac{p(D) \times TPR}{p(D) \times TPR + [1-(pD)] \times FPR}$$

For Thyroid Hormone Nonsuppression of Nodule

$$P = \frac{0.01 \times 0.91}{0.01 \times 0.91 + [1-0.1] \times 0.8} = \frac{0.091}{0.81}$$

$$= 0.112 \ (11.2\% \text{ posttest probability of disease})$$

For Malignant/Suspicious Fine-Needle Biopsy

$$P = \frac{0.01 \times 0.92}{0.1 \times 0.92 + [1-0.1] \times 0.2} = \frac{0.092}{0.272}$$

$$= 0.338 \ (33.8\% \text{ posttest probability of disease})$$

Probability of Disease if Test is Negative

$$P = \frac{p(D) \times FNR}{p(D) \times FNR + [1-p(D)] \times TNR}$$

For Thyroid Hormone Suppression of Nodule

$$P = \frac{0.1 \times 0.087}{0.1 \times 0.87 + [1-0.1] \times 0.2} = \frac{0.0087}{0.1887}$$

$$= 0.046 \ (4.6\% \text{ posttest probability of disease})$$

For Benign Fine-Needle Biopsy

$$P = \frac{0.1 \times 0.08}{0.1 \times 0.08 + [1-0.1] \times 0.8} = \frac{0.008}{0.728}$$

$$= 0.011 \ (1.1\% \text{ posttest probability of disease})$$

*Data rounded to nearest percent.
[†]p(D) = pretest probability of disease (10%); TPR = true-positive rate; FPR = false-positive rate; FNR = false-negative rate; TNR = true-negative rate.

analysis of the diagnosis of thyroid nodules. Table 5 shows that when thyroid hormone suppression is positive (i.e., the nodule fails to shrink), the posttest probability, or the likelihood of cancer being present, only rise to 11.2%. This compares unfavorably with FNB. When a nodule has a suspicious or malignant cytology by FNB, the posttest probability of malignancy rises to 33.8%. Conversely, when the test is negative (i.e., a nodule is judged to shrink to a critical degree in response to thyroid hormone suppression), the likelihood of cancer being present is 4.6%. This also compares unfavorably with a benign cytology by FNB which results in a 1.1% probability that the nodule is malignant. These observations have important cost implications.

Using these data, one can estimate the relative costs of either thyroid hormone suppression or FNB as the initial diagnostic test to select patients for surgery (Table 6). If 1,000 patients with thyroid nodules were evaluated and all patients with a positive test were taken to surgery, thyroid hormone suppression would result in almost a fourfold larger number of thyroidectomies than would FNB (623 operations for suppression vs. 157 for FNB; see Table 6). Thus, the total cost would be fourfold greater for thyroid hormone suppression than for FNB. Since about 10,000 thyroid cancers are diagnosed annually in the United States,[2] the total annual health care cost would be over $15.5 million if thyroid hormone suppression were used as the initial diagnostic test, compared with about $4 million if FNB were used.

Thus, the published data considered collectively show that both tests have about the same sensitivity, but vary substantially in specificity. As a result, surgery will be recommended to an unnecessarily large number of patients who have been given thyroid hormone suppression. The specific problems associated with thyroid hormone suppression can be appreciated by considering several individual studies.

Many older studies used rough measurements of nodule size to assess thyroid hormone suppression. In 1963, Badillo et al.[10] reported the responses of 56 patients who were given liothyronine (T$_3$) for 3 months in a well-designed, prospective, double-blind, crossover, placebo study. The thyroid lesions were described simply as euthyroid goiters that were either diffuse, multinodular or uninodular. Calipers were used to measure goiter or nodule size, but only rarely did both examiners record identical measurements for the same thyroid mass, and occasionally the discrepancy between paired observations was as great as 30%. Using this approach, the authors concluded that a measurable decrease in the goiter size occurred in about one half of the patients who completed the study. However, most of the decreases in thyroid mass observed over the 3-month period were relatively modest, between 20% and 30%. When given thyroid hormone, only 1 of 16 patients (6.3%) with a single thyroid nodule, and only 4 of 50 patients (8%) in the entire study group, experienced a 50% or greater decrease in the goiter or nodule diameter. Moreover, spontaneous reductions in nodule size occurred in 10% of the patients during placebo therapy. It is clear that data gathered by physical examination are too crude to adequately evaluate the

TABLE 6.
Cost Analysis Using Either Thyroid Hormone Suppression or Fine-Needle Aspiration Biopsy (FNB) as the Initial Diagnostic Test for Thyroid Nodules

	Nonsuppressible with Thyroid Hormone	Malignant/Suspicious by FNB
Total cases	1,000	1,000
Number to surgery*	623	157
Total cost of surgery†	$1,557,500	$392,500
Number of cancers resected‡	97	85
Cost per cancer resected	$16,057	$4,618

*Based upon the assumption that all nonresponders and all patients with malignant/suspicious cytology are taken to surgery. From the previous tables, 62.3% of those given L-thyroxine will be nonresponders (see Table 1) and 15.7% with FNB will have malignant/suspicious cytology (see Table 3).
†Based upon an estimated total cost of $2,500 per thyroidectomy.
‡Number of cancers resected estimated at 15.6% for nonresponders to L-thyroxine (see Table 1), e.g., 0.156 × 623 = 97, and at 54.4% for FNB (see Table 2), e.g., 0.544 × 57 = 85.

change in nodule size during thyroid hormone therapy. If one defines a 50% or greater reduction in nodule size as being a "response" (a definition which is used by many authors[5]), surgery would be recommended for most patients given thyroid hormone suppression.

Thyroid carcinomas sometimes appear to shrink during thyroid hormone suppressive therapy when physical examination alone is used to measure the nodule's response. We found that 11 of 83 patients (13.3%) with papillary thyroid carcinoma demonstrated an initial decrease in nodule size, but eventually were taken to surgery because the nodule either failed to disappear completely or showed renewed growth with continued follow-up over a period of about a year.[11] Hill et al.[12] reported that 4 of 31 patients (13%) who initially experienced a decrease in nodule size in response to thyroid hormone suppression ultimately were found to have thyroid cancer. One patient had complete disappearance of the nodule, but with continuing follow-up, the nodule reappeared and a papillary thyroid carcinoma metastatic to regional nodes was resected. Getaz et al.[13] also reported that 1 of 24 patients (4.2%) with a thyroid carcinoma had complete disappearance of a nodule in response to thyroid hormone, as judged by physical examination and ^{123}I scintillation scan. Surgery was recommended to a large number of patients in this study (61 of 85 [71.8%]), only 9.8% (6 of 85) of whom eventually were shown to have thyroid carcinoma. There is almost no information concerning the potential adverse effects of long delays in diagnosis when thyroid hormone suppression is used diagnostically. Relatively short delays in diagnosis do not alter outcome with papillary thyroid carcinoma,[2] but this may not apply to longer postponement or more aggressive tumors.

Thyroid hormone therapy itself is not entirely innocuous. When doses sufficient to suppress TSH are used, it may cause symptoms of thyrotoxicosis. Badillo et al.[10] reported that 53% of their patients treated daily with 75 µg of liothyronine reported symptoms of thyrotoxicosis consisting of tremor, palpitation, nervousness, sweating, heat intolerance, or weight loss of 2.2 lbs or more.

Evidence Against the Use of Thyroid Hormone for the Long-Term Management of Thyroid Nodules

Although thyroid hormone frequently is used over an extended period to suppress nodular growth or to prevent the appearance of new nodules after thyroidectomy, there is scant evidence that it is actually efficacious in this regard. Table 7 summarizes the data from four careful studies[3,7-9] that address this issue. Three of the four are prospective, randomized studies, two of which were controlled with placebos. Although the endpoints in each study differ, nodule size or goiter volume were measured carefully with ultrasonography during thyroid hormone suppression. It is apparent from Table 7 that new nodules appeared with the same frequency, or that the nodule or goiter volume changes were the same, both with and without thyroid hormone suppression. Thus, carefully controlled studies raise serious questions as to the efficacy of long-term thyroid hormone suppression of thyroid nodules or goiters.

The recent report by Gharib et al.[3] is particularly revealing in this regard. These investigators studied 53 patients with solitary colloid nodules confirmed by FNB who were randomly assigned in a double-blind manner to receive placebo or L-thyroxine for 6 months. High-resolution ultrasonography was used to measure the size of the nodules, while suppression of TSH release was confirmed by a thyrotropin-releasing hormone (TRH) test. They found that 6 months of therapy did not significantly decrease the diameter or volume of the nodules in the treated group as compared with the placebo group (Fig 1). There is no compelling evidence that therapy for longer periods will have a more favorable outcome.

Some have suggested that patients previously exposed to head or neck irradiation may represent a special group in regard to long-term thyroid

TABLE 7.
Response to Thyroid Hormone Following Thyroidectomy of Fine-Needle Biopsy (FNB) in Clinically Euthyroid Patients*

Author	Persson				Hegedus		Gharib		McGowen	
Type of study	Retrospective/nonrandomized after thyroidectomy				Prospective/randomized after thyroidectomy		Prospective/randomized/blinded/placebo after FNB		Prospective/randomized/blinded/placebo after FNB	
Endpoint measured	New thyroid nodules				Thyroid volume		Change in nodule size		Cyst recurrence	
Therapeutic groups	L-T$_4$ Continuous	L-T$_4$ Initially	None	All Groups	L-T$_4$ Continuously	None	L-T$_4$	Placebo	L-T$_4$/L-T$_3$	Placebo
Number of patients	138	30	29	197	52	58	28	25	10	10
Age (average years)	NA†	NA	NA	52	40	40	42	48.2	45.3	39.9
Male/Female	NA	NA	NA	31/166	6/46	6/52	2/26	3/22	4/6	2/8
(%) female	—	—	—	(84%)	(88%)	(90%)	(93%)	(88%)	(60%)	(80%)
Diagnosis n(%)										
Multinodular	NA	NA	NA	155 (79%)	21 (19.1%)	21 (19.1%)	0	0	0	0
Solitary Nodule‡	NA	NA	NA	42 (21%)	22 (20%)	28 (20%)	28 (100%)§	25 (100%)§	0	0
Diffuse goiter	NA	NA	NA	—	3 (2.7%)	3 (2.7%)	0	0	0	0
Cyst	NA	NA	NA	—	6 (5.5%)	6 (5.5%)	0	0	10 (100%)	10 (100%)
Follow-up (years)	5	6	4.2	5	1	1	0.5	0.5	10 months	9 months
New nodules										
Number	8¶	2	1	11	NA	NA	NA	NA	6¶	5
Percent	(5.8)	(6.7)	(3.5)	(5.6)	—	—	—	—	(60)	(50)
Thyroid/nodule volume change (average mL)	NA	NA	NA	NA	2¶	3	0.5¶	0.2	NA	NA

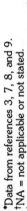

*Data from references 3, 7, 8, and 9.

†NA = not applicable or not stated.

‡Solitary by physical exam, none were hyperfunctional.

§All were colloid nodules by fine-needle biopsy, but by ultrasonography 43% were solid, 38% were solid with cystic spaces, 19% were primarily cystic, and 49% had multiple nodules.

¶Not statistically different (*P* = n.s.) compared to no treatment or placebo therapy.

hormone suppression. However, in a study of 42 previously irradiated patients with thyroid abnormalities, DeGroot et al.[14] found that the thyroid abnormality disappeared in 13 of 34 (38%) who were given thyroid hormone, compared with 5 of 8 (63%) who experienced complete regression of their abnormality without therapy. The situation may be different in patients with the elevated serum TSH concentrations that are sometimes seen following x-ray therapy. In addition to efficacy, the other main problem with long-term thyroid hormone treatment of thyroid nodules is the possibility of occult thyrotoxicosis.

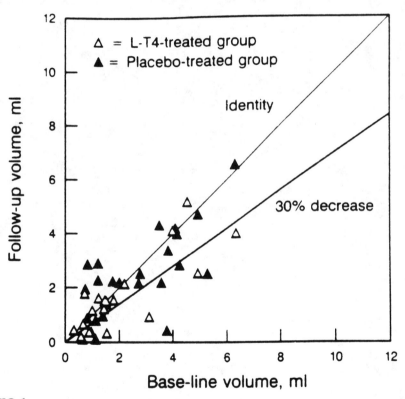

FIG 1.
Nodule volume at follow-up ultrasonography in relation to volume at baseline in 28 L-thyroxine–treated and 25 placebo-treated patients. Both the line of identity and that showing a hypothetical 30% decrease in size serve as reference lines and are not fitted to the data. Some of the *open triangles* represent more than one patient. (From Gharib H, James EM, Charboneau J, et al: *N Engl J Med* 1987; 317:70–75. Used by permission.)

The Danger of Subclinical Thyrotoxicosis During Long-term Thyroid Hormone Suppressive Therapy

The explicit goal of L-thyroxine therapy in the management of thyroid nodules is to suppress serum TSH concentrations. This raises questions about the dosage of thyroid hormone necessary to achieve this goal, the proper thyroid function test to monitor, and the long-term consequences of TSH suppression, particularly in elderly patients who are prone to develop thyroid nodules.

Controversy exists over which thyroid function test, or battery of tests, is most appropriate for monitoring patients being treated with L-thyroxine.[15] Although the availability of new, sensitive TSH assays has sharpened the monitoring of L-thyroxine therapy, this test also has increased the awareness of the potential for subclinical thyrotoxicosis in patients being treated with L-thyroxine. However, the significance of TSH suppression in patients taking L-thyroxine remains controversial. The main question is whether TSH suppression always signals subclinical thyrotoxicosis. In patients taking L-thyroxine, when the serum TSH is undetectable, both the serum total thyroxine (T_4) and total triiodothyronine (T_3) may be elevated, T_4 alone may be high, or both may be normal. In others, the serum TSH may be low but detectable, while both T_4 and T_3 are normal. There is evidence that all these thyroid function test permutations indicate various degrees of subclinical thyrotoxicosis.[15] Before considering the evidence for thyrotoxicosis during L-thyroxine therapy, the dosage of L-thyroxine necessary to suppress serum TSH concentrations should be considered.

Fish et al.[16] assessed the replacement dosage of L-thyroxine in hypothyroid patients by titrating the dose at monthly intervals using 25-μg increments until the serum TSH fell into the same range as normal controls. The mean replacement L-thyroxine dosage used to achieve these results was 112 ± 19 μg/day (or 1.63 ± 0.42 μg/kg/day), which was significantly less than the dose of an earlier formulation of thyroid hormone (169 ± 66 μg/day) used in a similar study by these authors.[16] The median replacement L-thyroxine dosage was 125 μg per day, and all patients required between 75 and 150 μg per day of L-thyroxine to normalize serum TSH concentrations. When the serum TSH fell within the normal limits, patients taking L-thyroxine had serum free T_4 concentrations significantly above those for euthyroid controls (Fig 2). The mean free thyroxine index in the treated hypothyroid patients was 11.3 ± 1.5 μg/dL compared with 8.7 ± 1.1 μg/dL for controls ($P < .001$). At the same time, serum T_3 concentrations were not significantly different in the two groups. When TSH suppression is the endpoint, even greater doses of L-thyroxine are required, and free hormone concentrations are raised even more. There is evidence that this results in subclinical thyrotoxicosis.

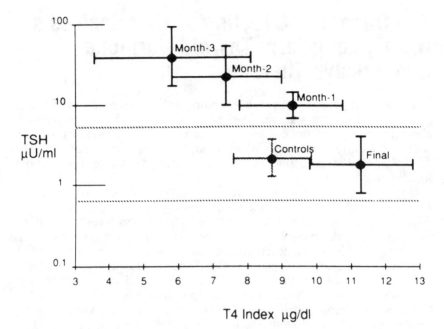

FIG 2.
Free thyroxine index in controls and in patients during months of titration, as a function of TSH concentration. Values are expressed by month, counting backward from the final dose. The *bars* represent 1 SD from the mean; the normal range lies between the *hatched lines*. (From Fish LH, Schwartz HL, Cavanaugh J, et al: *N Engl J Med* 1987; 316:764–770. Used by permission.)

Bartalena et al.[17] evaluated 452 clinically euthyroid patients, 272 of whom had diffuse or nontoxic nodular goiters. TSH suppression required L-thyroxine dosages between 1.9 and 2.3 µg/kg/day in goitrous patients (compared with 1.63 ± 0.42 µg/kg/day in the study by Fish et al.[16]). The L-thyroxine dosage associated with an undetectable basal serum TSH, without a TSH rise in response to TRH, averaged 2.1 ± 0.3 µg/kg/day. Younger patients required higher doses of L-thyroxine than did older patients. During thyroid hormone replacement, serum thyroid hormone concentrations were significantly higher ($P < .001$) than normal.* Of the goitrous patients with suppressed serum TSH concentrations, almost one half had both free T_4 and free T_3 indexes or free T_4 alone above the normal limits. Thus, there is good documentation that patients in whom serum TSH is suppressed require

*In this study, the mean serum total T_4 was 18.4 ± 4.7 µg/dL (normal 9.5 ± 2.1), the free T_4 was 18.4 ± 4.7 pg/mL (normal 9.5 ± 2.1), the free T_4 index was 12.1 ± 3.1 (normal 7.5 ± 1.3), the total T_3 was 174 ng/dL (normal 159 ± 28), the free T_3 was 4.9 ± 1.6 pg/mL (normal 4.0 ± 0.8), and the free T_3 index was 186 ± 48 (normal 156 ± 21), all of which were significantly higher ($P < .001$) than normal.

substantially higher than normal L-thyroxine doses and often have clearly elevated serum thyroid hormone concentrations.

There is mounting proof that there are physiological consequences of subclinical thyrotoxicosis in patients being treated with thyroid hormone. Ross[15] recently reviewed the evidence that patients being treated with thyroid hormone often have physiological abnormalities consistent with thyrotoxicosis, including an elevated heart rate, shortened systolic time intervals, a reduced isovolumetric contraction time, increases in sex-hormone binding globulin, a rise in liver enzymes and creatine kinase, and other occult biochemical abnormalities typical of thyrotoxicosis. Perhaps most unsettling is the possibility that osteoporosis may occur with greater than usual frequency in patients receiving long-term L-thyroxine therapy. Ettinger and Wingerd[18] retrospectively studied 151 hypothyroid women taking thyroid hormone and found that the use of 3 or 4 grains of desiccated thyroid daily was associated with a lower combined cortical thickness of the second metacarpal bone than the use of 1 or 2 grains daily ($P < .01$). The free T_4 index was inversely related to the combined cortical thickness, but this relation was not linear.

Ross and associates[19] retrospectively studied 28 white premenopausal women with regular menses who had taken L-thyroxine for 5 or more years. Thyroid hormone had been prescribed to shrink goitrous thyroid tissue or to prevent the growth of abnormal thyroid tissue. Eleven had Hashimoto's thyroiditis, 5 had multinodular goiters, 7 had solitary nodules, 4 had papillary or follicular thyroid carcinoma, and 1 had a lingual thyroid. Their mean serum total T_4 was 13.5 ± 2.6 µg/dL (normal 8.0 ± 2.4), their free T_4 index was 4.4 ± 1.0 (normal 2.4 ± 0.8), and their serum T_3 concentration was 154 ± 26 ng/dL (normal 132 ± 32). Basal TSH was undetectable (< 0.08 µU/mL) in 23 patients, did not rise after TRH in 13 patients, and rose only slightly in 10 patients. The bone mineral density of the nondominant radius was determined by direct photon absorptiometry. Women who had taken L-thyroxine for 10 or more years and who average 37 ± 4 years of age had a 9% reduction in bone density ($P < .01$) compared with normal premenopausal age-matched control subjects averaging 35 ± 6 years of age (Fig 3). These authors concluded that prolonged suppressive therapy with L-thyroxine may result in mild subclinical thyrotoxicosis with adverse effects on bone.

Paul and associates[20] retrospectively studied axial skeleton bone density in 31 postmenopausal clinically euthyroid women who had been treated with L-thyroxine for a minimum of 5 years for hypothyroidism, thyroid carcinoma, or the suppression of nontoxic goiter. Bone densities in these women were compared with those of 31 age- and weight-matched controls. Compared with controls, women being treated with thyroid hormone had significantly higher ($P < .001$) serum total T_4 concentrations (10.4 ± 0.4 vs. 7.4 ± 0.2 µg/dL) and serum free T_4 indexes (9.4 ± 0.4 vs. 6.8 ± 0.2), and significantly lower ($P < .001$) serum TSH concentrations (0.9 ± 0.2 vs. 2.1

± 0.3 µU/mL). Bone density in women being treated with L-thyroxine (Fig 4) was 12.8% lower at the femoral neck and 10.1% lower at the femoral trochanter compared with controls, but lumbar spine bone density was the same in both groups. The authors concluded that long-term L-thyroxine therapy may predispose women to decreased bone density at the hip and may increase the risk of age-related bone loss.

While not the result of prospective randomized trials, these data are nonetheless alarming, considering that the majority of patients with thyroid nodules are postmenopausal women. It is clear that TSH suppression requires larger than normal replacement doses of L-thyroxine, and that this commonly results in abnormal thyroid function tests and subclinical thyrotoxicosis in many patients. This potential risk, in my view, far outweighs the possible benefit of long-term thyroid hormone suppression in patients with benign thyroid disease.

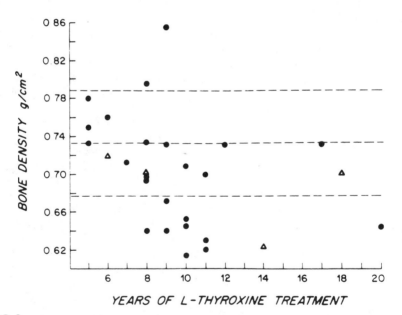

FIG 3.
Bone density in 28 premenopausal women taking L-thyroxine for 5 or more years. The normal mean ± the standard deviation (SD) for bone density in premenopausal women is indicated by the *dashed lines*. Patients with absent or subnormal responses of serum TSH concentration to the intravenous administration of TRH are indicated by *circles*, and women with normal TSH responses to TRH are indicated by *triangles*. (From Ross DS, Neer RM, Ridgway EC, et al: *Am J Med* 1987; 82:1167–1170. Used by permission.)

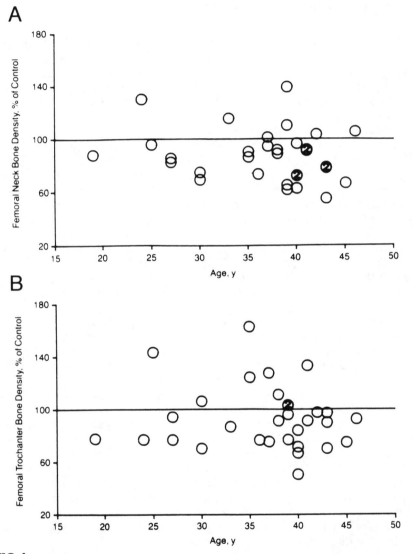

FIG 4.
Bone density in L-thyroxine–treated women plotted as percentage of bone density in age- and weight-matched controls. **A,** femoral neck bone density was lower in 74% of treated women compared with controls. **B,** femoral trochanter bone density was lower in 71% of treated women compared with controls. *Numbers within circles* indicate the number of patients with that bone density. (From Paul TL, Kerrigan J, Kelly AM, et al: *JAMA* 1988; 259:3137–3141. Used by permission.)

Conclusion

There is considerable theoretical and actual evidence against using thyroid hormone suppression of TSH for either the diagnosis or the long-term management of benign thyroid nodules in euthyroid patients. The basic premise that the growth of benign nodular thyroid tissue is dependent upon TSH stimulation may be flawed. Both in vivo and in vitro observations support the contention that TSH is not the principal factor promoting the growth of benign thyroid nodules.

As a diagnostic test, thyroid hormone suppression is clearly inferior to FNB. Although both techniques are equally sensitive in the diagnosis of thyroid cancer, thyroid hormone suppression has a much lower specificity than FNB (20% vs. 80%). The posttest probability of cancer if a nodule is nonsuppressible with L-thyroxine (a positive test) is much lower than that with FNB yielding malignant or suspicious cytology (11% vs. 34%). The ultimate cost of diagnosis using thyroid hormone suppression as the initial diagnostic test is much greater than with FNB because of the large number of positive tests with suppression. To excise all thyroid cancers detected each year in the United States, the total cost would be over $15.5 million using thyroid hormone suppression as the first diagnostic test, compared with about $4 million using FNB.

Considerable evidence supports the fact that larger than normal doses of L-thyroxine are necessary to suppress serum TSH concentrations, resulting in abnormal thyroid function tests in most patients. There is mounting proof that this results in subclinical thyrotoxicosis, which has potentially serious long-term consequences. The most important of these is accelerated bone loss resulting in osteoporosis, a particularly worrisome issue since so many thyroid nodules occur in postmenopausal women.

There is no evidence from properly controlled, prospective studies using modern techniques such as ultrasonography to indicate that long-term thyroid hormone suppression is more effective than placebo therapy in shrinking or preventing thyroid nodules or goiters in euthyroid patients. Benign thyroid nodules pose virtually no risk to the patient, while chronic thyroid hormone suppression therapy has potential long-term hazards. Thyroid hormone therapy should be reserved for patients with either hypothyroidism or differentiated thyroid cancers (these patients show lower recurrence rates with TSH suppression).[11]

Thus, considered in light of diagnostic accuracy and cost, the evidence weighs heavily against the routine use of thyroid hormone in the diagnostic evaluation of thyroid nodules. In addition, the potentially serious risks of long-term L-thyroxine therapy far outweigh its meager benefits in patients with benign nodular thyroid disease. Because of this, I believe the routine use of thyroid hormone in the management of euthyroid patients with benign nodular disease should be abandoned.

References

1. Rojeski M, Gharib H: Nodular thyroid disease: Evaluation and management. *N Engl J Med* 1988; 313:428–35. *A comprehensive review of the diagnosis and management of thyroid nodules is presented.*

2. Mazzaferri EL, de los Santos E, Keyhani SR: Solitary thyroid nodule: Diagnosis and management. *Med Clin North Am* 1988; 72:1178–1211. *This is a comprehensive review of the pathology, diagnosis and management of thyroid nodules.*

3. Gharib H, James EM, Charboneau J, et al: Suppressive therapy with levothyroxine for solitary thyroid nodules. *N Engl J Med* 1987; 317:70–75. *A prospective, randomized, placebo-controlled study of thyroid hormone suppression of colloid thyroid nodules is reported.*

4. Molitch ME, Beck JR, Dreisman M, et al: The cold thyroid nodule: An analysis of diagnostic and therapeutic options. *Endocr Rev* 1984; 5:185–199. *This report presents a decision analysis review of the diagnosis of thyroid nodules.*

5. Ashcraft MW, van Herle AJ: Management of thyroid nodules. 1:History and physical examination, blood tests, x-ray tests, and ultrasonography. *Head Neck Surg* 1981; 1:216–227. *A comprehensive review of the world literature on the diagnosis of thyroid nodules is given.*

6. Westermark B, Karlsson FA, Walinder O: Thyrotropin is not a growth factor for human thyroid cells in culture. *Proc Natl Acad Sci USA* 1979; 76:2022–2026. *This study shows that TSH does not promote thyroid cell growth in vitro.*

7. Person CP, Johanson HJ, Westermark K, et al: Nodular goiter — is thyroxine medication of any value? *World J Surg* 1982; 6:391–396. *This is a retrospective study showing that L-thyroxine does not alter the appearance of new thyroid nodules following thyroidectomy.*

8. Hegedus L, Hansen JM, Veiergang D, et al: Does prophylactic thyroxine treatment after operation for non-toxic goiter influence thyroid size? *Br Med J* 1987; 294:801–803. *This is a prospective study showing that L-thyroxine does not alter the growth of the thyroid remnant following subtotal thyroidectomy.*

9. McCowen KD, Reed JW, Fariss BL: The role of thyroid therapy in patients with thyroid cysts. *Am J Med* 1980; 68:853–855. *This study shows that L-thyroxine does not alter the recurrence patterns of thyroid cysts.*

10. Badillo J, Shimaoka K, Lessmann EM, et al: Treatment of nontoxic goiter with sodium liothyronine. *JAMA* 1963; 184:29–36. *This is an early placebo-controlled study of thyroid suppression with liothyronine.*

11. Mazzaferri EL, Young RL, Oertel JE, et al: Papillary thyroid carcinoma: The impact of therapy in 576 patients. *Medicine* 1977; 56:171–196. *This is a retrospective study of a large cohort of patients showing that thyroid hormone therapy may influence the growth of papillary thyroid carcinoma.*

12. Hill LD, Beebe HG, Hipp R, et al: Thyroid suppression. *Arch Surg* 1974; 108:403–405. *A retrospective review showing that thyroid carcinoma may initially shrink in response to thyroid hormone suppression is presented.*

13. Getaz EP, Shimaoka K, Razack M, et al: Suppressive therapy for postirradiation thyroid nodules. *Can J Surg* 1980; 23:558–560. *This is a study of thyroid hormone suppression in patients previously exposed to head or neck external irradiation.*

14. DeGroot LJ, Reilly M, Rinnameneni K, et al: Retrospective and prospective study of radiation-induced thyroid disease. *Am J Med* 1983; 74:852–862. *This is a study of thyroid hormone suppression in patients previously exposed to head or neck irradiation.*

15. Ross DS: Subclinical hyperthyroidism: Possible danger of overzealous thyroxine replacement therapy. *Mayo Clin Proc* 1988; 63:1223–1229. *A careful review of the physiological effects of subclinical thyrotoxicosis resulting from L-thyroxine replacement therapy is included.*

16. Fish LH, Schwartz HL, Cavanaugh J, et al: Replacement dose, metabolism, and bioavailability of levothyroxine in the treatment of hypothyroidism. *N Engl J Med* 1987; 316:764–770. *This is a recent review of the usual replacement dosage of L-thyroxine in the treatment of hypothyroidism.*

17. Bartalena L, Martino E, Pacchiarotti A, et al: Factors affecting suppression of endogenous thyrotropin secretion by thyroxine treatment: Retrospective analysis in athyreotic and goitrous patients. *J Clin Endocrinol Metab* 1987; 64:849–855. *This is a retrospective study of the L-thyroxine dosage and thyroid function tests in patients being treated with thyroid hormone.*

18. Ettinger B, Wingerd J: Thyroid supplements: Effect on bone mass. *West J Med* 1982; 6:473–476. *A retrospective review of the effects of thyroid hormone on the metacarpal bone cortical thickness is presented.*

19. Ross DS, Neer RM, Ridgway EC, et al: Subclinical hyperthyroidism and reduced bone density as a possible result of prolonged suppression of the pituitary-thyroid axis with L-Thyroxine. *Am J Med* 1987; 82:1167–1170. *This is a retrospective review of bone density in women treated long-term with L-thyroxine.*

20. Paul TL, Kerrigan J, Kelly AM, et al: Long-term L-Thyroxine therapy is associated with decreased hip bone density in premenopausal women. *JAMA* 1988; 259:3137–3141. *A retrospective review of bone density in women treated with L-thyroxine is provided.*

Rebuttal: Affirmative

Manfred Blum, M.D.
Don Zwickler, M.D.

While we strive for the ideal or perfect answer to a problem in clinical medicine, we rarely find it. In the issue of the diagnosis and management of patients with a thyroid nodule, we do not see a competition between two opposing views: fine-needle biopsy (FNB) vs. the use of thyroid hormone. Rather, we submit that there is a need to use the available diagnostic and therapeutic tools in concert and safely.

Dr. Mazzaferri has taken the point of view that "The routine use of thyroid hormone in the management of euthyroid patients with benign nodular disease should be abandoned." He feels that we should rely only on the results of FNB. In contrast, our analysis of the currently available data suggests a moderate approach. Thyroid hormone continues to be useful in diagnosis when FNB cannot be used or gives equivocal or imperfect results, and in long-term management.

We feel that it is not appropriate to abandon the use of suppressive therapy for five reasons: (1) thyrotropin (TSH) *is* a growth factor for thyroid cells and tumors that is reciprocally responsive to thyroid hormone; (2) this therapy remains essential in the management of thyroid carcinoma, a situation that cannot be unequivocally excluded by FNB in patients with a solitary nodule or even multiple nodules; (3) some thyroid nodules shrink during suppressive therapy and by and large those are benign; (4) we suspect that without suppressive therapy, the slow growth of nodules and goiters (especially after surgery) over the years will result in a considerable population of patients with large thyroid masses and goiters that will require surgery in the future, as was the case years ago before thyroid therapy was used; and (5) when FNB does not show malignancy, then growth of a thyroid mass when TSH is suppressed should alert the clinician to the possibility of tumor and the need to reconsider management.

It is prudent, as it always has been, to select patients for this therapy rather than to employ it routinely, and to avoid untoward effects. The patient should not be permitted to become significantly thyrotoxic; the clinical state, TSH (by the new sensitive assays), and T_4 should be monitored when suppression is used. Furthermore, a prospective, properly controlled study is needed to see if osteoporosis is a consequence of cautious suppressive therapy.

185

Even if TSH Is Not the Sole Growth-Promoting Factor for Thyroid Cells, It Is One of the Factors, Especially for Thyroid Cancer

The data suggesting that TSH is not a potent growth factor are seriously flawed. As discussed by Dr. Mazzaferri, Westermark and others[1] reported in 1979 that thyrotropin is not a growth factor in human thyroid cells when examined in vitro in tissue culture. They showed that TSH reduced ^{3}H thymidine incorporation and the proliferation of thyroid cells but not of glial cells. The TSH, which was impure, did not have zero effect, it had a negative effect. Yet the cells "maintained a thyrotropin-sensitive adenylate cyclase system." The observations are interesting, but their relevance to a balanced, living organism is unclear and recent observations give new perspective. Perhaps TSH by itself is not a sufficient growth factor. It has been recognized that other factors, including IgF-1, exert a necessary synergistic role with TSH. Investigations are in progress to examine the growth-stimulating ability of TSH at a molecular level.[2-4] Furthermore, the carefully designed study by Matte strongly supports the in vivo growth-promoting effect of TSH after hemithyroidectomy.[5]

A. B. Schneider and his group reported at the 1988 meeting of the American Thyroid Association that therapy with thyroid hormone is effective in reducing the recurrence of benign thyroid lesions in patients with a history of exposure to therapeutic x-ray after surgery for benign thyroid nodules. Recurrences while the patients took suppressive therapy had an increased likelihood of being malignant. Most importantly, Lindsay and Chaikoff[6,7] and others subsequently demonstrated the enhanced growth of thyroid tumors under the influence of elevated TSH and the prevention of tumor growth when TSH was suppressed with thyroid hormone in vivo. This was shown first in the Long-Evans strain of rats and then in several other species. Thus, even if the preparation of TSH used had an isolated negative effect in vitro on the proliferation of benign thyroid cells in a defined tissue culture, it is difficult to challenge that TSH has a trophic role in vivo in thyroid nodules and especially in thyroid cancers, which are the subject of our major concern. We believe that this concept may translate into patient management in the case of patients who appear to have a benign nodule on FNB but, in fact, have an undetected thyroid malignancy. In this group, TSH suppression is a reasonable adjunct to needle biopsy.

There Is Need for a Multifaceted Approach

In defending his position, Dr. Mazzaferri emphasizes a comparison between FNB and suppressive therapy with respect to specificity, diagnostic yield, and long-term consequences. In the short term, FNB appears to be more cost-effective and superior to suppressive therapy as a diagnostic tool. There is no reason to doubt that contention when the aspiration is performed and interpreted properly and leads to a diagnosis of cancer. However, since thyroid cancer is rare and slow-growing, the outcome may not be known for many years when cancer is not found at the time of FNB. In the long term, unfortunately, we must devote a considerable portion of our attention to those patients with a negative biopsy because there are so many of them and a few do have cancer. Repeated FNB at intervals is part of the answer. However, we contend that thyroid suppression is another important aspect. It is helpful diagnostically in confirming the results of cytology when the condition is benign and shrinks. More importantly, it can alert the clinician to the possibility of an erroneous diagnosis when a nodule grows in spite of suppressive therapy. False-negative results do occur with FNB when there is a solitary nodule, and it is perilous for the patient and physician to ignore that.

There are questions about FNB that have not been answered to our satisfaction. Its accuracy, specificity, and utility has been determined mainly from studies in which there was a solitary nodule in an otherwise completely normal gland. There are meager data that validate the technique when there is a dominant nodule in a multinodular thyroid. In this situation, many clinicians perform the procedure for purposes of reassurance and usually are rewarded with equivocal or suspicious results. We also are not sure about the accuracy of FNB in average rather than in highly expert clinical hands.

We make no claim that all nodules shrink or that FNB is not a considerable diagnostic advance. Rather, we just do not see any reason to abandon something that we think has been useful.

The Efficiency of Suppressive Therapy

Analysis of the numerous studies that have examined the efficiency of suppressive therapy in shrinking nodules is difficult, confusing, and open to interpretation. We agree with Dr. Mazzaferri that an assessment of thyroid size on clinical grounds is inadequate and that high-resolution ultrasound is more accurate and objective. We also agree that the lack of uniformity of suppressive regimens precludes a definitive analysis of these data. However, we are not convinced by the conclusions that were drawn from the Gharib et al. analysis of the situation, as discussed previously.[8] We are concerned about the adequacy of the therapy and long-term compliance as well as about the inclusion of nodules that appear to be autonomous and therefore are not expected to shrink with suppressive therapy. We previously have addressed the possible effect on outcome of differences between the protocols that use thyroxine or triiodothyronine as the suppressive agent. We reiterate that we do not advocate the use of triiodothyronine for long-term management, and that even a "flat" thyrotropin-releasing hormone (TRH) test at one point in time does not necessarily reflect long-term patient compliance.

We are concerned about, but not strongly moved by, the concept that carcinoma initially may shrink with suppression only to regrow later and lead to a dangerous delay in diagnosis. The decision analysis that was reported by Molitch substantially put that issue to rest; morbidity and mortality are unrelated to the approach used in diagnosing thyroid nodules, whether it be suppressive therapy, FNB followed by suppressive therapy, or direct surgery.[9] Furthermore, in this scenario the easily diagnosable cancers would have been uncovered by FNB and, without suppressive therapy, the ones that were "missed" by aspiration might have escaped rapid detection among the many enlarging benign nodules being followed.

The argument that thyroid hormone that is administered for months to a year does not influence the size of a nodule is not persuasive either, since the growth of thyroid nodules is slow. To demonstrate the effect of thyroid hormone in preventing significant growth could take many years. If one considers a 20-year-old patient with a small nodule, the effect of thyroid medication may not be detected even after 5 or 10 years. A demonstrable therapeutic effect in preventing growth may not be observable until 30 or more years later, well within the life expectancy of the individual. Is it appropriate to do a yearly FNB on all those people? Are there enough cytologists for that? Will patients allow it, or even return for observation? There is also uncertainty about long-term suppressive therapy. However, we already have experience with that treatment, know that it can be done, and know what precautions to take. Furthermore, we suspect that treatment with thyroid hormone and careful regulation of the dose would be more likely to motivate patients to submit to regular medical visits than would observation without medication.

Slow Growth of Untreated Nodules May Lead to an Increased Need for Thyroid Surgery in the Elderly

Another aspect of the question relates to the behavior of benign thyroid nodules. It appears to be the natural course of events that these nodules enlarge slowly over many years. One may question whether progressive, slow growth of a thyroid nodule or a multinodular goiter over many years could escape detection during the brief period of one physician's observation. We also do not know if there will be an increased incidence of sudden, obstructing thyroid hemorrhage without suppressive therapy. The use of the medication would remove the variable of TSH as a growth factor. The growth of a nodule when TSH is not suppressed may be a functional event, while growth in the absence of TSH is more likely to be an indication of neoplasia, either benign or malignant. There is reasonable clinical evidence that thyroid hormone can retard that tendency, thereby reducing the need for surgical intervention late in life, or at another inopportune time, when obstruction of the thoracic inlet may occur. We do not know how often this will occur, but we do know that huge nodules and goiters were more common in the past than they are now. While it is possible that the natural history of thyroid disorders has changed for other reasons, we submit that the most likely pertinent variable is the recent widespread use of suppressive therapy with thyroid hormone.

Ideally, a long-term (perhaps 30 or more years), prospective, double-blind, randomized study, using a large number of patients with nonfunctioning nodules that are cytologically benign would be necessary to validate the use of diagnostic and therapeutic suppressive therapy. However, priorities are such that this investigation is not likely to take place. In its absence, it is reasonable to look retrospectively with a critical and analytical eye, and to recall the great number of patients with very large thyroid masses who were seen previously, a problem rarely encountered during the past decade. Our concern should not be only the immediate cost-effectiveness of needle biopsy as the solitary diagnostic tool. Rather we must be mindful also of the long-term implications of a global approach to patient management and of the undesirable and costly potential of large thyroid masses and surgery, if it were to turn out that suppressive therapy was effective after all.

Can We Tolerate the Risks of Suppressive Therapy?

The consideration of risks and benefits always has been integral to medical management. We have been cognizant of the cardiovascular risks. The use of suppressive therapy has been tempered in the elderly and in those with heart disease. The potential for osteoporosis expands our criteria for treating cautiously, rather than for abandoning treatment. A recent review of the literature by Wartofsky[10] offers worthy criticisms of the publications that were discussed by Dr. Mazzaferri and reflects our views on the subject. Central to the issue is that clinical hyperthyroidism may be associated with decreased density of the bone mineral, especially cortical bone. It is not clear if this defect occurs even with moderate over-replacement of thyroid hormone. The risk of bone fracture does not appear to be increased in these patients.[11,12]

Summary

We conclude from an analysis of the available information that the prudent diagnostic approach to a patient with a solitary thyroid nodule is FNB and surgery if malignancy is found. When FNB is not permitted, cannot be done, or gives equivocal results, suppressive therapy continues to play a role because TSH is a growth factor, especially for cancer. The growth of a presumed benign mass when TSH is suppressed should lead to reconsideration of the diagnosis and altered management. It is our concern that abandoning suppressive diagnostic therapy and long-term management may eventuate in large thyroid growths and avoidable surgery late in life. However, the treatment must be monitored carefully. For patients who have had malignant thyroid disease, we employ the least amount of thyroid hormone that suppresses TSH and for those with benign disorders or indefinite diagnoses, thyrotoxicosis should be avoided. Given these precautions, we believe that (1) few, if any, clinically significant thyroid carcinomas will be missed; (2) thyroid carcinomas that escape detection by the initial FNB will be discovered in a timely fashion; (3) the slow growth of thyroid nodules and goiters during the life of a patient will be minimized; (4) needless surgery in the elderly will be avoided; (5) there probably will be no appreciable change in bone mineral density and, almost certainly, no increased incidence of fractures; and (6) long-term cost-effectiveness will be achieved. We submit that this approach should be continued unless clear evidence of a serious adverse effect is uncovered.

References

1. Westermark B, Karlsson FA, Walinder O: Thyrotropin is not a growth factor in human thyroid cells in culture. *Proc Natl Acad Sci USA* 1979; 76:2022–2026.
2. Tramontano D, Chin WW, Moses AC, et al: Thyrotropin and dibutyryl cyclic amp increases levels of c-myc and c-fos MRNA in cultured rat thyroid cells. *J Biol Chem* 1986; 261:3919.
3. Tramontano D, et al: Insulin-like growth factor I stimulates the growth of rat thyroid cells in culture and the stimulation of DNA synthesis induced by TSH and Graves' 1g6. *Endocrinology* 1986; 119:340.
4. Yamashita S, Ong J, Fagin JA, et al: Expression of the myc cellular proto-oncogene in human thyroid tissue. *JCEM* 1986; 63:1170.
5. Matte R, Ste-Marie LG, Comtois R, et al: The pituitary thyroid axis after hemithyroidectomy in euthyroid man. *JCEM* 1981; 53:337–380.
6. Lindsay S, Chaikoff IL: The effects of irradiation on the thyroid gland with particular reference to the induction of thyroid neoplasms. A review. *Cancer Res* 1964; 24:1099.
7. Goldberg RC, Lindsay S, Nichols CW, et al: Induction of neoplasms in thyroid

glands of rats by subtotal thyroidectomy and by injection of one microcurie of I-131. *Cancer Res* 1964; 24:35–43.

8. Gharib H, James EM, Charboneau J: Suppressive therapy with levothyroxine for solitary thyroid nodules. *N Engl J Med* 1987; 317:70–75.

9. Molitch ME, Beck JR, Dreisman M, et al: The cold thyroid nodule: An analysis of diagnostic and therapeutic options. *Endocr Rev* 1984; 5:185–199.

10. Wartofsky L: Osteoporosis: A growing concern for the thyroidologist. *Thyroid Today* 1988; 4:1–11.

11. Cooper DS: Thyroid hormone and the skeleton. A bone of contention (editorial). *JAMA* 1988; 259:3175.

12. Ahmann AJ, Solomon B, Duncan WE, et al: Normal bone mineral density in premenopausal women on suppressive doses of 1-thyroxine (abstracted). Presented at the Annual Meeting of the American Thyroid Association, 1987.

Rebuttal: Negative
Ernest L. Mazzaferri, M.D.

Drs. Blum and Zwickler conclude that fine-needle biopsy (FNB) is very useful in the diagnosis of the solitary "cold" nodule, pointing out that it may be the only procedure required to establish the correct diagnosis of malignancy, a supposition with which I completely concur. They emphasize that FNB has certain limitations, an assertion which is true. Beyond these broad points, however, our opinions regarding the diagnosis of thyroid nodules diverge substantially.

I would take issue with several of their arguments regarding the limitations of FNB. That sampling errors occur, especially with small nodules or those that are very large, hemorrhagic, or deep in the neck, is well appreciated and simply must be taken into account when attempting to perform FNB or interpret cytology results. Like any procedure, an appreciation of its limitations only enhances its usefulness. Drs. Blum and Zwickler argue that results are suboptimal when FNB is performed by clinicians who are not "experts," and that the results often are inconclusive when interpreted by inexperienced cytologists. While there is certainly some truth to this, the implication that only experts at large referral hospitals can use this technique effectively simply is not accurate. When the technique was first widely publicized in this country, its proponents offered the admonition that adequate proficiency was necessary at the institutions utilizing the technique, advice with which one can hardly disagree.[1] Initially, it was suggested that to gain adequate proficiency in FNB, each operator should perform 100 to 200 biopsies for familiarization, followed by not less than 10 biopsy specimens each week, or about 500 biopsies a year — a truly gargantuan experience.[1] Few medical centers satisfy these criteria. Moreover, the efficacy of FNB in smaller institutions performing substantially fewer biopsies has been well established. Asp and his associates[2] reviewed their experience at Fitzsimons Army Medical Center, a 550-bed teaching hospital, where 155 biopsy specimens were obtained over 3½ years. In their hands, the sensitivity of FNB was 100%, the specificity was 47.4%, and the accuracy was 73%. They found the surgical yield to be 26% in those who underwent surgery without FNB compared to 64% in patients evaluated with this technique. Nowadays it can hardly be argued that FNB is such a specialized technique that only a relatively few large referral centers can use it effectively.

Drs. Blum and Zwickler argue further that there is a high number of nonspecific results from FNB, and that uncertainty exists about the management of nodules that yield suspicious cytology. They refer to nonspecific, suspicious, and inconclusive cytology results. However, they fail to distin-

192

guish clearly between *inadequate* and *suspicious* cytologic specimens. The former (generally less than about 5%) simply are specimens with inadequate material for accurate diagnosis that require repeat aspiration biopsy, while the latter imply the real possibility of cancer. More than 60% to 80% of all FNB cytologic specimens are benign, about 5% are frankly malignant, and the remainder (between 20% and 40%) are suspicious. Malignant lesions should be excised promptly, while benign lesions should be followed carefully (without thyroid hormone therapy in my view) and rebiopsied if further suspicion of malignancy arises. There is *not* uncertainty, as stated by Drs. Blum and Zwickler, regarding how nodules with suspicious cytology should be handled. Most authorities agree that lesions with suspicious cytology should be considered potentially malignant and should be excised promptly, since about 20% harbor a malignancy. There is no firm evidence from carefully controlled clinical studies that thyroid hormone suppression enhances the diagnostic accuracy in this subset of patients, as implied by Drs. Blum and Zwickler.

Drs. Blum and Zwickler express the "need to do something for a patient who cannot have a FNB or who refuses to have one." While I agree that this is a troublesome situation, one can argue, based on the data already presented, that the "something" should be careful patient counseling with conscientious follow-up.

The argument is made that clinical factors such as the patient's history, the nodule's physical characteristics, and its radioisotopic scanning properties are important in the assessment of a thyroid nodule. This certainly is a reasonable generality. However, only a few patients have clinical evidence for malignancy that is overwhelming and, for the majority, clinical evaluation alone does not adequately distinguish between malignant and benign disease. For instance, Drs. Blum and Zwickler suggest that firmness to palpation is a good physical finding suggesting malignancy in a nodule. Yet it is widely recognized that many papillary carcinomas are soft, cystic lesions, while benign adenomas are commonly quite firm lesions that sometimes even become rock-hard when they develop calcification. A thyroid gland involved with Hashimoto's thyroiditis is palpably quite firm, and may demonstrate alarming nodularity that sometimes seems to infiltrate the thyroid, or may even adhere to surrounding tissues. Thus, a nodule's physical characteristics are commonly quite misleading. Indeed, even classic findings of malignancy such as hemoptysis, tracheal compression, and hoarseness due to vocal cord paralysis can occur with benign thyroid disease.[1] The strongest argument underscoring the frailty of simple clinical assessment for diagnosing thyroid nodules is the array of tests (including thyroid hormone suppression) that have evolved over the years in an attempt to refine the diagnostic accuracy of these disorders.

In short, FNB remains the most accurate diagnostic test for thyroid nodules. It is readily available, safe, and clearly the most accurate and cost-effective means of diagnosing malignancy. For FNB to be utilized optimally, physicians must understand the procedure — not only its strengths and weaknesses, but also the technical aspects of obtaining diagnostic material. Its time has come.[3] Physicians should learn how to use FNB in the everyday practice of medicine.

Drs. Blum and Zwickler mention that there is still no consensus about the value of thyroid hormone suppression in the diagnosis of thyroid nodules. This is a strong argument *against* its efficacy, considering the many years that thyroid hormone suppression has been used in this regard. They recommend using liothyronine (T_3) for evaluating thyroid nodules, pointing out that the hormone's side effects are more evanescent that those of L-thyroxine and that symptoms abate quickly when liothyronine is withdrawn. They acknowledge, however, that it is difficult to avoid mild thyrotoxicosis in the process, and state further that mild thyrotoxicosis actually may be required during the diagnostic trial. I simply do not believe that it is proper and am not comfortable as a physician with creating one disease (albeit a minor one and probably not consequential in most younger patients) to diagnose another. Intrinsic to my concern is the fact that many patients with thyroid nodules are elderly individuals in whom even slight thyrotoxicosis may lead to atrial fibrillation, anxiety, tremors, and other irritating and noxious symptoms. Over the years, I have developed a deep respect for thyrotoxicosis in the elderly, even when it is mild and transient.

Regarding the chronic use of thyroid hormone in the management of thyroid nodules and benign goiters, Drs. Blum and Zwickler indicate that its long-term benefits and risks have not been evaluated adequately. I agree. They offer the caveat that it is prudent to avoid "very high levels of thyroid hormones," especially when treating benign disease. Again, I agree. However, if one acknowledges that the basic goal of using thyroid hormone for benign thyroid disease is to suppress TSH secretion, then avoiding high serum thyroid hormone levels is in conflict with this goal. I don't believe that the two ideas are compatible. Either TSH is suppressed effectively and the patient sustains mild chronic subclinical thyrotoxicosis with its attendant potential problems, or the suppressive therapy misses its mark and TSH remains elevated.

In summary, there is compelling evidence that FNB is the most accurate, safe, and cost-effective test to diagnose thyroid nodules. Thyroid hormone suppression as a diagnostic test is laden with problems, including arbitrary protocols, vague endpoints, and potentially serious side effects. Added to these problems is the high rate of false-positive responses and subsequent high cost of surgery which often is advised for the many patients whose nodules fail to shrink. The issue of long-term thyroid hormone suppressive therapy for euthyroid patients with benign thyroid lesions has become clouded by new and potentially serious concerns regarding its potentially harmful effects. These worrisome issues should give thoughtful clinicians considerable reluctance about prescribing long-term, and in many cases lifetime, thyroid hormone to treat benign conditions for which it may be not only ineffective, but potentially harmful.

References

1. Van Herle AJ, Rich P, Ljung BE, et al: The thyroid nodule. *Ann Intern Med* 1982; 96:221–232.
2. Asp AA, Georgitis W, Waldron EJ, et al: Fine needle aspiration of the thyroid: Use in an average health care facility. *Am J Med* 1987; 83:489–493.
3. Bottles K, Miller TR, Cohen MB, et al: Fine needle aspiration biopsy: Has its time come? *Am J Med* 1986; 81:525–531.

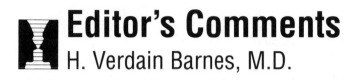

Editor's Comments
H. Verdain Barnes, M.D.

The discovery of one or more thyroid nodules is perplexing for most patients and their physicians. The most common concerns revolve around the issue of cancer and the nodule's effect or potential effect on their appearance. Although it is generally agreed that papillary, mixed papillary/follicular, and follicular thyroid carcinomas are typically slow-growing and relatively nonvirulent as malignancies, the phychological impact on the patient of possibly having cancer is often no less than that for more aggressive cancers. Consequently, the personal concern of the patient often outweighs the level of our medical concern. The same may be true when the patient has a primary cosmetic concern. The need for a confident diagnosis and an effective method of management is clear. A significant component in both areas has been thyroid hormone (TH) therapy. Recently, questions regarding the effectiveness of TH for diagnosis and therapy have come to the fore, hence the issue of this debate by two internationally know thyroidologists, Drs. Blum and Mazzaferri, and Dr. Blum's colleague Dr. Zwickler.

The major issues addressed by our debators are: (1) what is the best current method available for diagnosis, (2) is there a role for TH in diagnosis and/or management, and (3) what are the potential adverse consequences of using TH therapy?

In principle, our authors agree that the technique of fine-needle aspiration biopsy (FNB) has the greatest potential of all current methods of providing an accurate diagnosis. In my judgment, few thyroidologists would quarrel with this conclusion. Our authors, however, do no agree as to whether TH suppression has value in diagnosis. Dr. Mazzaferri says no. Drs. Blum and Zwickler argue that when the FNB cannot be accomplished or has an equivocal result, TH suppression can be a valuable and useful adjunct in the diagnostic assessment. They do not suggest that the result allows a definitive diagnosis if the nodule decreases in size, increases in size, or is unchanged. However, they do view the nodule that increases in size during suppressive therapy to be more highly suspect for thyroid cancer. They clearly define the method they use for this diagnostic/therapeutic trial (a 3-month course of triiodothyronine). The concern about using T_3 therapy in the elderly is appreciated by all debators. Based on the data presented in their position statements and responses, plus my own experience, I am not persuaded that TH suppression is useful as an adjunct in diagnosis. I am convinced, however, that the appearance of new nodule or the growth of an existing nodule during thyroid hormone therapy demands histological assessment.

Our debators also disagree regarding the use of TH in managing the euthyroid patient's benign thyroid nodule. Dr. Mazzaferri cites recent data suggesting that thyroid-stimulating hormone (TSH) is not a primary thyroid growth-stimulating factor, as well as clinical studies showing a small or no response of thyroid nodules to TH suppression therapy. He also points to the potential adverse consequences of clinical or subclinical hyperthyroidism on bone. He concludes that TH therapy today should be reserved for those patients with a nodule who are hypothyroid. Drs. Blum and Zwickler argue that the data cited by Dr. Mazzaferri are flawed and cite evidence that "TSH is a growth factor for thyroid cells and tumors that is reciprocally responsive to thyroid hormone," and that the data supporting significant bone loss are not conclusive. From the clinical perspective, they content that some thyroid nodules, albeit probably a relatively small percentage, shrink or disappear during suppressive TH therapy and that "...by and large those are benign." Further, they believe that a larger percentage of thyroid nodules become dormant and that the formation of a new, clinically definable nodule is often thwarted or prevented. Recent data from Fogelfel et al.[1] again suggest that TH therapy reduces the risk of benign nodule recurrences in postoperative patients with a history of head and neck irradiation during childhood, especially females. However, this was not true for thyroid cancer. In this editor's view, the evidence to date is not sufficiently clear to make an unequivocal statement.

Our debators disagree regarding the degree of concern one should have about the potential adverse effects of the excess circulating thyroid hormone needed for adequate suppressive therapy. However, they agree that major TH excesses resulting in clinically apparent hyperthyroidism should be avoided in benign thyroid disease. Dr. Mazzaferri summarizes current data on the physiological effects of "subclinical hyperthyroidism" as well as on the effect of excess TH on bone density. He concludes from these data and his own experience that the potential long-term risks of TH do not justify "...its meager benefits in patient management." Therefore, he believes that the use of TH in euthyroid patients with a benign thyroid nodule should be abandoned as a routine management modality. Drs. Blum and Zwickler recognize the potential risks of TH suppression, but do not view the data to be as alarming, especially with mild subclinical hyperthyroidism.

Our debators do appear to agree that the most accurate current method of monitoring TH therapy is a highly sensitive TSH assay. In this editor's view, an important question not yet adequately addressed is whether any benefit TH may have on the development or growth of a benign nodule requires maximal TSH suppression?

After reviewing the data and views presented by our debators, this editor concludes that (1) FNB is the diagnostic technique of choice for thyroid nodule evaluation and diagnostic TH suppression is rarely, if ever, a useful adjunct; (2) TH therapy still has a role in the long-term management of benign nodule disease in many, if not most, euthyroid patients; and (3) we must be cognizant of the potential long-term effects of subclinical hyperthyroidism and await the results of prospective randomized trials using more sophisticated and reproducible bone density measurements before eliminating TH therapy from our armamentarium.

Reference

1. Fogelfel L, Wiviott MBT, Shore-Freedman E, et al: Recurrence of thyroid nodules after surgical removal in patients irradiated in childhood for benign conditions. *N Engl J Med* 1989; 320:835–840.

When Is Bicarbonate Appropriate in Treating Metabolic Acidosis, Including Diabetic Ketoacidosis?

Chapter Editor: H. Verdain Barnes, M.D.

Perspective 1: R. D. Cohen, M.D.
Professor of Medicine and Director, Medical Unit, The London Hospital Medical College, University of London, London, England

Perspective 2*: Abbas E. Kitabchi, M.D., Ph.D.
Professor of Medicine and Biochemistry, Director, Division of Endocrinology and Metabolism and Clinical Research Center, University of Tennessee College of Medicine, Memphis, Tennessee

Mary Beth Murphy, R.N., M.S.
Clinical Nurse Specialist, Division of Endocrinology and Metabolism and Clinical Research Center, University of Tennessee College of Medicine, Memphis, Tennessee

*The work of the investigators described in this manuscript was supported in part by AM-05497 from the National Institutes of Health; RR-00211 General Clinical Research Center, National Institutes of Health; a Research Grant from The Juvenile Diabetes Foundation International; and the Abe Goodman Fund for Diabetic Research..

Editor's Introduction

Metabolic acidosis is a common clinical problem. Acute metabolic acidosis, such as diabetic ketoacidosis (DKA) and lactic acidosis, are life-threatening conditions which require immediate intervention. Whether the therapeutic regimen should include bicarbonate is the crux of this debate.

Over the past quarter century, there has been an ongoing debate about the advantages and disadvantages of bicarbonate therapy in modest to severe DKA. For the majority of physicians, the question has been answered effectively in the past 5 to 7 years by the careful studies which have come from the laboratory of one of our debators, Dr. Abbas E. Kitabchi of the University of Tennessee College of Medicine. His data support the view that bicarbonate is not needed in the DKA patient whose pH is between 6.9 and 7.3. Our other debator, Dr. R.D. Cohen of the University of London-Medical Unit, agrees that based on the outcome variables typically measured during therapy, there is no substantial improvement when sodium bicarbonate is used. In taking a more global perspective on metabolic acidosis, he suggests that based on the etiology of the acidosis, other alkalinizing agents merit consideration in therapy. In addition, he prompts us to consider cellular-level dynamics in DKA and other acidosis as well as the variables typically measured during therapy.

Do we have an unequivocal answer to the bicarbonate question in DKA? You be the judge.

H. Verdain Barnes, M.D.

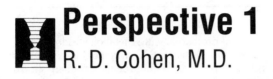

Perspective 1
R. D. Cohen, M.D.

The use of sodium bicarbonate in the treatment of metabolic acidosis has become increasingly controversial over the past decade, principally due to the provocative experimental studies of Dr. Allen Arieff and his colleagues[1-5] and to the different interpretations placed on them. The present writer has acted as "moderator" on a number of panels devoted to this issue and welcomes this opportunity to reflect on the arguments mobilized on either side, typified by the review by Stacpoole[6] (broadly "against" bicarbonate or, more precisely, demanding a more rigorous examination of its value) and the riposte of Narins and Cohen.[7] Some shrewd suspicion of the true state of the argument may be gleaned from the fact that both of these reviews conclude that the onus of proof regarding the value or harmfulness of bicarbonate therapy rests with the other side.

What are the basic reasons for these uncertainties? The most significant is that almost no carefully controlled studies have been done of the *outcome* of treatment for clinical metabolic acidosis. The reasons for this are several, a major one being that it is very difficult to design such studies. This is because these patients are usually acutely ill and in a wide variety of different metabolic states at the start of therapy due to the diversity of the preceding natural history of their disease. This applies even within specific categories of metabolic acidosis, e.g., diabetic ketoacidosis (DKA) or type A lactic acidosis. The result is that any groups randomly selected as part of a treatment trial are likely to have so much "internal noise" as to make it difficult to demonstrate a clear difference between the groups in the outcome measures used. The situation is quite different in the carefully designed comparisons between bicarbonate, saline, and other treatments of metabolic acidosis performed by Arieff and his colleagues in animal models. By virtue of the study design, these animals were in a relatively uniform state at the start of treatment.

The second major reason for the controversy is that many writers equate metabolic acidosis with lowered arterial pH (pH_a). The fallacy here is that, despite conventional definitions based on blood measurements, metabolic acidosis is a complex syndrome of derangements of cellular metabolism and organ function and there is no convincing evidence to suggest that these derangements are tightly linked to the disturbance of pH_a itself. For instance, there is good evidence[8] that the deterioration of myocardial contractility observed in experimental acidosis is related more closely to a decline in intracellular pH (pH_i) than to a fall in pH_a. Similarly, the inhibition of gluconeogenesis from lactate that has been observed in rat liver subjected to metabolic or respiratory acidosis[9] is related most closely to pH_i changes. It is also clear that the pH_i in different organs often is not predictable from pH_a and, furthermore, any relationship between pH_a and pH_i that exists varies between organs. Thus, we recently have shown[10] that there is a gross lowering of hepatic pH_i in rats with severe metabolic acidosis due to ammonium chloride ingestion or hydrochloric acid infusion. In contrast, there is scarcely any lowering of hepatic pH_i in diabetic ketosis of similar severity. Given that there are adverse clinical effects of acidosis, we need to treat the whole syndrome, not "whitewash" the arterial pH. It is certainly logically possible that the final outcome would be improved if physicians were not so generally obsessed with the need to correct abnormal blood variables.

The final reason for the controversy is a tendency for writers on this subject to use the phrases "bicarbonate therapy" and "alkali therapy" interchangeably. However, as we shall see, there are many forms of potential alkali therapy other than bicarbonate. There are the obvious ones like "carbicarb" (an equal mixture of sodium bicarbonate and sodium carbonate[11]) and TRIS buffer (tromethamine, or THAM), and the less obvious ones like sodium dichloracetate (DCA) for lactic acidosis and rehydration and insulin for diabetic ketoacidosis. The latter therapy suppresses ketogenesis and increases peripheral ketone body metabolism, both of which are processes resulting in amelioration of the acidosis. DCA effectively disinhibits pyruvate dehydrogenase and provides an oxidative sink for lactate. When a simple organic acid anion, charged at all ordinary pH values, is fully metabolized to neutral products (such as CO_2 and water or glucose), protons (H^+) are consumed, leading to alkalinization.[9] It should be noted that this form of alkalinization, which takes place initially in cells (rather than in the blood, as when giving $NaHCO_3$), will be more likely to result in a rise in pH_i in tissues metabolizing organic anions. More detailed investigations of the effects of methods of alkalinization other than bicarbonate administration are overdue.

Having outlined the fundamental problem, I shall now attempt to deal with some of the more detailed arguments that have been deployed on both sides of the controversy.

The Validity of the Experimental Models Employed by Arieff et al.

Arieff and his colleagues used two main models, both in dogs: phenformin-induced lactic acidosis in diabetic animals and hypoxic lactic acidosis induced by breathing hypoxic atmospheres. The basic findings were that bicarbonate therapy (compared with NaCl) resulted in a decline of cardiac output, liver blood flow, and hepatic pH_i, and in an elevation of blood lactate related to an increase in gut lactate production. Whereas DCA produced an improvement in cardiac output in phenformin-induced lactic acidosis, $NaHCO_3$

caused a further decline. DCA increased liver pH_i, and lowered blood lactate and gut lactate production; opposite effects were observed with $NaHCO_3$. There was a marked improvement in short-term survival in the DCA-treated animals.

These models have been criticized by Narins and Cohen[7] on the grounds that the administration of $NaHCO_3$ as the only therapy in these severely ill dogs was doomed to failure because the underlying hypoxia and heart disease (due to phenformin cardiotoxicity) were left untreated; therefore, $NaHCO_3$ therapy has been artificially disadvantaged. Furthermore, it might be said that clinical phenformin-induced lactic acidosis has now vanished (since phenformin has been removed from the market) and hypoxic hypoxia is scarcely the commonest form of clinical lactic acidosis, so it could be argued that these studies are relatively unimportant to clinical practice. I do not accept these criticisms. The purpose of using animal models of disease is to reveal pathophysiological phenomena and mechanisms which eventually might lead to the improvement of treatment. This seems to me to be precisely what Arieff and colleagues have done. What they have clearly shown is that certain aspects of the hemodynamic and biochemical situation are worsened by $NaHCO_3$ compared with saline and are improved by DCA, pointing to the possibility that similar events could occur clinically. All they claim at the conclusion of their papers is that their results suggest that the clinical use of $NaHCO_3$ should be reevaluated.

There are, however, certain other problems with these studies. The first is a technical matter, concerned with the method used for measurement of hepatic pH_i. This method uses the distribution between intracellular and extracellular spaces of the weak acid dimethadione (DMO), a distribution that depends on the pH gradient between the two compartments. To delineate the extracellular space so that the intracellular compartment can be calculated from the total tissue water, the authors use the chloride ion as a measure of the extracellular compartment. Unfortunately, a good deal of chloride is intracellular in the liver, due to a low potential across the hepatocyte plasma membrane. Furthermore, this potential is variable under different conditions, so apparent changes in pH_i may merely reflect alterations in membrane potential. In addition, the calculation of pH_i from the DMO distribution requires a knowledge of extracellular pH (pH_e). This is relatively simple under ordinary conditions, but in low flow states (e.g., phenformin-lactic acidosis) where there could be gross pH_e changes from one end of the capillary (or sinusoid) to the other, the value of pH_e for use in the calculation becomes rather indeterminate. At the least, Arieff's findings with respect to pH_i require confirmation by an independent technique.

Another problem with Arieff's studies is related to species differences. The acidotic dog appears to be extraordinarily resistant to the elevation of pH_a by bicarbonate and in none of the studies by Arieff's group is more than a very small amelioration of pH_a achieved. Perhaps this is related to the stimulation of gut lactate production in the dog by $NaHCO_3$ in a manner rather reminiscent of the situation in the rare tumor-associated lactic acidosis, where bicarbonate infusion may merely increase glycolytic production of lactic acid. Some patients with phenformin-induced lactic acidosis likewise were very resistant to bicarbonate, while some appeared to do very well with it. It was always impossible to be certain[12] whether the infusion of saline would have had the same effect and whether spontaneous improvement was occurring unrelated to $NaHCO_3$ therapy. Nevertheless, the obvious resistance of the dog to $NaHCO_3$ does raise the question of the relevance of these studies to humans.

Similarly, my colleagues Drs. Richard Iles and John Beech (unpublished), using ^{31}P-magnetic resonance spectroscopy, have shown very recently that $NaHCO_3$ treatment in vivo of rats with diabetic ketoacidosis or NH_4Cl acidosis results in a rise in hepatic pH_i, despite elevation of Pco_2. In parallel experiments on livers from similar animals perfused with acidotic media, the introduction of bicarbonate raised Pco_2 and lactate uptake. These types of acidosis are different from those studied by Arieff and his colleagues but raise the question of species-specific and/or "type of acidosis"–specific responses to $NaHCO_3$.

Matters Concerning Pco_2

It is now well established that mixed venous Pco_2 ($P_{\bar{v}}co_2$) may be grossly raised in low flow states in both man and animals while arterial Pco_2 (P_aco_2) is normal or low. Thus, in the observations of Weil et al.,[13] $P_{\bar{v}}co_2$ averaged 74 mm Hg (9.9 kPa) compared with a P_aco_2 of 32 mm Hg (4.3 kPa) during resuscitation from clinical cardiac arrest. The gross elevation of $P_{\bar{v}}co_2$ reflects similar or even grosser elevations of Pco_2 in the venous blood of individual organs. This elevation has two components. The first is due to the proportional decrease in an organ blood flow rate exceeding that of aerobic metabolism in that organ. The second component is due to the titration of tissue and local blood bicarbonate by protons principally derived from the increased glycolysis which in the steady state produces H^+ stoichiometrically with lactate ions. The titrated bicarbonate may be partly exogenous, of course, if $NaHCO_3$ therapy has been given.

Now it is widely stated[5,13] that the raised Pco_2 derived from HCO_3 titration acidifies the cells (i.e., lowers pH_i) in individual organs, and it has been hypothesized that this may be at least one factor in the deleterious effect of bicarbonate. This hypothesis requires critical examination. Let us consider the intravenous infusion of bicarbonate into a patient with a low flow state and resulting type A lactic acidosis. Some of the bicarbonate will be titrated on the venous side with a consequent rise in Pco_2. But, according to the observations quoted earlier,[13] Pco_2 will be reduced to normal or below by the time the segment of blood infused with bicarbonate has reached the arterial side. The bicarbonate concentration, however, will remain elevated.

Suppose this blood now enters the coronary arteries of a heart sharing in the general low flow state and therefore producing lactate and accompanying protons. The bicarbonate may either (1) enter the myocardial cell (e.g., on the general anion transporter) and be titrated by intracellular H^+ or, (2) remain in the extracellular compartment and be titrated by H^+ leaving the cells. Therefore, CO_2 will be released, elevating Pco_2, but pH_i will *rise*. There is no way in which CO_2 thus derived can lower pH_i, because carbonic acid is a much weaker acid than lactic acid and its conjugate base, bicarbonate, will always accept protons produced in association with lactate. The fact that Pco_2 rises is merely a sign of effective buffering. So from this point of view, if raising pH_i is a desirable objective, the more bicarbonate the better!

The hypotheses that the harmful effect of $NaHCO_3$ could be due to falls in pH_i caused by raising tissue Pco_2 by titration is therefore physicochemically invalid. However, if the initial raised Pco_2 at the site of infusion has not been dissipated by the time the segment of blood has reached the heart, then the bicarbonate-induced elevation of P_aco_2 could have some effect in lowering cardiac pH_i. This caveat has some bearing on the situation in the liver. For blood reaching the liver via the hepatic artery, the same arguments apply as for the heart. However, portal vein blood has passed through the gut circulation. Arieff's group showed that gut lactate production was stimulated by bicarbonate infusion and that, in partial consequence of this, portal vein Pco_2 was raised. This would have the effect of acidifying the liver cell.

It follows from the previous arguments that if CO_2 produced by titration of administered bicarbonate is responsible for deterioration of cardiac function, then it must be either because it has raised P_aco_2 or because CO_2 has some deleterious effect not directly related to pH. The matter is of importance, since in a recent paper[5] Bersin and Arieff have used their hypoxic dog lactic acidosis model to compare the effect of $NaHCO_3$ and "carbicarb" ($NaHCO_3/Na_2CO_3$ mixture). "Carbicarb" has the property of buffering protons with minimal change in Pco_2. $NaHCO_3$ had the usual deleterious affect on cardiac output, blood pressure, and arterial lactate. In contrast, "carbicarb" raised cardiac output and had little effect on blood lactate. "Carbicarb" increased whole body oxygen delivery and consumption; $NaHCO_3$ did the opposite. In these experiments, P_aco_2 was fixed at 37 mm Hg (4.9 kPa). P_vco_2 did not change with "carbicarb," although a small but significant rise was seen with $NaHCO_3$. It should be remembered that these were not low flow states, except after the administration of $NaHCO_3$, since hypoxia of the degree induced somewhat raises cardiac output. Bersin and Arieff hypothesized that the Pco_2 in the coronary capillaries and sinus was considerably higher than the P_vco_2 in the $NaHCO_3$ experiments, and that this was the reason for the obvious difference in the hemodynamic state from that seen with "carbicarb." If they are right, then, as argued earlier, the deleterious effect of raised Pco_2 originating from the titration of bicarbonate cannot be mediated through a direct effect on cardiac pH_i.

I have tried to emphasize that the previous arguments apply only to that component of elevated tissue Pco_2 in ischemia which is derived from the titration of bicarbonate. However, the other major component (i.e., that derived from residual aerobic respiration) does have an effect in lowering pH_i, and insomuch as this is so, any infused agent reaching the organ which "buffers" CO_2, (such as "carbicarb") could have a beneficial effect on cardiac function, which in this case would be mediated by elevating pH_i. Furthermore, even though a raised Pco_2 derived from bicarbonate titration denotes a pH_i raising effect, any subsequent lowering of tissue Pco_2 by a CO_2 buffering agent would result in a further elevation of pH_i, with possible benefit, and it may be that this is a component of "carbicarb" action.

Arguments About the Blood Titration Curve

Narins and Cohen[7] point out how extremely sensitive blood pH is at low concentrations of plasma bicarbonate to further depression by a comparatively small decrement in bicarbonate. They imply that it is important to raise pH out of this dangerously unstable range by giving bicarbonate. For reasons outlined earlier, I am unconvinced of this logic. First, it aims treatment at the blood, rather than at the syndrome. Second, there is an implicit assumption that bicarbonate is the right way to achieve this "rescue from the brink." There is no clear evidence that pH_a rather than, for instance, cardiac pH_i, is the critical variable. If it were the latter, then it is at least conceivable that $NaHCO_3$ would worsen matters, whereas "carbicarb," TRIS, or DCA might improve them.

Diabetic Ketoacidosis

There seems to be a general consensus that it is unnecessary to treat DKA with bicarbonate unless pH_a is less than 7. Below this value, there is disagreement. A study by Lever and Jaspan[14] retrospectively compared the course and outcome in 95 episodes of diabetic ketoacidosis (DKA) in patients in two hospitals, one in the United States and one in the United Kingdom. In each of the hospitals, some patients were treated with $NaHCO_3$ in addition to the usual insulin and rehydration. They found no difference in the rate of recovery of blood glucose, bicarbonate, pH, or neurologic status between the group that was treated with bicarbonate and the one that was not. Superficially, the groups were well matched in terms of severity of acidosis and quantity of bicarbonate administered. Many of the patients had an initial pH_a of less than 7.0. Although this study is valuable, its limitations were well recognized by the authors; it was retrospective, the indications for bicarbonate were not defined, and it was in no sense randomized. Therefore, the possibility of a positive or negative effect of bicarbonate being missed cannot be excluded. Hale and colleagues[15] compared blood pH, ketones, lactate, and glucose in groups receiving or not receiving bicarbonate. Although the pH_a rise was faster in the bicarbonate groups, the recovery of blood ketones, lactate, and the lactate/pyruvate ratio (for what that is worth) was delayed. Whether these delays have any clinical importance is not apparent.

Whether alkalinizing therapies other than bicarbonate or insulin have a clearer beneficial effect on DKA is completely unknown. I have already referred to the behavior of hepatic pH_i in experimental DKA. This is an example of the quantitatively individual control of pH_i in different organs. Basically, cells have three principal ways of controlling their internal pH: ordinary physicochemical buffering, altering the rate of production or consumption of weak acids, and changing the rate of transit of H^+ (or HCO^-_3 or OH^-) across the plasma membrane. How the various alkalinization strategies might interact with these pH_i control mechanisms is poorly understood. The maintenance of a relatively high pH_i in DKA may be an example of the second of these mechanisms. Thus, the high rate of lactate conversion to glucose in DKA driven by the hormone and metabolic environment may maintain a normal pH_i. In turn, the near-normal pH_i may allow lactate consumption to continue, for it has been shown that hepatic intracellular acidosis inhibits gluconeogenesis from lactate.[9]

Conclusion

It must be obvious from this discussion that, in general, the only reasonable conclusion that can be drawn about the advisability of $NaHCO_3$ therapy in metabolic acidosis is that *we simply do not know*. There are one or two exceptions; for example, it is generally agreed that $NaHCO_3$ is advisable in severe diarrheal states (e.g., cholera[16] and certain types of renal tubular acidosis,[17] albeit with certain vital precautions concerning prior treatment of hypokalemia). But for the majority of metabolic acidoses there is no position that can be justified by the available data other than an admission of ignorance.

I have sometimes felt in this affair like a spectator in a court of law, listening to the advocates on each side marshal the evidence in favor of their case. However, the disciplines of law and science are fundamentally different in that in science (including clinical science), each player is expected to perceive all sides of the case. Of course, it is uncomfortable for a physician not to have a proven recipe for action, but this scenario occurs so many times in medicine that it is virtually routine. In fact, the way that physicians act in such circumstances is to acquaint themselves with the broad spectrum of accepted clinical practice and choose some position within that spectrum, which in the present context encompasses both the giving and withholding of bicarbonate in metabolic acidosis. If anyone is worried about the medicolegal aspects of taking one side or another, we have in this particular case the assertion of both sides that the onus of proof rests on the other —

comforting for the physician in the middle, but hardly a satisfactory situation for the patient with metabolic acidosis.

This brings us to possible ways out of the present impasse. I have remarked that the clinical diversity of patients with each type of metabolic acidosis is a major stumbling block to proper comparative trials of different therapies. One possible approach is to seek ways of matching the trial groups other than, or in addition to, the current conventional ones. In particular, the use of arterial pH as a stratifier seems unlikely to be especially helpful, and the question arises as to whether individual organ pH_i would be more logical both as an initial stratifier and as a variable to follow during alternative therapeutic regimes in the different types of metabolic acidosis. The reason for this suggestion is twofold. First, at least in the heart and liver, certain important functional and metabolic processes are closely related to cell pH_i. Second with the advent of magnetic resonance spectroscopy it is practicable in theory to follow pH_i in individual organs noninvasively and continuously during different therapies and to correlate the results with hemodynamic and metabolic changes. A major problem is the care of seriously ill patients while undertaking magnetic resonance spectroscopy investigations; however, a few centers are attempting to overcome this difficulty. Finally, the prolonged obsession with bicarbonate as the only alkalinizing strategy needs to be discarded and the other agents referred to earlier assessed.

References

1. Arieff AI, Park R, Leach W, et al: Systemic effects of NaHCO$_3$ in experimental lactic acidosis in dogs. *Am J Physiol* 1982; 242:F586–F591.
2. Park R, Arieff AI, Leach W, et al: Treatment of lactic acidosis with dichloroacetate in dogs. *J Clin Invest* 1982; 70:853–862.
3. Graf H, Leach W, Arieff AI: Metabolic effects of sodium bicarbonate in hypoxic lactic acidosis in dogs. *Am J Physiol* 1985; 249:F630–F635.
4. Graf H, Leach W, Arieff AI: Effects of dichloroacetate in the treatment of hypoxic lactic acidosis in dogs. *J Clin Invest* 1985; 76:919–923.
5. Bersin RM, Arieff AI: Improved hemodynamic function during hypoxia with carbicarb, a new agent for the management of acidosis. *Circulation* 1988; 77:227–233. *The above five papers demonstrate adverse effects of bicarbonate in hypoxia-induced and phenformin-induced lactic acidosis, and more advantageous effects of dichloracetate and 'carbicarb'.*
6. Stacpoole PW: Lactic acidosis: The case against bicarbonate therapy. *Ann Intern Med* 1986; 105:276–279.
7. Narins RG, Cohen JJ: Bicarbonate therapy for organic acidosis: The case for its continued use. *Ann Intern Med* 1987; 106:615–618. *The above two papers review the pro and con arguments for the use of bicarbonate.*
8. Steenbergen C, Deleeuw R, Rich T, et al: Effects of acidosis and ischaemia on contractility and intracellular pH of rat heart. *Circ Res* 1977; 41:489–858. *This is a demonstration of the probable prime importance of intracellular pH in determining cardiac effects of acidosis.*

9. Cohen RD, Guder WG: Carbohydrate metabolism and pH, in Häussinger D (ed): *pH Homeostasis: Mechanisms and Control.* London, Academic Press, 1988, pp 403–426.
10. Beech JS, Williams SR, Cohen RD, et al: Gluconeogenesis and the protection of hepatic intracellular pH during diabetic ketoacidosis in rats. *Biochem J* 1989; 263:737–744.
11. Filley GF, Kindig WB: Carbicarb, an alkalinizing ion - generating agent of possible clinical usefulness. *Trans Am Clin Climatol Assoc* 1984; 96:141–153. *The theory behind the use of "carbicarb" in metabolic acidosis is presented.*
12. Cohen RD, Woods HF: *Clinical and Biochemical Aspects of Lactic Acidosis.* Oxford, Blackwell, 1976. *The above three references are general reviews of the basic physiology and clinical background to the present paper.*
13. Weil MH, Rackow EC, Trevino R, et al: Difference in acid-base state between venous and arterial blood during cardiopulmonary rescuscitation. *N Engl J Med* 1986; 315:153–156. *This study demonstrates grossly elevated mixed venous P_{CO_2} but virtually normal arterial P_{CO_2} in patients undergoing cardiopulmonary resuscitation.*
14. Lever E, Jaspan JB: Sodium bicarbonate therapy in severe diabetic ketoacidosis. *Am J Med* 1983; 75:263–268.
15. Hale PJ, Crase J, Nattrass M: Metabolic effects of bicarbonate in the treatment of diabetic ketoacidosis. *Br Med J* 1984; 289:1035–1038. *Descriptions of the clinical and biochemical effects (and lack of) of bicarbonate in diabetic ketoacidosis are given.*
16. Harvey RM, Enson Y, Lewis ML, et al: Haemodynamic effects of dehydration and metabolic acidosis in Asiatic cholera. *Trans Assoc Am Physicians* 1966; 79:177–186. *This is a classical description of an apparently beneficial effect of bicarbonate.*
17. Cohen RD: Renal tubular acidosis, in Weatherall DJ, Ledingham JGC, Warrell DA (eds): *Oxford Textbook of Medicine,* 2nd ed. Oxford, Oxford University Press, 1987.

Perspective 2

Abbas E. Kitabchi, Ph.D., M.D.
Mary Beth Murphy, R.N., M.S.

Diabetic ketoacidosis (DKA) is an acute complication of diabetes most frequently noted in the insulin-dependent form of this disease. The symptom complex consists of hyperglycemia, ketosis, acidosis, and loss of water and electrolytes (Fig 1). The most frequent precipitating factors are severe infection, omission of insulin injection in insulin-dependent diabetes, or previously undiagnosed diabetes brought about by a stressful event.

Although the pathophysiological basis of DKA is complex, numerous studies over the last decade have defined the course of metabolic derangements in this state more clearly. The primary hormone derangement is insulin lack which leads to hyperglycemia as a result of excess hepatic glucose output through glycogenolysis and gluconeogenesis. Additionally, decreased glucose utilization by peripheral tissues increases hyperglycemia; however, the former mechanism plays the more prominent role. In the presence of a net effective reduction of insulin (the major antilipolytic hormone) and

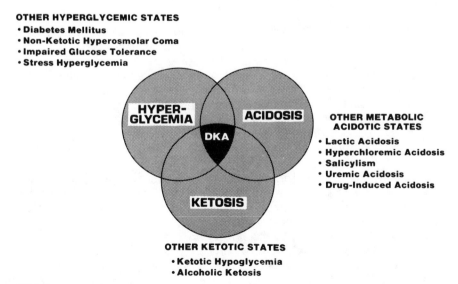

OTHER HYPERGLYCEMIC STATES
• Diabetes Mellitus
• Non-Ketotic Hyperosmolar Coma
• Impaired Glucose Tolerance
• Stress Hyperglycemia

HYPER-GLYCEMIA   ACIDOSIS

DKA

KETOSIS

OTHER METABOLIC ACIDOTIC STATES
• Lactic Acidosis
• Hyperchloremic Acidosis
• Salicylism
• Uremic Acidosis
• Drug-Induced Acidosis

OTHER KETOTIC STATES
• Ketotic Hypoglycemia
• Alcoholic Ketosis

FIG 1.
Symptoms complex in diabetic ketoacidosis associated with hyperglycemia, metabolic acidosis, and ketotic states.

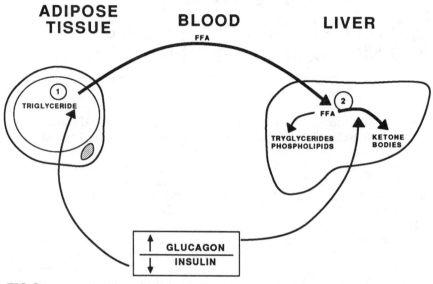

FIG 2.
Bihormonal model for the regulation of ketogenesis. Site 1 represents the primary site of insulin action in the adipocyte, while site 2 indicates the locus of glucagon acyltransferase. (From McGarry JD: *Diabetes* 1979; 28:517–523. Used by permission.)

increased catecholamine levels (the major lipolytic hormone in humans), depot fat (triglyceride) is broken down into free fatty acids and glycerol.

However, accelerated lipolysis is not the only explanation for the ketogenesis in DKA. As the ratio of insulin/glucagon is decreased, ketogenesis is increased through the stimulation of carnitine acyltransferase, and enzyme located in the wall of the hepatic mitochondria. This enzyme accelerates the entry of fatty acids across the mitochondrial membrane to be oxidized into keto acids (Fig 2). Additionally, levels of malonyl coenzyme A (CoA), an intermediate in the biosynthesis of fatty acids, are decreased during DKA. Malonyl CoA inhibits carnitine acyltransferase, thereby stimulating fatty acid synthesis.[1] Additionally, ketone body utilization is decreased in the peripheral tissues, resulting in an excess of keto acids in the circulation. Since ketone bodies must be excreted by the body in a neutralized form, bicarbonate reserve is reduced and acidosis results.

With the decreased ratio of insulin/glucagon and the stimulation of the hypothalamic pituitary axis (mainly cortisol), proteolysis is stimulated and protein synthesis is decreased in the muscle, leading to an accumulation of amino acids (mainly alanine) in the circulation. Alanine serves as an important substrate for gluconeogenesis. Thus, increasing proteolysis, glucose production, and lipolysis bring about the acute metabolic derange-ments characteristic of diabetic ketoacidosis: loss of electrolytes, volume depletion, and transient impaired renal function. These interrelated events are depicted in Figure 3.

One of the most controversial issues in the management of DKA is whether to withhold or administer alkali for correction of the acidosis.[2,3] The controversy exists because no rational basis for the use of alkali has been elucidated. Questions regarding safety, efficacy, and dosing remain unan-swered. Arguments in favor of the use of sodium bicarbonate (HCO_3) center around the premise that if acidosis is attended by morbidity and mortality, then reversal of the acidosis by the administration of HCO_3 should decrease morbidity and mortality, specifically with reference to cardiovascular func-tion.

Animal studies on the effect of acid-base derangements on myocardial function have given conflicting conclusions as a result of the nature of the cardiac dysfunction studied, the type of model used, and the mechanism of induction of acidosis.[4] Previously reported results from a subgroup of patients in our bicarbonate study, described later in this paper, showed that treatment with sodium bicarbonate was not attended by myocardial depres-sion. Therefore, our findings suggest that alkali therapy is not necessary in maintaining cardiac function during recovery from DKA in young patients with significant cardiac reserve. Arguments against HCO_3 therapy state that alkali may be harmful by causing paradoxical central nervous system (CNS) acidosis, intracellular acidosis, hypokalemia, cerebral edema, and peripheral hypoxia.

Paradoxical Central Nervous System (CNS) Acidosis

The intravenous administration of HCO_3 may cause a paradoxical fall in cerebrospinal fluid (CSF) pH. Posner and Plum[5] explained that sodium bicarbonate diffuses slowly across the blood-brain barrier with consequent minimal effect on spinal fluid pH. However, the increase in plasma pH decreases the respiratory drive, causing a relative hypoventilation with a consequent rise in blood Pco_2 which readily diffuses across the blood-brain barrier, causing the CSF pH to drop even further. Therefore, although the serum is being alkalinized rapidly, a paradoxical acidosis exists in the cerebrospinal fluid which may prolong or induce obtundation.

We[2] studied 21 adult patients with severe diabetic ketoacidosis in a randomized prospective protocol in which variable doses of sodium bicar-bonate (based on initial arterial pH levels ranging from 6.9 to 7.14) were administered to 10 patients (treatment group) and withheld from 11 patients (control group). Bicarbonate was administered to the treatment group

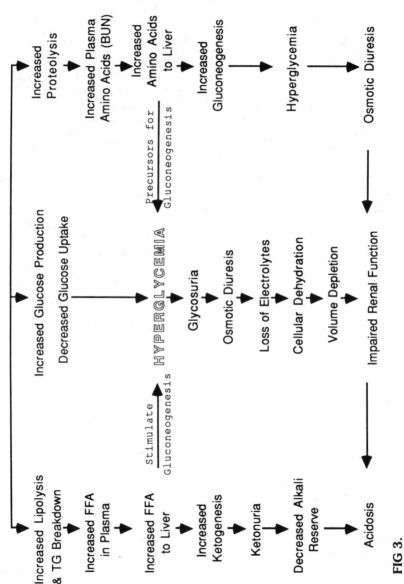

FIG 3.
Metabolic consequences of insulin deficiency and increased counter-regulatory hormones.

according to the following schedule: 133.8 mEq of intravenous bicarbonate if the initial arterial pH was 6.9 to 6.99; 89.2 mEq of intravenous bicarbonate if the pH was 7.0 to 7.09; and 44.5 mEq of intravenous bicarbonate if the pH was 7.1 to 7.14. The bicarbonate was infused intravenously over 30 minutes and repeated every 2 hours until the pH reached 7.15 or more. Other treatment methods were performed as previously described in other publications. Venous blood samples were obtained at regular intervals and lumbar punctures were performed at baseline, at 6 to 8 hours after therapy, and at 12 to 24 hours after therapy.

Cerebrospinal fluid chemistry data were of particular interest because both the bicarbonate and the pH values were significantly higher there than in the blood and because the levels of glucose and ketone bodies were significantly lower there than in the blood. These findings show that the blood-brain barrier effectively protects the CNS against ketoacidosis (Table 1). Although we noted a slight drop in cerebrospinal fluid pH in the treatment group after 6 to 8 hours of bicarbonate administration (0.05) compared with the control group (0.01), the differences were not statistically significant.

To assess the responses of various chemical components of CSF during therapy in the two groups, regression analyses of the levels of glucose, bicarbonate, pH, lactate, and ketones were obtained at three time points (0, 6 to 8, and 12 to 14 hours). Table 2 demonstrates that there were no significant differences in the slopes of these variables between the two groups. Although no significance was shown, it should be noted that the rate of decline for total ketones, lactate, and bicarbonate was greater for the treatment group. This may be secondary to the lack of adequate numbers of

---

TABLE 1.
Comparison: Initial Plasma/Cerebrospinal Values*

	Number of Samples	Plasma[†]	Cerebrospinal Fluid[†]	P Value[‡]
Glucose (mg/dL)[§]	14	503 ± 42	368 ± 27	<.001
Bicarbonate (mEq/L)	12	3.7 ± 0.6	7.7 ± 0.55	<.001
Arterial pH	11	7.01 ± 0.03	7.26 ± 0.02	<.001
Total ketones (mM)	11	10.9 ± 1.2	7.6 ± 0.66	<.05
Osmolality (mOsm/kg)	12	324 ± 7.7	320 ± 9.8	NS[¶]

*Data from Morris LR, Murphy MB, Kitabchi AE: *Ann Intern Med* 1986; 105:836–840.
[†]Mean ± standard error of the mean.
[‡]Paired *t*-test.
[§]To convert glucose to mM, divide by 18.
[¶]NS = Not significant.

TABLE 2.
Linear Regression of Cerebrospinal Fluid Chemistries in Patients on Two Forms of Therapy During Recovery From Diabetic Ketoacidosis*

Parameter	Estimates of Slopes (95% Confidence Limit on Slope)					
	Bicarbonate Therapy		No Bicarbonate Therapy		Differences	P Value†
	Slope	95% Confidence Limit	Slope	95% Confidence Limit	95% Confidence Limit	
Glucose	-8.7	(-15.6, -1.8)	-10.7	(-16.5, 4.9)	(-6.7, 10.6)	NS‡
Bicarbonate	0.31	(0.03, 0.59)	0.47	(0.23, 4.9)	(-0.5, 0.19)	NS
pH	0.004	(-0.004, 0.01)	0.002	(-0.003, 0.006)	(-0.006, 0.010)	NS
Total ketones	-0.28	(-0.43, -0.12)	-0.13	(-0.41, 0.15)	(-0.43, 0.14)	NS
Lactate	-0.68	(-1.4, 0.07)	0.098	(-1.4, 1.6)	(-2.21, 0.65)	NS

*Data from Morris LR, Murphy MB, Kitabchi AE: *Ann Intern Med* 1986; 105:836-840.
†Significance determined by comparison of 95% confidence intervals of slope estimates.
‡NS = Not significant.

observations. More frequent assessments of CSF fluid would have been of great scientific value, but were not done because of ethical considerations.

Intracellular Acidosis

Similarly, intracellular acidosis in the peripheral tissues is exacerbated by the same differential permeability of CO_2 and HCO_3 across the cell membrane. Presumably, a lowered intracellular pH would result in a decrease in function of various intracellular enzyme processes, contributing to overall pathophysiology.[6] We made no attempt to assess intracellular pH in peripheral tissues to confirm such a phenomenon in our patients.

Hypokalemia

Electrolyte disturbances also may be associated with bicarbonate administration, especially if it is performed rapidly. In the initial presentation, the patient may have a normal, low, or high serum potassium concentration. Ketone bodies accompany hydrogen ions into the cell, which leads to potassium depletion intracellularly, then to subsequent elevations in the plasma. However, with the ensuing diuresis, potassium levels will begin to fall, resulting in intracellular and extracellular potassium depletion. Bicarbonate administration enhances the shifts in potassium, leading to wider wings in the serum concentration.[7] We evaluated the decline in serum potassium levels by comparing the slopes of the linear regression over time to determine if the amount of bicarbonate supplementation (mean 120.4 ± 7.7 mEq) increased the frequency of hypokalemia (potassium < 3.3 mEq/L). This comparison showed that there was no significant difference between the treatment and control groups. However, to avoid rapid shifts in potassium, we infused bicarbonate slowly over 30 minutes in the treatment group and added potassium to the intravenous solutions by the end of the first hour, unless otherwise indicated.

Cerebral Edema

The administration of sodium bicarbonate may induce rapid changes in the osmolarity of the intravascular space and cause rapid shifts of fluid from the intracellular space to the extracellular space in the cerebrum, leading to prolongation of the comatose state.[8,9] Therefore, at critical points in the treatment of DKA, fluid management should be aimed at restoring both intracellular and extracellular deficiencies.

Average water loss in DKA is between 5 and 10 liters, average sodium loss is 400 to 700 mmol, and average potassium loss is 250 to 700 mmol.[7] This level of fluid loss could lead to shock; therefore, the first priority of fluid replacement is to restore intravascular volume. Hillman suggests that a "relatively" hypotonic saline solution should be used in restoring intravascular volume because the fluid lost in DKA is similar to half-normal saline. Furthermore, he states that when losses are replaced by isotonic fluid alone, intravascular volume is restored but a gross expansion of the interstitial compartment (ISC) occurs with no replacement of the intracellular compartment (ICC) (Fig 4). Therefore, he recommends the administration of colloid to reverse hypovolemic shock and hypotonic solution to replace the ICC and ISC losses.[10]

Peripheral Hypoxia

Because phosphate is an intracellular electrolyte, it follows a path similar to that of potassium in that it is shunted into the intravascular compartment and then lost in the ensuing diuresis. Therefore, intracellular phosphate depletion occurs, leading to a deficiency in 2,3-diphosphoglycerate (2,3-DPG) and altered hemoglobin affinity for oxygen. Additionally, alterations in 2,3-DPG levels in DKA will affect the oxygen delivery to peripheral tissues. A lower pH decreases hemoglobin affinity for oxygen through the action of 2,3-DPG. In metabolic acidosis, the oxygen-hemoglobin dissociation curve shifts to the right and the P_{50} increases, which indicates that more oxygen is available to the tissue. With persistent acidosis, phosphate depletion occurs and 2,3-DPG synthesis is inhibited, thereby increasing hemoglobin affinity for oxygen and resulting in peripheral hypoxia.[6] Because acidosis shifts the oxygen dissociation curve to the right, more oxygen is available to the tissue. However, when bicarbonate is administered, the curve is shifted back to the left, resulting in increased hemoglobin affinity for oxygen and the potential for peripheral hypoxia and subsequent lactic acidosis.

Using a randomized protocol and giving one standard dose of 150 mEq of bicarbonate regardless of initial pH, Hale and colleagues recently showed a similarity in the responses of patients with or without bicarbonate in the treatment of DKA.[11] However, these authors only measured biochemical changes (including glucose and pH) for the first 2 hours of therapy, and did not measure any of the biochemical changes in the cerebrospinal fluid. In our study of 21 patients using variable doses of bicarbonate, overall recovery parameters in the treatment group as compared to the control group were not affected by the omission or administration of bicarbonate (Fig 5).

Therefore, we conclude on the basis of our studies that the administration of bicarbonate in severe diabetic ketoacidosis (arterial pH 6.9 to 7.14) does not affect recovery outcome variables compared to those of a control group. Further studies need to be done on patients with arterial pH levels of less than 6.9.

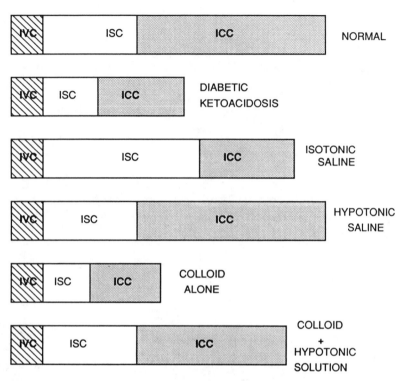

FIG 4.
The *top diagram* represents normal fluid distribution. The nature of the fluid and electrolyte loss in diabetic ketoacidosis is such that there is equal fluid loss from each compartment. When these losses are replaced with isotonic saline alone, it can be seen that although the IVC is restored, there is gross expansion of the ISS and no replacement of the ICC. Because hypotonic saline is similar to the fluid lost, there is accurate replacement of all compartments. However, because of the large distribution volume of hypotonic saline, the intravascular space is correspondingly resuscitated at a slow rate. To overcome this disadvantage, colloid could be given initially to reverse the hypovolemic shock and hypotonic solution could be given concurrently to replace the other two spaces. *IVC*-intravascular compartment; *ISC*-interstitial compartment; *ICC*-intracellular compartment. (From Hillman K: *Intensive Care Med* 1987; 13:3–4. Used by permission.)

At present, our recommended protocol for the management and follow-up of DKA patients includes the following guidelines:

 1. A rapid but careful history and physical examination should be performed, with special attention to (1) the patency of the airway, (2)

mental status, (3) the cardiovascular and renal state, (4) the source of infection, and (5) the state of dehydration.

2. The initial biochemical evaluation should consist of immediate emergency room assessment of urine ketones and glucose and blood ketones and glucose. Additionally, stat. orders should consist of a plasma glucose, blood gases, serum electrolytes, blood urea nitrogen (BUN), amylase, a complete blood cell count, and a urinalysis. Chest films, an electrocardiogram, and appropriate bacterial cultures are also obtained, if indicated.

3. As soon as the initial blood chemistries are drawn, give 1 L of 0.45% or 0.9% sodium chloride solution in the first hour with subsequent fluid therapy depending on the state of hydration.

4. With the confirmation of the diagnosis of DKA, give a priming dose of 0.3 to 0.4 units of regular insulin per kilogram of body weight (one half as intravenous [IV] push and one half intramuscularly [IM] in the deltoid area). However, insulin should be given solely as an intravenous priming bolus of 10 units followed by 7 units of regular insulin per hour

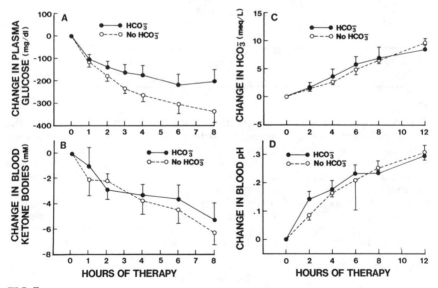

FIG 5.
Changes in blood chemistry values during treatment of patients with diabetic ketoacidosis with or without bicarbonate. Ten patients received bicarbonate therapy *(solid circles)* and 11 patients received no bicarbonate therapy *(open circles)*. No significant differences between the treatment groups were seen by any variable measured. (From Morris LR, Murphy MB, Kitabchi AE: *Ann Intern Med* 1986; 105:836–840.)

of intravenous infusion if the patient is severely dehydrated, hypotensive, or unconscious.

5. Determine the plasma glucose level hourly and the electrolytes and blood gases every 2 to 6 hours as needed. If the plasma glucose does not fall by 10% in the first hour, repeat the initial priming dose of insulin.

6. After satisfactory glucose decrement, give 7 units of regular insulin per hour as IM intermittent injection or IV infusion until the plasma glucose level reaches 200 mg/dL.

7. As soon as the plasma glucose reaches 200 mg/dL, switch to 5% glucose, 0.45% NaCl if the serum sodium is over 145 mEq/L or to 5% glucose, 0.9% NaCl if the serum sodium is under 145 mEq/L. Use a rate of 100 to 300 mL/h depending on the state of hydration. Give insulin at a rate of 10 units per 2 hours until DKA is completely controlled (plasma glucose < 200 mg/dL, HCO_3 > 15 mEq/L, and pH > 7.3).

8. If the initial potassium level is under 3.5 mEq/L, potassium supplementation should be provided at a rate of 40 mEq/L with the initial insulin therapy. Give 20 mEq of potassium per liter after the first liter of solution if the potassium level is over 3.5 mEq/L but under 5.5 mEq/L and the urinary output is adequate. Give no potassium if levels are greater than 5.5 mEq/L.

9. No bicarbonate is necessary unless the arterial pH is less than 7.0 or the bicarbonate levels are less than 5 mEq/L. For an arterial pH of less than 7.0 but greater than 6.9, administer 44 mEq of $NaHCO_3$ over 30 minutes intravenously with 10 mEq of potassium supplement, unless contraindicated. For an arterial pH of less than 6.9, give 88 mEq of $NaHCO_3$ with potassium supplement over 30 minutes. This regimen should be continued every 2 hours until the pH is above 7.0.

10. Ancillary measures include stomach aspiration in unconscious patients, oxygen therapy for a Po_2 greater than 80 mm Hg, plasma expander for consistent hypotension, and antibiotic therapy as needed.

11. Avoid the excessive use of 0.9% NaCl, as hyperchloremic acidosis may ensue.

12. Continue to look for precipitating factors, monitor the patient's clinical condition, and assess the management frequently.

13. Continue close monitoring of the plasma glucose after DKA is controlled. After the IV/IM insulin regimen is discontinued, plasma glucose levels frequently elevate and may lead to a relapse of DKA. Therefore, we recommend the following insulin regimen for patients after DKA is under control:

(A) give regular insulin subcutaneously every 4 hours based on plasma glucose levels (150 to 200 mg/dL, 5 units regular insulin; 201 to 250 mg/dL, 10 units regular insulin; 251 to 300 mg/dL, 15 units regular insulin; and > 300 mg/dL, 20 units regular insulin), but do not give insulin if the plasma glucose is less than 150 mg/dL (do repeat the plasma glucose every 2 hours); and (B) as soon as the patient can take food, give 10 to 15 units of intermediate insulin twice daily and continue regular insulin before each meal based on the aforementioned plasma glucose algorithm.

References

1. McGarry JD: New perspectives in the regulation of ketogenesis. *Diabetes* 1979; 28:517–523. *A comprehensive review of ketogenesis is presented.*
2. Morris LR, Murphy MB, Kitabchi AE: Bicarbonate therapy in severe diabetic ketoacidosis. *Ann Intern Med* 1986; 105:836–840. *A prospective randomized study comparing bicarbonate versus no bicarbonate therapy in diabetic ketoacidosis is reported.*
3. Assal J, Aoki T, Manzano F, et al: Metabolic effects of sodium bicarbonate in the management of diabetic ketoacidosis. *Diabetes* 1974; 23:405–411. *The authors studied bicarbonate and no bicarbonate therapy in diabetic ketoacidosis, demonstrating that bicarbonate did not vary the clinical course but may be needed if prompt correction of acidosis is necessary.*
4. Ng M, Levy M, Zieske H: Effects of changes of pH and carbon dioxide tension on left ventricular performance. *Am J Physiol* 1967; 213:115–120. *This article discusses the adverse effects on cardiac function occurring following bicarbonate administration in animals in acidotic and alkalotic states.*
5. Posner J, Plum F: Spinal fluid pH and neurological symptoms in systemic acidosis. *N Engl J Med* 1967; 277:605–613. *This is one of the original articles that suggested that bicarbonate therapy may cause paradoxical central nervous system acidosis.*
6. Alberti K, Darley J, Emerson P, et al: 2.3-DPG and tissue oxygenation in uncontrolled diabetes mellitus. *Lancet* 1972; 26:391–395. *These investigators suggest that bicarbonate therapy in diabetic ketoacidosis may be harmful by causing intracellular acidosis in peripheral tissues.*
7. Atchley DW, Loeb RF, Richards DW Jr, et al: On diabetic acidosis: A detailed study of the electrolyte balance following the withdrawal and re-establishment of insulin therapy. *J Clin Invest* 1933; 12:297. *This is a comprehensive review of electrolyte changes following insulin cessation and initiation.*
8. Ohman J, Marliss E, Aoki T, et al: The cerebrospinal fluid in diabetic ketoacidosis. *N Engl J Med* 1971; 284:283–289. *This article discusses problems encountered with bicarbonate therapy in diabetic ketoacidosis.*
9. Bureau M, Begin R, Berthiaume Y, et al: Cerebral hypoxia from bicarbonate infusion in diabetic acidosis. *J Pediatr* 1980; 96:968–973. *This is an investigation of the effects of bicarbonate therapy in metabolic acidosis in animals concluding that bicarbonate therapy decreases cerebral oxygen availability, affecting cerebral function.*
10. Hillman K: Fluid resuscitation in diabetic emergencies-a reappraisal. *Intensive Care Med* 1987; 13:4–8. *A comparison of various fluid therapies and their advantages and disadvantages in diabetic emergencies is presented.*
11. Hale P, Crase J, Nattrass M: Metabolic effects of bicarbonate in the treatment

of diabetic ketoacidosis. *Br Med J* 1984; 289:1035–1038. *A 2-hour randomized study comparing bicarbonate use and omission in the treatment of diabetic ketoacidosis is described.*

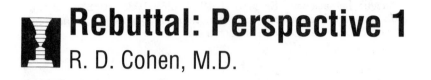

Rebuttal: Perspective 1
R. D. Cohen, M.D.

Dr. Kitabchi and Ms. Murphy have taken "terms of reference" in this debate somewhat different to those I have adopted. Whereas I have discussed the use of bicarbonate therapy in the general context of metabolic acidosis, they have restricted themselves to diabetic ketoacidosis (DKA). Therefore, the comments which follow are confined in the main to DKA.

Dr. Kitabchi and Ms. Murphy focus on the paradoxical acidification of the cerebrospinal fluid (CSF) during the treatment of DKA with bicarbonate as described by Posner and Plum[1] and Ohman et al.[2] They reproduce recent data from Dr. Kitabchi's group demonstrating that there is no significant difference in the time course of CSF, pH, bicarbonate, ketones, lactate, and glucose in bicarbonate-treated patients compared with those not so treated. They also show the time courses of similar variables in blood or plasma during the treatment and state again that there is no statistical difference. Their overall conclusion is that bicarbonate therapy in DKA patients (with an initial arterial pH of 6.9 to 7.14) does not affect recovery outcome variables.

The outcome variable which is of prime importance is patient survival, coupled with restoration to normal mental and physical health. DKA still has an appreciable mortality, even in the best centers. Next in importance may be the rate at which the patient is restored to normal neuropsychiatric and hemodynamic status. In the original paper[3] from which the data given in Dr. Kitabchi and Ms. Murphy's paper were derived, it is stated that there was no difference in the rate of recovery of mental status between the groups studied. Hemodynamic data were not given, but reference was made to an abstract[4] which indicated that neither DKA nor its treatment was associated with depression of cardiac function. These data are difficult to assess in the present debate, since only nine patients were involved and no information is given in this short report concerning the actual treatment employed. The incidence of hypokalemia, an important cause of mortality during the treatment of DKA, was similar in the two groups. Kitabchi and Murphy's conclusion that bicarbonate therapy has little effect on outcome variables in DKA of the severity studied is broadly in line with the current consensus view, and I agree with it. Some caution is needed, however, since arterial pH is frequently less than 6.9 in patients with DKA and the above conclusion does not necessarily apply in such cases. It is easy to see how these extremely acidotic patients could be made either better or worse by bicarbonate; we do not know which!

Dr. Kitabchi and Ms. Murphy pay special attention to changes in CSF pH, glucose, and other biochemical measurements, presumably because of suggestions that changes in these variables might be related to the neuro-psychiatric state. Posner and Plum[1] initially had proposed that a CSF pH of 7.24 or below was likely to be associated with impairment of consciousness, a suggestion based on a very small number of cases and one which was not borne out by subsequent observations.[2,5] The original suggestion of Posner and Plum also was invoked to explain the deterioration of neuropsychiatric status occasionally seen during the treatment of DKA, because of the paradoxical acidification of the CSF observed during treatment. However, the observations of Ohman et al showed that CSF pH fell during treatment, in some cases to below 7.26, notwithstanding which all patients improved neurologically. A much more likely cause of neurological deterioration during treatment is osmotic disequilibrium due to blood osmolality declining faster than CSF and brain osmolality, with subsequent cerebral edema and raised intracranial pressure as clearly demonstrated by Clements et al.[5] Fulop et al.[6] showed that there was no relationship at presentation between arterial pH and the depth of coma, but that in contrast there was a reasonable correlation between blood glucose (and plasma) osmolality and coma grade. These observations make it unlikely that CSF acid-base status is a major contributor to neurological problems arising before or during treatment, with or without bicarbonate. In view of the previous studies, it is not clear how the present CSF observations can provide further help in deciding the issue of the value of bicarbonate therapy, since no data are given on CSF pressure changes, which may have a major influence on consciousness. Besides osmotic disequilibrium, diffuse intravascular coagulation has to be considered as a possible cause of disturbed consciousness in DKA, though this is more often a feature of hyperosmolar nonketoacidotic coma than of DKA.

I find it a little surprising that Kitabchi and Murphy found no significant difference in the rate of fall of plasma glucose between the two treatment groups (see Fig 5), and I wonder whether the statistical technique they employed had sufficient power to detect a real difference. Superficially, at least, it does appear that the bicarbonate-treated group experienced a slower fall in plasma glucose than did the control group. If this is indeed so, it could be construed as one argument in favor of bicarbonate, since a slow rate of fall of plasma glucose is less likely to precipitate osmotic disequilibrium problems. In this context, I note that Kitabchi and Murphy give no guidance on permissible rates of decline of blood glucose in their protocol for the management DKA. It is common practice in the United Kingdom to set 5 mmol/L/hr (90 mg/dL/hr) as a maximum rate of decline. The rate of insulin dose is tailored on the basis of frequent estimation of blood glucose to keep within this limit and frequently is considerably less than 7 units of soluble insulin per hour.

Of further note regarding their protocol, Dr. Kitabchi and Ms. Murphy administer bicarbonate if the arterial pH is less than 7.0. This is common practice. I think it should be emphasized that if bicarbonate is administered, then it should be in the form of the isotonic solution (1.4%) rather than the hypertonic (8.4%). Administration of the latter is likely to exacerbate the already substantial risks associated with the hyperosmolar state.

Returning to the main part of Kitabchi and Murphy's paper, they assume that treatment with bicarbonate will exacerbate "intracellular acidosis" because of the differential permeability of CO_2 and HCO_3^- across cell membranes, thereby contributing to overall pathophysiology. It must be reemphasized that intracellular pH (pH_i) is controlled in a quantitatively different fashion between different organs and under different pathological circumstances and that, in the absence of specific data, it is difficult to make any general statement about the behavior of intracellular pH. In my own position paper, I have outlined the general mechanisms by which cells control their internal pH in the face of external perturbations; these mechanisms almost certainly vary from organ to organ both in their absolute and relative efficacy. I have quoted experimental evidence that liver pH_i in DKA is unusually resistant to the effects of extracellular acidosis, and that bicarbonate infusion into acidotic rats or liver perfusions appears to raise hepatic pH_i, despite elevating PCO_2. My guess is that the behavior of cardiac pH_i may be a critical factor in determining the overall value of bicarbonate therapy in metabolic acidosis, a speculation similar to that of Arieff and his colleagues.

The argument about the effects of bicarbonate on the position of the oxygen dissociation curve and the potential for tissue anoxia arising from left shifts is a well known one and is a theoretical possibility. It is more likely to be important if alkalinization is effected at a time when the patient still has circulatory insufficiency, since compensation for the left shift by increased tissue perfusion would be less likely to occur then. However, I am unaware of any direct evidence that this effect is of clinical importance. There are two other well-known acid-base–related phenomena which occur during the treatment of DKA. First, there is the phenomenon of persistent hyperventilation, which may be present for some 24 hours after the correction of any metabolic acidosis and could be due to persistent CSF acidosis. Second, "alkaline overshoot" arises in patients with organic acidosis (e.g., DKA or lactic acidosis) who have been treated with substantial amounts of bicarbonate. During recovery, organic acid anions are metabolized to bicarbonate which, together with the administered bicarbonate, may give rise to metabolic alkalosis. Again, there is little evidence that either persistent hyperventilation or alkaline overshoot has major clinical consequences.

Finally, Dr. Kitabchi and Ms. Murphy have confined their discussion to bicarbonate therapy, as is not unreasonable given the terms of reference of this discussion. However, I would like to reiterate the importance of further experimental and clinical observations of the effects of alternative alkalinizing agents.

References

1. Posner J, Plum F: Spinal fluid pH and neurological symptoms in systemic acidosis. *N Engl J Med* 1967; 277:605–613.
2. Ohman JL, Marliss EB, Aoki TT, et al: The cerebrospinal fluid in diabetic ketoacidosis. *N Engl J Med* 1971; 284:283–290.
3. Morris LR, Murphy MB, Kitabchi AE: Bicarbonate therapy in severe diabetic ketoacidosis. *Ann Intern Med* 1986; 105:836–840.
4. Awdeh M, Morris L, Terkeurst J, et al: Myocardial function in patients with diabetic ketoacidosis. *Diabetes* 1979; 28(suppl):411.
5. Clements RS, Blumenthal SA, Morrison AD, et al: Increased cerebrospinal fluid pressure during treatment of diabetic ketosis. *Lancet* 1971; 2:671–675.
6. Fulop M, Tannenbaum H, Dreyer N: Ketotic hyperglycaemic coma. *Lancet* 1973; 2:635–639.

Rebuttal: Perspective 2

 Abbas E. Kitabchi, Ph.D., M.D.
Mary Beth Murphy, R.N., M.S.

Dr. Cohen's analysis of the bicarbonate controversy appropriately discusses the merits and demerits of bicarbonate for the entire spectrum of acidosis, whereas our charge was to discuss particularly the demerit of bicarbonate therapy in diabetic ketoacidosis (DKA). In our initial position paper we examined both sides of the issue, looked at the data of proponents and opponents of bicarbonate therapy, and came to a conclusion similar to that of Dr. Cohen that, except for two prospective randomized studies,[1,2] there are no comparative data available on the efficacy of bicarbonate therapy in DKA.

We also agree with Dr. Cohen that the models used in the majority of all studies of bicarbonate therapy have been experimental models and, although they are offered as useful pathophysiological models, extension of their application to man is not always warranted. Obviously, this dearth of data in clinical studies in humans is particularly distressing in metabolic acidotic conditions where hemodynamic instability adds insult to injury, precluding a careful, methodical approach to such investigation. The use of well-defined population, such as DKA patients, with specific exclusion and inclusion criteria would narrow the range of investigation so that more specific questions could be addressed. However, even those studies performed in such a subgroup of patients have been lacking. The two DKA studies which we reported last year[2] that agreed with the study of Hale et al.[1] (with the exception that Hale's study employed a shorter follow-up period) have not addressed the more specific questions raised by Dr. Cohen, such as the use of other alkalinizing agents ("carbicarb," sodium dichloracetate, THAM) in the treatment of DKA.

In considering these other treatment modalities, one is struck by the conspicuous absence of any data on the use of sodium dichloracetate (DCA) or THAM in human studies of DKA. This is understandable, since insulin therapy is the gold standard in this condition and no practical experience could be obtained through the use of these agents in vivo in DKA. However, the question of "carbicarb" is a more practical and cogent one, particularly in those DKA conditions associated with a low arterial pH. To our knowledge, Arieff has not studied the efficacy of "carbicarb" on DKA (personal communication, 1989). Such an investigation may be useful if it is coupled with an assessment of the intracellular pH of various organs and arterial pH measurement. An assessment of the intracellular pH of various organs was not possible prior to the advent of magnetic resonance imaging (MRI), but the current availability of this sophisticated technique makes the performance of such studies more plausible now. Until such time as they are performed, however, prudence and clinical judgment must dictate the use of bicarbonate therapy in DKA patients with an arterial pH below 6.9.

There has been almost unanimous agreement among workers in the field that no patient with a pH equal to or greater than 7.10 needs bicarbonate therapy.[3] Two recent studies suggest further that DKA patients with a pH in the range of 6.9 to 7.14 do not benefit from the use of bicarbonate either. However, those patients in DKA with a pH of less than 6.9 or with cardiovascular instability are somewhat different. In general, these patients are more severly decompensated and have a greater vulnerability to acid-base disturbance. This is the subgroup of patients in whom a thorough comparative study of bicarbonate and "carbicarb" would be of interest, since at this time it would be difficult if not impossible to convince any institutional review board to authorize the withholding of alkalinizing agents in patients with a pH below 6.9. A study of bicarbonate vs. "carbicarb" would provide a means whereby these two agents could be compared through the measurement of intracellular pH vs. arterial pH at specific time points correlated with the clinical condition of the patients.

As to Dr. Cohen's more specific comments regarding our paper, the following points deserve further explanation and discussion:

1. Although we agree that the real outcome variable in patients is survival, it is also important to note that in this day and age of modern medicine, very few centers experience a mortality greater than 2% or 3% in DKA patients. Notwithstanding Dr. Cohens' comments about a high mortality rate of patients with DKA, this is not the experience of the majority of centers in the United States.[4]

2. In our earlier attempt to study the efficacy of bicarbonate and its effects on the cardiovascular status of DKA patients, we were faced with the difficulty of structuring the protocol so that stable conditions could be maintained. Therefore, clinical judgment dictated adherence to rigid criteria, including an age limit to preclude other age-related diseases as well as cardiac instability. Therefore, the number of patients whose blood pH ranged from 6.9 to 7.14 remained below the ideal number for comparative measurement.[5]

3. As to cerebrospinal fluid (CSF) pressure, only limited data are available for six patients in each group. Bicarbonate therapy did not change the pressure from baseline 6 to 8 or 12 to 24 hours (213 vs. 225 vs. 250, respectively) as compared to the group that did not receive bicarbonate therapy (160 vs. 102 vs. 131, respectively). Although these values are based on a small number of subjects, significance was not reached. However, the two groups demonstrated differing trends — the no bicarbonate therapy appeared to suggest a more desirable improvement in CSF opening pressure compared to the bicarbonate group.

4. Regarding the rate of glucose decline in our study of bicarbonate

therapy, it is important to point out that the acceptable rate was taken as 10% of the initial glucose value in the first hour followed by 50 to 80 mg/dL in the subsequent 2 to 6 hours.[6] Using these criteria, the rate of decline was not calculated to be significantly different between the two groups. However, there was a tendency for a greater fall in serum glucose in the group that did not receive bicarbonate therapy than in the group that did, but this was not clinically significant. Furthermore, greater overlap surely must have contributed to the nonsignificant status of the two groups of results also.

5. Regarding the use of bicarbonate, it is important to point out that it was used as a 7.5% solution at the rate of 100 mL/hr with 15 mEq of potassium chloride. It is interesting to note that there was no mortality in either group and the amount of morbidity or mental obtundation was not significantly different between the two groups. We noted no deterioration of mental status in the two groups of patients during the entire follow-up period.

6. The issue of intracellular pH has been adequately addressed above and deserves greater attention with the advent of MRI as a means of measuring organ pH during the course of therapy.

7. As stated earlier, the use of different alkalinizing agents in the acidotic state is a moot question in DKA patients with a pH of 6.9 or greater, since insulin and saline is the gold standard for therapy. The use of such therapy with frequent monitoring of the patient has decreased mortality to less than 1.0%. The only group in which comparative study may be of interest in DKA patients with a pH below 6.9. To our knowledge, no study has reported on the comparative efficacy of bicarbonate vs. no bicarbonate in this group, let alone "carbicarb" vs. bicarbonate. The only situation in which a comparative study is justified is in severely acidotic patients where the data on the use of bicarbonate have not been forthcoming and the condition is associated with a greater degree of morbidity.

In conclusion, the available comparative data on alkaline therapy in acidosis in general and in DKA in particular compel one to evaluate all claims regarding the merit of such therapy with caution. Since the mortality rate in well-managed DKA patients with a pH of 6.9 or greater is below 1.0% with the use of insulin and saline, the use of bicarbonate in this group would not be appropriate. However, in DKA patients with a pH lower than 6.9, clinical judgment dictates the careful use of bicarbonate therapy until comparative studies regarding the use of this agent become available. Based on these considerations, we recently have provided an algorithm for the management of patients with DKA that includes the use of bicarbonate in patients with severe acidosis, i.e., a pH of less than 6.9.[6]

References

1. Hale PJ, Crase J, Nattrass M: Metabolic effects of bicarbonate in the treatment of diabetic ketoacidosis. *Br Med J* 1984; 289:1035–1038.
2. Morris LR, Murphy MB, Kitabchi AE: Bicarbonate therapy in severe diabetic ketoacidosis. *Ann Intern Med* 1986; 105:836–840.
3. Kitabchi AE, Murphy MB: Diabetic ketoacidosis and hyperosmolar hyperglycemic nonketotic coma, in Rizza RA, Green D (eds): *Medical Clinics of North America,* vol 72. Philadelphia, WB Saunders, 1988, pp 1545–1563.
4. Kitabchi AE: Low-dose insulin therapy in diabetes ketoacidosis: Fact or fiction, in DeFronzo R (ed): *Diabetes Metabolism Reviews.* New York, John Wiley & Sons, 1989, pp 337–363.
5. Awdeh M, Morris L, Terkeurst J, et al: Myocardial function in patients with diabetic ketoacidosis. *Diabetes* 1979; 28(suppl):411.
6. Kitabchi AE, Rumbak MJ: Management of diabetic emergencies. *Hosp Pract* 1989; 24:129–160.

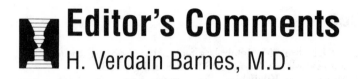

Editor's Comments
H. Verdain Barnes, M.D.

Diabetic ketoacidosis (DKA) is a prime example of metabolic acidosis, a potential complication of several diseases which is a therapeutic challenge for the clinician. In the initial planning for this debate, our intent was to focus on the use of bicarbonate in the treatment of DKA. Dr. Abbas E. Kitabchi, an internationally recognized investigator and scholar in this area, kindly agreed to provide the negative position statement. After contacting several other leaders in the field, the consensus was that an affirmative position for the use of bicarbonate therapy in DKA was not truly defensible based on available data. Some months after Dr. Kitabchi and Ms. Murphy's position paper was received, Dr. R.D. Cohen, an internationally recognized authority in the area of metabolic acidosis, agreed to write an analysis of the bicarbonate controversy from the more global perspective of metabolic acidosis. The result, I believe, can best be described as a "modified debate" (more of a response than a position paper debate) which focuses for the reader the strengths and weaknesses of the data available, the problems encountered by investigators, and the key directions for the future.

In their position paper, Dr. Kitabchi and Ms. Murphy succinctly summarize the pathophysiology of DKA, their work on the use of bicarbonate in DKA, and an approach to DKA therapy. Based on the evaluation parameters used, the studies of Dr. Kitabchi et al. have demonstrated that bicarbonate therapy has no statistically significant effect on overall outcome in young diabetics with severe DKA (arterial pH 6.9 to 7.14).

Dr. Cohen agrees in general with their position in regard to DKA, but he raises several concerns about metabolic acidosis. First, he points out the complexities of intracellular pH, particularly the fact that different organs may respond differently in varied pathophysiological settings. For example, the intracellular pH in rat livers during ketoacidosis appears to be unusually resistant to the effects of extracellular acidosis, while there may be less resistance in other organs. Furthermore, it appears that the response of an organ's intracellular pH may be different depending on the pathogenesis of the acidosis. Dr. Cohen concludes by hypothesizing that the status and response of the heart's intracellular pH may be "a critical factor in determining the overall value of bicarbonate therapy in metabolic acidosis," a point with which I agree. With the advent of magnetic resonance spectroscopy, this now can be more accurately assessed. Such data may be extremely helpful, since our debaters agree that the extrapolation of animal data to humans is not necessarily appropriate and therefore cannot drive our clnical decisions in humans.

In his position paper, Dr. Cohen effectively summarizes the data available on the use of other potentially more advantageous alkalinizing agents such as "carbicarb," DCA, and THAM in metabolic acidosis. There are no data regarding the use of these drugs in DKA and, as Dr. Kitabchi and Ms. Murphy point out, "carbicarb" could be a practical consideration. Hopefully, this as well as intracellular pH will be focuses for future investigation. In addition, Dr. Cohen's position paper analyzes Pco_2 and blood titration curve concerns in relation to metabolic acidosis. His points in this regard are well taken.

In summary, as this editor views the debators' position statements and responses, the following can be stated. First, in view of overall outcome, current data confirm that for young diabetics with ketoacidosis there is no benefit derived from bicarbonate therapy and also apparently no proven harm. Second, there are no data addressing the use of bicarbonate in DKA patients whose arterial pH is less than 6.9. Consequently, in this setting it remains prudent until such data are available to administer enough bicarbonate to raise the pH to over 6.9. Third, in severe diarrhea with acidosis, as well as in selected types of renal tubular acidosis, bicarbonate therapy appears to be appropriate. Finally, additional data need to be generated regarding intracellular pH and the use of other alkalinizing agents in metabolic acidosis. The former should allow physicians to better understand intracellular pathophysiology and physiology in metabolic acidosis therapy and recovery. The latter may provide us with an alternative(s) to bicarbonate and better facilitate cellular and clinical outcomes. It appears that the debate is not really over, nor should it be given the data currently available. Again, as has been true in many debates in these volumes, the physician must use his or her balanced clinical judgment in tailoring therapy for the individual patient. This debate assists us in preparing to make a more "balanced judgment."

Is 5-Aminosalicylic Acid (5-ASA) a Breakthrough or Ballyhoo?

Chapter Editor: Gary Gitnick, M.D.

Affirmative: Stephen Hanauer, M.D.
Associate Professor of Medicine, University
of Chicago Medical Center, Chicago, Illinois

Negative: Allen L. Ginsberg, M.D.
Professor of Medicine, George Washington
University School of Medicine and Health
Sciences, Washington, District of Columbia

Editor's Introduction

With the realization that 5-aminosalicylic acid is actually the active ingredient in sulfasalazine (or Azulfidine), interest rapidly developed in determining whether 5-ASA could be utilized as an effective therapeutic agent independent of the carrier molecule sulfapyridine. The latter has been shown to be responsible for many of the side effects attributed to sulfasalazine. The availability of technology that allowed for the development of a 5-ASA product free of sulfapyridine resulted in a variety of products being developed by many drug companies. This in turn led to the obvious question of whether 5-ASA is a breakthrough or just ballyhoo. The following debate undertakes to review the arguments which favor and those which negate the utilization of this agent.

Gary Gitnick, M.D.

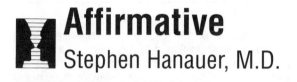
Affirmative
Stephen Hanauer, M.D.

5-ASA: A Breakthrough

5-ASA (5-aminosalicylic acid, mesalamine, mesalazine) clearly is a breakthrough in the treatment of inflammatory bowel disease (IBD). As the effective moiety of sulfasalazine, 5-ASA has been the mainstay of therapy for mild to moderate colitis and for the maintenance of ulcerative colitis (UC) in remission. In specialized delivery forms, 5-ASA offers enhanced efficacy for many IBD patients without the adverse consequences of the sulfa moiety in sulfasalazine. In the laboratory, 5-ASA is a tool with which the pathophysiological mechanisms of intestinal inflammation can be evaluated.

As is true of many scientific discoveries, therapy with 5-ASA proceeded with a combination of an hypothesis and a great deal of serendipity. Dr. Nanna Svartz observed a similar inflammatory response in the joints of patients with rheumatoid arthritis and in the wall of the intestine of patients with UC. Additional observations led to the theory that both diseases were bacterial in origin and sulfasalazine was developed initially to deliver both an antibacterial (sulfapyridine) and an anti-inflammatory agent (5-ASA) into the connective tissue of the gut wall and joints.[1]

Dr. Svartz' initial studies with UC patients supported the effectiveness of sulfasalazine and subsequent clinical trials confirmed its efficacy in acute mild to moderate ulcerative colitis,[2,3] its dose-response in the maintenance of UC in remission,[4] and its activity in mild to moderate colonic Crohn's disease.[5] It was not until 3 decades later that Peppercorn, Goldman, and Das elucidated the pharmacokinetics of sulfasalazine, disproving the concept of systemic connective tissue deposition of the drug and revealing the requirement for bacterial azo-reduction of the parent compound and inverse concentrations of sulfapyridine and 5-ASA within the colonic lumen and plasma.[6,7] These observations led to the appreciation of the toxicity caused by sulfapyridine and the colonic delivery of 5-ASA. However, it was not revealed until the pioneering clinical trial of Azad Khan, Juan Piris, and Sidney Truelove that 5-ASA was the active moiety of sulfasalazine and that sulfasalazine was a delivery system protecting 5-ASA from proximal absorption for delivery to the colon.[8] It then became apparent that 5-ASA was active topically, would not be released from the parent compound with rapid colonic transit (e.g., severe disease), and would not reliably release 5-ASA into the small intestine (accounting for the reduced efficacy in Crohn's disease). These background absorption and metabolic studies then led to the development of specific pharmacological delivery systems for 5-ASA.

Upon this foundation, the modern era of IBD therapy is evolving. Although the specific cause and, hence, cure for IBD is still unknown, we now can provide more effective therapy with a much improved safety profile. Campieri extended the rectal applicability of 5-ASA by demonstrating the heightened efficacy of 4-gm enemas compared to hydrocortisone enemas.[9] Subsequent clinical studies have confirmed the response of patients with distal colitis to the high-dose 5-ASA enemas, allowing the recruitment of previously refractory patients[10] and the elimination or reduction of treatment with concomitant sulfasalazine and steroids with their associated toxicity.[11] The door now has opened for another major clinical innovation: targeted, site-specific delivery of a locally active, nonsystemic agent. These technologies eventually will be applicable to alternative therapies, most conspicuously nonsystemic steroids, although the methodologies will be applicable to many pharmaceutical agents.

In the treatment of UC, we now have the ability to delivery 5-ASA to the rectum via suppositories or to the distal colon by enema. To date, both alternatives are the most effective, least toxic treatment for the largest proportion of patients with IBD. The oral delivery of 5-ASA via an alternative azo-bond attached to either an inert vehicle (e.g., Balsalazide)[12] or another molecule of 5-ASA (olsalazine)[13] provides pancolonic distribution of 5-ASA without an additional systemic burden of salicylate or a toxic carrier molecule. The improved efficacy of high-dose enemas suggests that we now will be able to utilize and evaluate further the dose-response of ulcerative colitis to 5-ASA without concerns over toxicity. Recent studies of oral doses of 5-ASA up to and above 4.8 gm, equal to 12 gm of sulfasalazine, have been utilized without significant toxicity.[14]

Up until now, patients with small-bowel Crohn's disease have been deprived of the therapeutic benefit of 5-ASA, accounting for the equivocal efficacy of sulfasalazine in ileal Crohn's disease. Slow-release (Pentasa) and delayed-release (Asacol, Claversal, Rowasa) preparations now will provide the ability to select a delivery system that will target the release of 5-ASA to the site of inflammation in individual patients, thereby amplifying the dose while limiting undesirable absorption or fecal wastage.[15] Indeed, preliminary studies have begun to show promising results with 5-ASA in selected populations of patients with Crohn's disease including, for the first time, the prolongation of remission in patients with clinically inactive Crohn's disease.[16]

5-ASA is metabolized rapidly by the intestinal epithelium to acetyl-5-ASA, which does not have the same apparent efficacy as the native molecule.[17] Hence, one must choose the clinicopathological situations where 5-ASA is likely to have a therapeutic benefit via luminal delivery. For example, 5-ASA is much more likely to be effective for the mucosal/submucosal inflammation that occurs in mild to moderate UC rather than the severe, transmural UC or Crohn's disease. Thus, one would predict that 5-ASA will be more effective for the treatment of mild, mucosal Crohn's disease or for the prevention of postoperative relapses. The investigators and evaluators of clinical studies must choose their patient populations, specific products, doses, and durations of therapy carefully before conclusions can be drawn about the "global" efficacy of these preparations in the treatment of IBD.

Another arena for breakthrough with 5-ASA will be in the laboratory where basic mechanisms of intestinal inflammation are being investigated. Indeed, 5-ASA is providing clues about the process of intestinal inflammation. Perhaps because of its pharmacokinetics and rapid metabolism, the intestinal mucosal milieu is the only recognized application for 5-ASA. Here, investigators can utilize the aberrant observations of enhanced prostaglandin release with active mucosal inflammation with the discrepant finding of the exacerbation of IBD with other nonsteroidal anti-inflammatory agents that specifically inhibit the cyclooxygenase system.[18] This has led to concentration upon the lipoxygenase system and the ability of leukotrienes to regulate local inflammatory events and the recruitment of circulating inflammatory and immunological participants into the eventual pathological sequence of Crohn's disease or UC.[19,20]

5-ASA is a tool with which to explore further the intercellular relationships between immune and inflammatory components and the intracellular regulation of inflammatory precursors. The observations of Stenson and coworkers[21] that 5-ASA is an inhibitor of leukotriene synthesis has led to the development and eventual testing of other inhibitors and antagonists of the lipoxygenase cascade. Further studies will be required to determine how individual components respond to an initial injury (or specific types of injuries), how these cells can be regulated (by 5-ASA or other inhibitors), and what the differences are between the specific cellular events in UC and Crohn's disease.

Drs. Eugene Chang and Terrence Barrett, working with a cell line of intestinal macrophages provided by Lloyd Mayer, have recognized that the indigenous gut macrophage is capable of producing leukotriene B_4, a potent chemotactic agent and stimulator of leukocytes.[22] One might hypothesize that the inhibition of these inhabitant cells may account for the prophylactic properties of 5-ASA in quiescent UC. Hence, when the inhibition ceases the initiation process (which is still to be determined) stimulates the macrophage to recruit circulating inflammatory cells to produce the cascade of tissue destruction that we interpret as "active" UC. Further studies will help to ascertain the local regulation of inflammation by manipulations of single cell functions and interactions between cells in UC and Crohn's disease. 5-ASA also is a potent scavenger of oxygen free radicals which are generated by inflammatory cells and can amplify further release of arachidonic acid metabolites.[23] The reduction of reactive oxygen species of 5-ASA contrasts with 4-ASA which does not affect arachidonic metabolism in human neutrophils or production of free oxygen radicals.[24]

As we await the basic laboratory studies related to 5-ASA and its mechanisms of action, our patients are already reaping the rewards of this breakthrough. The 4-gm 5-ASA enemas have been shown to produce clinical responses in 90% of Italian patients.[25] We have been able to achieve remissions in 75% of refractory patients, many of whom have had active symptoms for years without any benefit from sulfasalazine or corticosteroids.[26] Best of all, these benefits have come with fewer adverse effects than have been observed in patients treated with placebos.

Studies in UC comparing oral 5-ASA compounds vs. sulfasalazine continue to demonstrate equal efficacy with a marked improvement in adverse effects.[27–29] Even in patients who have tolerated sulfasalazine, there are fewer reports of adverse events after a change to 5-ASA. One would expect that this would improve patient compliance and reduce the likelihood of relapse. Interestingly, changing to a 5-ASA alternative has restored the fertility of many male patients who were infertile on sulfasalazine.[30] Therefore, 5-ASA should replace sulfasalazine as the drug of choice for patients desiring a family.

The argument that 5-ASA cannot be a breakthrough because it is not a "new" agent will not suffice. The ability to optimize therapy and target site-specific treatment with 5-ASA, and its improved safety profile are all breakthroughs. The ability to reverse male infertility while maintaining UC in remission and to control refractory proctosigmoiditis with 5-ASA are breakthroughs. The ability to prevent relapses in Crohn's disease is a breakthrough. The ability to manipulate the inflammatory cascade and the recognition of the importance of leukotrienes in gut inflammation are breakthroughs. Finally, the ability to manipulate individual gut inflammatory cells is a breakthrough.

While the saying, "it's more important to know that a drug works than how it works" certainly applies to 5-ASA, so too does the statement that "diseases that harm call for drugs that harm less." I am happy to proclaim that 5-ASA ushers us into this new era of drug therapy for IBD. To quote Hippocrates, "Healing is a matter of time, but it is sometimes also a matter of opportunity." Whether 5-ASA is a scientific or a therapeutic breakthrough, it is up to us, clinicians and basic researchers together, to utilize the opportunity it provides. There are many questions to be asked and investigated in IBD. Rather than resting on the laurels of this single breakthrough, we must forge ahead until the eventual cause and cure of this disease are identified.

References

1. Bachrach, WH: Sulfasalazine: I. An historical perspective. *Am J Gastroenterol* 1988; 83:487–496. *This fascinating manuscript provides an historical perspective of the development of sulfasalazine by an experienced gastroenterologist, friend of Dr. Svartz, and Food and Drug Administration official.*
2. Baron JH, Connell AM, Lennard-Jones JE, et al: Sulphasalazine and salicyla-

zosulphadimidine in ulcerative colitis. *Lancet* 1962; 1:1094–1096. *This is the report of an initial clinical trial documenting the benefit of sulfasalazine.*

3. Dick AP, Grayson MJ, Carpenter RG, et al: Controlled trial of sulphasalazine in the treatment of ulcerative colitis. *Gut* 1964; 5:437–442. *The first placebo-controlled trial of sulfasalazine is reported.*

4. Azad Khan AK, Howes DT, Piris J, et al: Optimum dose of sulphasalazine for maintenance treatment of ulcerative colitis. *Gut* 1980; 21:232–240. *This study provides documentation of the dose-response for sulfasalazine in ulcerative colitis maintenance therapy.*

5. Summers RW, Switz DM, Sessions JT, et al: National Cooperative Crohn's Disease Study: Results of drug treatment. *Gastroenterology* 1979; 77:847–869. *This is a randomized, controlled trial suggesting the efficacy of sulfasalazine in colonic Crohn's disease.*

6. Peppercorn MA: Sulfasalazine: Pharmacology, clinical use, toxicity, and related new drug development. *Ann Intern Med* 1984; 3:377–386. *This is an excellent review of sulfasalazine, its pharmacology, and its toxicity.*

7. Das KM, Eastwood MA, McManus JPA, et al: Adverse reactions during salicylazosulfapyridine therapy and the relation with drug metabolism and acetylator phenotype. *N Engl J Med* 1973; 289:491–495. *Clinical studies relating the intolerance to sulfasalazine with the sulfapyridine moiety are documented.*

8. Khan AKA, Piris J, Truelove SC: An experiment to determine the active therapeutic moiety of sulphasalazine. *Lancet* 1977; 2:892–895. *This is the first clinical trial to suggest 5-ASA is the active moiety of sulfasalazine.*

9. Campieri M, Lanfranchi GA, Bazzocchi G, et al: Treatment of ulcerative colitis with high-dose 5-aminosalicylic acid enemas. *Lancet* 1981; 2:270–271. *This is the initial report of the use of high-dose 5-ASA enemas in ulcerative colitis.*

10. McPhee MS, Swan JT, Biddle WL, et al: Proctocolitis unresponsive to conventional therapy: Responsive to 5-aminosalicylic acid enemas. *Dig Dis Sci* 1987; 32:76S–81S. *The response of refractory colitis to 5-ASA enemas is described.*

11. Hanauer SB, Schultz PA: Relapse rates after successful treatment of refractory colitis with 5-ASA enemas (abstract). *Gastroenterology* 1987; 92:1424. *The importance of maintenance therapy with topical treatment as well as oral treatment in ulcerative colitis is emphasized.*

12. Chan RP, Pope DJ, Gilbert AP, et al: Studies of two novel sulfasalazine analogs, Ipsalazide and Balsalazide. *Dig Dis Sci* 1983; 28:609–615. *Alternative delivery systems for 5-ASA to the colon are described.*

13. Sandberg-Gertzen H, Jarnerot G, Kraaz W: Azodisal sodium in the treatment of ulcerative colitis: A study of tolerance and relapse-prevention properties. *Gastroenterology* 1986; 90:1024–1030. *This is a study describing the efficacy of olsalazine in sulfasalazine-intolerant patients.*

14. Schroeder KW, Tremaine WJ, Ilstrup DM: Coated oral 5-aminosalicylic acid therapy for mildly to moderately active ulcerative colitis. *N Engl J Med* 1987; 317:1625–1629. *This is an initial study of Asacol in active ulcerative colitis suggesting a dose-response different from sulfasalazine.*

15. Hanauer SB: 5-ASA agents, in Peppercorn M (ed): *The Management of*

Inflammatory Bowel Disease. New York, Marcel Dekker Publishers, 1988. *This is a recent review of 5-ASA agents.*

16. Thomson ABR (on behalf of International Study Group, Edmonton, Canada): Claversal/Mesasal prevents relapse and maintains remission of inactive Crohn's disease. 1989; in press. *This is the first study to suggest a maintenance role of 5-ASA in Crohn's disease.*

17. Van Hogezand RA, Van Hees PAM, Van Gorp JPWM, et al: Double-blind comparison of 5-aminosalicylic acid and acetyl-5-aminosalicylic acid suppositories in patients with idiopathic proctitis. *Aliment Pharm Therapeutics* 1988; 2:33–40. *5-ASA may be more effective than acetyl-5-ASA because the latter is not absorbed across the epithelial lining.*

18. Hoult JRS: Pharmacological and biochemical actions of sulphasalazine: Section 1-Mode of action. *Drugs* 1986; 32:18–26. *The exact mode of action of sulfasalazine and 5-ASA is, as yet, undetermined.*

19. Allgayer H, Stenson WF: A comparison of effects of sulfasalazine and its metabolites on the metabolism of endogenous vs. exogenous arachidonic acid. *Immunopharmacology* 1988; 15:39–46. *A description of the effects of sulfasalazine and 5-ASA on the arachidonic acid cascade is given.*

20. McDermott RP, Stenson WF: The immunology of idiopathic inflammatory bowel disease. *Hosp Pract[off]* 1986; 15:97–116. *This is a description of multiple (secondary) immunological perturbations in inflammatory bowel disease.*

21. Stenson WF, Lobos E: Sulfasalazine inhibits the synthesis of chemotactic lipids by neutrophils. *J Clin Invest* 1982; 69:494–497. *The effects of sulfasalazine and 5-ASA on neutrophil chemotaxis are documented.*

22. Barrett TA, Musch MW, Vaitla R, et al: Differential regulation of lipoxygenase and cyclooxygenas metabolism of arachidonic acid in isolated rabbit colonic macrophages. *Gastroenterology* 1989; 96:A29. *The possible site of 5-ASA activity may be the macrophage.*

23. Miyachi Y, Yochioka A, Imamura S, et al: Effect of sulphasalazine and its metabolites on the generation of reactive oxygen species. *Gut* 1987; 28:190–195. *Another possible mechanism of 5-ASA is the scavenging of oxygen free radicals.*

24. Nielsen OH, Ahnfelt-Ronne I: 4-aminosalicylic acid, in contrast to 5-aminosalicylic acid, has no effect on arachidonic acid metabolism in human neutrophils, or on the free radical 1,1-diphenyl-2-picrylhydrazyl. *Pharmacol Toxicol* 1988; 62:223–226. *Differential effects of 4-ASA and 5-ASA in experimental conditions.*

25. Campieri M, Lanfranchi GA, Brignola C, et al: High-dose 5-aminosalicylic acid enemas in the treatment of ulcerative colitis. *Ann Intern Med* 1984; 5:164–171. *The combined experience of the Italian group in treating patients with 5-ASA enemas is reported.*

26. Hanauer SB: 5-ASA enema therapy. *Neth J Med* 1989; 35:S11–S20. *This is a review of 5-ASA topical therapies.*

27. Riley SA, Mani V, Goodman MJ, et al: Comparison of delayed-release 5-aminosalicylic acid (Mesalazine) and sulfasalazine as maintenance treatment for patients with ulcerative colitis. *Gastroenterology* 1988; 94:1383–1389. *This a study which demonstrates equivalency between sulfasalazine and Asacol.*

28. Mulder CJ, Tytgat GN, Weterman IT, et al: Double-blind comparison of slow-release 5-aminosalicylate and sulfasalazine in remission maintenance in ulcerative colitis. *Gastroenterology* 1988; 95:1449–1453. *Comparable efficacy between Pentasa and sulfasalazine to maintain remissions in ulcerative colitis is reported.*
29. Rachmilewitz D (on behalf of an international study group): Coated mesalazine (5-aminosalicylic acid) versus sulphasalazine in the treatment of active ulcerative colitis: A randomized trial. *Br Med J* 1989; 298:82–86. *Comparable efficacy between sulfasalazine and Claversal in active ulcerative colitis is reported.*
30. Cann PA, Holdworth CD: Reversal of male infertility on changing treatment from sulphasalazine to 5-aminosalicylic acid. *Lancet* 1984; 1:119. *Reversible sperm abnormalities with substitution of 5-ASA for sulfasalazine is demonstrated.*

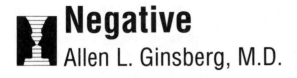

Negative

Allen L. Ginsberg, M.D.

5-ASA: More Ballyhoo than Breakthrough

I have been asked to argue the position that 5-aminosalicylic acid (5-ASA) is more ballyhoo than breakthrough. A breakthrough is defined in Webster's Dictionary as "a *sudden* advance in knowledge or technique." Ballyhoo is defined as "(1) a noisy, attention-getting demonstration or talk or (2) flamboyant, exaggerated, or sensational advertising or propaganda." 5-ASA unquestionably is not a breakthrough therapy for Crohn's disease. Although 5-ASA undoubtedly will be useful in the therapy of some patients with ulcerative colitis, it is little more than the recycling of an old drug in a new, less toxic form. The hoopla surrounding 5-ASA and the excited anticipation of its approval represent more ballyhoo than scientific breakthrough.

Any discussion of 5-ASA should start with a brief discussion of sulfasalazine, since 5-ASA is merely the active component of this established drug. Dr. Nanna Svartz[1] synthesized sulfasalazine and reported it to be useful in the treatment of rheumatoid arthritis and ulcerative colitis in 1942. It is now widely accepted that sulfasalazine is useful primarily in maintaining remission in ulcerative colitis. It is also of value in the treatment of mild to moderate colitis, especially when used as adjunctive therapy in combination with corticosteroids.

Data demonstrating the effectiveness of sulfasalazine in Crohn's disease have been harder to obtain. Many questioned its usefulness at all in this disease until 1979 when the National Cooperative Crohn's Disease Study[2] demonstrated it to be effective in Crohn's colitis. Efficacy in small intestinal Crohn's disease could not be demonstrated and sulfasalazine was ineffective in preventing relapses after surgery. After 46 years, the Food and Drug Administration still has not recognized or approved sulfasalazine for use in Crohn's disease. Thus, although sulfasalazine has a recognized role in the therapy of some patients with Crohn's disease, it does not fit the definition of a breakthrough, because it does not represent a sudden, major therapeutic advance.

In a landmark paper by Azad Khan, Juan Piris, and Sidney Truelove in 1977,[3] 5-ASA was demonstrated to be the active moiety of sulfasalazine. At that time it was anticipated that we would be able to treat patients with large amounts of the active component of sulfasalazine and avoid the toxicity of the sulfapyridine moiety. Expectations were raised regarding the development of wonderful new drugs that would reduce the morbidity of inflammatory bowel disease and alter the natural history of this disorder. In repsonse, the pharmaceutical industry has given us olsalazine (Dipentum), mesalamine (Asacol, Pentasa, Salofalk, Claversal, and Rowasa), and 4-ASA (Colony1). However, it is reasonable to question the benefits our patients have received 11 years after 5-ASA was demonstrated to be the active component of sulfasalazine.

Crohn's Disease

A review of the published data on the use of 5-ASA in Crohn's disease is appropriate. Unfortunately, most of the meager published data are anecdotal and derived from the open and uncontrolled use of 5-ASA preparations. The trials comparing 5-ASA to sulfasalazine that have been performed show no difference in effectiveness between the two agents. The only published placebo-controlled trial to date shows 5-ASA to be no more effective than placebo. The scanty available data are summarized below.

Rasmussen et al.[4] treated 18 patients who were suffering from active Crohn's disease. Sulfasalazine and corticosteroids were discontinued for a 2-week wash-out period. Patients then were treated with 1.5 g of Pentasa for 6 weeks. The clinical course was estimated to have improved in 13 patients, remained unchanged in 2 and become worse in 3. The Crohn's Disease Activity Index (CDAI) decreased from a median of 226 to 99. This open pilot study led to a 16-week, double-blind, placebo-controlled, multicenter study of 67 patients with Crohn's disease[5] in which no difference was found between treatment with 1.5 g of Pentasa and with placebo.

Maier[6] compared therapy with 3 g of sulfasalazine to therapy with 1.5 g of Salofalk in 30 patients with Crohn's disease in an 8-week trial. Twelve of the 15 patients who received sulfasalazine improved compared to 13 of the 15 patients who received Salofalk. No differences were discernible between the two treatment groups.

In an open trial, Donald and Wilkinson[7] treated with Asacol seven patients who had active Crohn's colitis and were allergic to or intolerant of sulfasalazine. They reported that four of the seven patients with poor disease control on the initiation of Asacol achieved a remission during 6 months of therapy.

The only mention of 5-ASA therapy of Crohn's disease in the recent literature is an abstract[8] that reports a patient with Crohn's colitis who was treated with Asacol. The patient developed pancreatitis which was thought to be a complication of the Asacol. Two rechallenges each led to the recurrence of symptoms and a rise in the serum amylase level.

In summary, there are no data to suggest that 5-ASA in any form represents a therapeutic breakthrough in the management of Crohn's disease. However, a small subset of patients who are allergic to or intolerant of sulfasalazine may obtain a similar clinical benefit from 5-ASA.

Ulcerative Colitis

In 1977 Azad Khan et al.[3] demonstrated that 5-ASA enemas and sulfasalazine enemas were equally effective in producing clinical, sigmoidoscopic, and histological improvement in patients with distal colitis and proctitis. In that study over 60% of patients had clinical and sigmoidoscopic improvement and 29% had pronounced histological improvement whether treated with 5-ASA or sulfasalazine enemas. Sulfapyridine enemas were found to be ineffective. In the ensuing 11 years these findings have been confirmed by Campieri et al.[9] and Sutherland et al.[10] and ultimately even the Food and Drug Administration has recognized the safety and efficacy of 5-ASA enemas. It is not my intention to belittle the safety and efficacy of 5-ASA and 4-ASA enemas. They clearly are of great value in some patients with distal colitis and proctitis. However, they do have serious limitations which can be itemized as follows:

1. A large, multicenter, placebo-controlled trial[10] reported improvement in only 55% of patients using a disease activity index based on clinical and sigmoidoscopic findings and physicians' overall assessment. That means that nearly half the patients were not helped by the purported breakthrough drug for which we waited 11 years.
2. Most patients must take adjunctive sulfasalazine in addition to the 5-ASA enemas in order to achieve the desired therapeutic effect.[10–12]
3. More than 80% of patients treated with 5-ASA enemas relapse within 4 months of stopping enema therapy and, therefore, may require chronic maintenance enema therapy if their disease is to be controlled.[13,14]
4. The cost of 5-ASA enema therapy is outrageous ($50 a week).
5. 5-ASA enemas may be no more effective than sulfasalazine enemas.[3]

To date, there are no studies which demonstrate that any of the oral 5-ASA compounds are more effective than sulfasalazine. Side effects do appear to occur less frequently, and patients allergic to sulfapyridine often can tolerate the 5-ASA compounds. However, for the majority of patients with ulcerative colitis who have been taking sulfasalazine for years without adverse effects, the new compounds are not likely to offer any breakthrough benefits. Examples of the comparable efficacy of 5-ASA and sulfasalazine are most apparent when maintenance studies of patients in remission are reviewed (Table 1). When the overall trends in these studies are examined, there is even a suggestion that sulfasalazine may be marginally more effective.

5-ASA and 4-ASA compounds will play a role in the therapy of inflammatory bowel disease, especially in patients who are allergic to or intolerant of sulfasalazine. However, the concept that they represent a sudden major

TABLE 1.
Relapse Rate

Author	Sulfasalazine	5-ASA	Placebo	Trial Duration
Dissanayake and Truelove[15]	12.1% (2 g)		54.8%	6 months
Jewell and Ireland[16]	12.2% (2 g)	19.5% (olsalazine, 1 g)		6 months
Sandberg-Gertzen et al.[17]		23.1% (olsalazine, 1 g)	44.9%	6 months
Dew et al.[18]	20% (mean 2.3 g)	22% (Asacol, mean 2.7 g)		6 months
Riley et al.[19]	38.6% (median 2 g)	37.5% (Asacol, median 800 mg)		48 weeks

advance (i.e., a breakthrough) in the treatment of inflammatory bowel disease (particularly Crohn's disease) is a lot of "ballyhoo!"

References

1. Svartz N: Salazopyrin, a new sulfanilamide preparation. A. Therapeutic results in rheumatic polyarthritis. B. Therapeutic results in ulcerative colitis. C. Toxic manifestations in treatment with sulfanilamide preparations. *Acta Med Scand* 1942; 110:577–598. *This is the first description of the use of sulfasalazine.*
2. Summers RW, Switz DM, Sessions JT, et al: National Cooperative Crohn's Disease Study: Results of drug treatment. *Gastroenterology* 1979; 77:847–869. *The beneficial effect of sulfasalazine in Crohn's colitis is documented.*
3. Azad Khan AK, Piris J, Truelove SC: An experiment to determine the active therapeutic moiety of sulphasalazine. *Lancet* 1977; 2:892–895. *This is the first documentation that 5-ASA is the active component of sulfasalazine.*
4. Rasmussen SN, Binder V, Maier K, et al: Treatment of Crohn's disease with peroral 5-aminosalicylic acid. *Gastroenterology* 1983; 85:1350–1353. *This is a preliminary report suggesting that oral 5-ASA might be useful in Crohn's disease.*
5. Rasmussen SN, Lauritsen K, Tage-Jensen U, et al: 5-Aminosalicylic acid in the treatment of Crohn's disease: A 16 week double-blind, placebo-controlled, multicenter study with Pentasa. *Scand J Gastroenterol* 1987; 22:877–883. *This is a placebo-controlled trial of Pentasa which fails to document efficacy in Crohn's disease.*

6. Maier K, et al: Successful management of chronic inflammatory bowel disease with oral 5-aminosalicylic acid. *DMW* 1985; 110:363–368. *Sulfasalazine and Salofalk are equally effective in an 8-week trial in patients with Crohn's disease.*

7. Donald IP, Wilkinson SP: The value of 5-aminosalicylic acid in inflammatory bowel disease for patients intolerant or allergic to sulphasalazine. *Postgrad Med* 1985; 61:1047–1048. *Anecdotal reports of response to Asacol in patients with Crohn's colitis who are allergic to sulfasalazine are presented.*

8. Sachedina B, Cohen LB, Whlitley J, et al: Asacol induced pancreatitis (abstract). *Gastroenterology* 1988; 94:A622. *5-ASA has side effects, albeit rare.*

9. Compieri M, Lanfranchi GA, Brignola C, et al: 5-Aminosalicylic acid as a rectal enema in ulcerative colitis patients unable to take sulphasalazine. *Lancet* 1984; 1:403. *This study provides confirmation that 5-ASA enemas are effective in proctitis and left-sided ulcerative colitis.*

10. Sutherland LR, Martin F, Greer S, et al: 5-Aminosalicylic acid enema in the treatment of distal ulcerative colitis, proctosigmoiditis and proctitis. *Gastroenterology* 1987; 92:1894–1898. *This study provides confirmation that 5-ASA enemas are effective in proctitis and left-sided ulcerative colitis.*

11. Ginsberg AL, Steinberg WM, Nochomovitz LE: Deterioration of left sided ulcerative colitis after withdrawal of sulfasalazine (abstract). *Gastroenterology* 1985; 88:1395. *Aminosalicylate enemas are most effective in combination with oral sulfasalazine.*

12. Ginsberg AL, Beck LS, McIntosh TM, et al: Treatment of left sided ulcerative colitis with 4-aminosalicylic acid enemas: A double-blind, placebo-controlled trial. *Ann Intern Med* 1988; 108: 195–199. *4-ASA enemas are safe and effective in the treatment of proctitis and left-sided ulcerative colitis.*

13. Biddle WL, Greenberger J, Swan T, et al: 5-Aminosalicylic acid enemas: Effective agent in maintaining remission in left sided ulcerative colitis. *Gastroenterology* 1988; 94:1705–1709. *There is a high relapse rate after 5-ASA enemas are discontinued.*

14. Guarino J, Chatzinoff M, Berk T, et al: 5-Aminosalicylic acid enemas in refractory distal ulcerative colitis: Long-term results. *Am J Gastroenterol* 1987; 82:732–737. *Further data on the high relapse rate seen after the discontinuation of 5-ASA enemas are reported.*

15. Dissanayake AS, Truelove SC: A controlled therapeutic trial of long term maintenance treatment of ulcerative colitis with sulphasalazine. *Gut* 1973; 14:923–926. *Patients that discontinue sulfasalazine have four times the number of flare-ups of colitis as do those that continue maintenance therapy.*

16. Jewell DP, Ireland A: A comparative trial of Olsalazine and sulphasalazine for the maintenance treatment of ulcerative colitis in remission. *Gastroenterology* 1987; 92:1447. *Relapse rates are comparable in patients taking olsalazine and sulfasalazine.*

17. Sandberg-Gertzen H, Janerot G, Kraaz W: Azodisal sodium in the treatment of ulcerative colitis: A study of tolerance and relapse prevention properties. *Gastroenterology* 1986; 90:1024–1030. *Olsalazine is more effective than placebo in preventing relapses in patients with ulcerative colitis.*

18. Dew MJ, Harries AD, Evans N, et al: Maintenance of remission in ulcerative colitis with 5-aminosalicylic acid in high doses by mouth. *Br Med J* 1983; 287:23–24. *Sulfasalazine and Asacol are comparable as maintenance therapy in patients with ulcerative colitis.*
19. Riley SA, Mani V, Goodman MJ, et al: Comparison of delayed release 5-aminosalicylic acid (Mesalazine) and Sulfasalazine as maintenance treatment for patients with ulcerative colitis. *Gastroenterology* 1988; 94:1383–1389. *Confirmation that Asacol and sulfasalazine are comparable as maintenance therapy is offered.*

Rebuttal: Affirmative
Stephen B. Hanauer, M.D.

Dr. Ginsberg begins his argument by discussing sulfasalazine. Dan Quayle may be no Jack Kennedy, but 5-aminosalicylic acid (5-ASA) is certainly not sulfasalazine. Furthermore, 5-ASA does meet the Webster's Dictionary definition of "a sudden advance in knowledge or technique," for, as Dr. Ginsberg has discussed, recognition that 5-ASA is the active moiety of sulfasalazine has allowed immediate advances in our knowledge and techniques of administering a therapeutic moiety to specific sites along the gastrointestinal tract without complicating treatment with the harmful sulfa portion of the compound. The reason sulfasalazine has not been found to be effective in clinical trials of Crohn's disease is related to the inability of the drug to deliver therapeutic concentrations of the active moiety to the site of inflammation. Indeed, when 5-ASA is delivered to colonic Crohn's disease, the clinical trials have shown its efficacy.[1,2] Furthermore, as most experienced clinicians recognize, many patients with Crohn's disease respond to sulfasalazine both in its active phase and as a maintenance continuing therapy for those who have responded to it.

In 1988 and in the future we must be cautious when interpreting the results of clinical trials that have used inadequate sample sizes, poorly defined or inappropriate endpoints, and unspecified or inadequate drug doses or follow-up periods before concluding that 5-ASA possesses efficacy or a lack thereof in the treatment of inflammatory bowel disease. A number of the studies that Dr. Ginsberg has quoted are lacking on all these accounts.

The study by Rasmussen et al[3] used a small group of patients with minimally active Crohn's disease who were given very low doses of Pentasa. Although there was no statistical difference, the trend was certainly in favor of the active compound compared to the placebo. The study by Donald and Wilkinson[4] describes the success with Asacol. Furthermore, as I described previously, a study by Thompson presented at a Frankfurt symposium and currently in press describes the efficacy of Claversal at a dose of 1.5 g daily in preventing relapse in patients with inactive Crohn's disease.[5]

As far as ulcerative colitis is concerned, we must consider 5-ASA a breakthrough for two irrefutable reasons: (1) 5-ASA in enema form is able to induce remissions in 75% of previously refractory patients with distal ulcerative colitis,[6] and (2) 80% of patients who could not tolerate sulfasalazine are able to receive therapeutic benefit from 5-ASA without the sulfa moiety.[7] While I agree with Dr. Ginsberg that there are no studies which demonstrate a therapeutic advantage of 5-ASA over sulfasalazine, tolerance of the former is much greater and the side-effect profile is much reduced. In addition, 5-

ASA does not induce the sperm abnormalities that are recognized in 80% of males taking sulfasalazine.

Hence, I must reiterate that 5-ASA is a breakthrough because (1) it allows the therapeutic moiety of sulfasalazine to be delivered directly to the sites of inflammation, thereby enhancing therapeutic efficacy (i.e., enema for distal ulcerative colitis, small-bowel delivery for Crohn's disease); (2) it allows higher doses to be administered, which should increase efficacy; and (3) it markedly reduces the side-effect profile from sulfasalazine.

References

1. Nielsen OH, Bondesen S: Kinetics of 5-aminosalicylic acid after jejunal instillation in man. *Br J Clin Pharmacol* 1983; 16:738–740.
2. Klotz U, Maier KE, Fischer C, et al: A new slow-release form of 5-aminosalicylic acid for the oral treatment of inflammatory bowel disease: Biopharmaceutic and clinical pharmacokinetic characteristics. *Arzneimittelforschung* 1985; 35:636–639.
3. Rasmussen SN, Lauritsen K, Tage-Jensen U, et al: 5-Aminosalicylic acid in the treatment of Crohn's disease: A 16 week double-blind, placebo-controlled, multicenter study with Pentasa. *Scand J Gastroenterol* 1987; 22:877–883.
4. Donald IP, Wilkinson SP: The value of 5-aminosalicylic acid in inflammatory bowel disease for patients intolerant or allergic to sulphasalazine. *Postgrad Med* 1985; 61:1047–1048.
5. Goldstein F, Farquhar S, Thornton JJ, et al: Favorable effects of sulfasalazine on small bowel Crohn's disease: A long-term study. *Am J Gastroenterol* 1987; 82:848–853.
6. Willoughby CP, Aronson JR, Agback H, et al: Distribution and metabolism in healthy volunteers of disodium azodisalicylate, a potential therapeutic agent for ulcerative colitis. *Gut* 1982; 23:1081–1087.
7. Rao SS, Cann PA, Holdworth CD: Clinical experience of the tolerance of mesalazine and olsalazine in patients intolerant of sulphasalazine. *Scand J Gastroenterol* 1987; 22:332–336.

Rebuttal: Negative
Allen L. Ginsberg, M.D.

The discovery of sulfasalazine and its application in ulcerative colitis was a breakthrough. The use of 5-aminosalicylic acid (5-ASA), the active moiety of sulfasalazine, is not a breakthrough but merely the recycling of an old drug. Based on the published data, neither drug represents a breakthrough in the therapy of Crohn's disease.

Dr. Hanauer's presentation avoided data. The reason for this is because there are very few data, most of which are not very good. Dr. Hanauer talks about "preliminary studies [which] have begun to show promising results with 5-ASA in selected populations of patients with Crohn's disease." These studies are as yet unpublished in peer-reviewed journals and are unconfirmed. Until good, placebo-controlled, double-blind studies are published and confirmed, their trumpeting represents more ballyhoo than breakthrough.

Dr. Hanauer states, "another arena for breakthrough with 5-ASA will be in the laboratory where basic mechanisms of intestinal inflammation are being investigated." At present, none of these mechanisms have been established to play a clear role in the pathogenesis of inflammatory bowel disease. Until such time as we have data which lead to better treatment of disease, this argument represents ballyhoo or hope of things to come if a lucky lottery number is picked.

The discovery of penicillin was a breakthrough. The polio vaccine was a breakthrough. 5-ASA is more akin to a new cephalosporin or new H_2 blocker. The claim of "breakthrough" is ballyhoo!

▌Editor's Comments
Gary Gitnick, M.D.

The active ingredient in sulfasalazine is 5-aminosalicylic acid (5-ASA); the other component of the drug, sulfapyridine, is merely a carrier molecule. With the demonstration that the latter component is responsible for many of the adverse effects of sulfasalazine came the hope of developing a product with the anti-inflammatory activity of sulfasalazine without the drawbacks of sulfapyridine. Now, after several years in development, a variety of 5-aminosalicylic acid products is becoming available.

Dr. Hanauer believes that these products will constitute a real breakthrough. He maintains that the targeted, site-specific delivery of a locally active, nonsystemic anti-inflammatory agent will revolutionize our management of the inflammatory bowel diseases. These new agents will allow us for the first time to treat effectively Crohn's disease of the small bowel, a condition that responds poorly to sulfasalazine. Suppositories and enemas allow for more effective treatment of localized colonic disease. The editor agrees that the ability to target delivery may become a great advantage. The clinician will be able to use designer drugs, i.e., drugs developed specifically for small intestinal disease, colonic disease, or rectal disease.

Dr. Hanauer goes on to argue that 5-ASA will elucidate the steps in the inflammatory process. He argues that investigators can utilize the effects of 5-ASA to understand better prostaglandin release and its role in mucosal inflammation. This, in turn, may lead to a better understanding of the lipoxygenase system and the role of leukotrienes in the regulation of the inflammatory process. The editor disagrees with this concept. Certainly the inflammatory process is being actively investigated. Five scientific laboratories located throughout the world have been investigating and will continue to strive to understand the steps that lead to inflammation and the propagation of disease. The contribution of 5-ASA to this understanding has been relatively minor thus far and probably will not become much more significant in the future. On this point Dr. Hanauer's argument is purely speculative.

Finally, Dr. Hanauer points to studies in ulcerative colitis which compare oral 5-ASA to oral sulfasalazine. These studies demonstrate equal efficacy but fewer side effects with the 5-ASA product.

In contrast, Dr. Ginsberg argues that a breakthrough is "a sudden advance in knowledge or technique." He points out that although 5-ASA will be useful in the management of some patients, it is far from a breakthrough. He points to a plethora of uncontrolled anecdotal reports on the use of 5-ASA preparations in the management of Crohn's disease and to the lack of prospective, double-blind, controlled trials with significant numbers of patients yielding data of statistical significance. He notes a single trial comparing 5-ASA to placebo but questions the absence of studies comparing 5-ASA to sulfasalazine and other treatment regimens. In those small studies in which such comparisons have been made, efficacy has been approximately equal between 5-ASA and sulfasalazine. He agrees that "a small subset of patients who are allergic to or intolerant of sulfasalazine may obtain some clinical benefit."

Furthermore, he points out that, although 5-ASA enemas may play a role in the management of ulcerative colitis, this role should not be glorified. After 11 years of study, less than half of the patients in one large multicenter trial showed any responsiveness to them. Most patients must combine 5-ASA enemas with oral sulfasalazine to obtain therapeutic efficacy, and more than 80% of patients treated with 5-ASA enemas relapse within 4 months of stopping this therapy. Finally, the cost of this treatment is remarkably high. Although the drug will find its therapeutic role, its predominant benefit will be for those patients who are allergic to sulfasalazine. Even here Dr. Ginsberg maintains that we are not dealing with "a sudden major advance (i.e., a breakthrough)."

In the opinion of this editor, the available data are unconvincing and 5-ASA will have a limited role as an oral agent in the therapeutic armamentarium. It will be most useful for those patients who have important side effects. Fortunately, most patients are not allergic to sulfasalazine and will respond equally well to either medication given orally. The data are not yet in with regard to the efficacy of 5-ASA or 4-ASA enemas in colitis. Very preliminary data suggest a more important role than has been observed with other treatments. Convincing findings based on prospective, randomized, controlled trials yielding data of statistical significance are still lacking. Until such data are available, few will be convinced. Thus, for the time being, 5-ASA is a helpful adjunct in the management of the inflammatory bowel diseases. Let us not attribute to it more significance than the available data justify.

Should Malignant Polyps of the Colon and Rectum Be Treated Conservatively?

Chapter Editor: Thomas P. Duffy, M.D.

Affirmative: Kenneth W. Barwick, M.D.
Professor of Pathology, Department of
Pathology, Baptist Medical Center,
Jacksonville, Florida

Negative: Anton J. Bilchik, M.D.
Postdoctoral Associate, Gastrointestinal
Surgery Research Unit, Departments of
Surgery, Yale University School of
Medicine, West Haven Veterans
Administration Medical Center, West Haven,
Connecticut

Garth H. Ballantyne, M.D.
Associate Professor of Surgery,
Gastrointestinal Surgery Research Unit,
Departments of Surgery, Yale University
School of Medicine, West Haven Veterans
Administration Medical Center, West Haven,
Connecticut

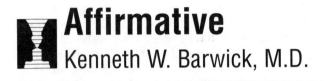

Affirmative
Kenneth W. Barwick, M.D.

It is now widely accepted that most carcinomas occurring in the colon and rectum develop from benign adenomas. Lines of evidence supporting this adenoma-carcinoma sequence are several and include pathological studies demonstrating the frequent presence of carcinoma within large adenomas and residual adenoma adjacent to small carcinomas, clinical studies demonstrating protection against carcinoma by removal of all endoscopically encountered adenomas, and epidemiological studies documenting spatial and temporal associations of adenomas and carcinomas. With acceptance of this sequence, it follows that all adenomas should be removed whenever they are discovered. In recent years, the widespread use of colonoscopy has allowed visualization of the entire colon and the removal of many adenomas with a diathermy snare. Both pedunculated and sessile polyps can be removed, although removal of the latter is technically more difficult and associated with a higher risk of perforation. There is much agreement regarding the management of patients with colorectal adenomas. Any detected adenoma should be removed completely in a patient without clinical contraindications. It is preferable to remove the lesion as a single fragment whenever possible, since piecemeal removal or biopsy ablation will prevent adequate pathological evaluation. Histological evaluation must determine the nature of the resected lesion, indicate the presence or absence of carcinoma, and assess the margins of resection. Finally, the patient should be placed into a surveillance program which is determined by clinical, endoscopic, and histological findings.

There is considerably less agreement regarding the management of that subset of patients in which the resected adenoma contains carcinoma, i.e., the malignant polyp. Even here, there is general agreement that adenomas containing noninvasive carcinoma (carcinoma in situ), can be treated safely by polypectomy alone. Conversely, if invasive carcinoma involving the resection line is present, transabdominal bowel resection generally is recommended. There is controversy, however, regarding the management of patients with histological findings intermediate to those just described, that is, with lesions containing invasive carcinoma not involving the lines of resection. Consideration of this group of patients is complicated at several levels, including definition of histological lesions, inadequate numbers of patients receiving standardized therapy, and lack of comparability of existing studies. Nonetheless, an increasing number of studies published in the last several years support, in the author's opinion, a conservative approach to most endoscopically removed malignant polyps, provided certain histological criteria are present. Of the several criteria that have been defined which indicate an increased risk of recurrence and thereby argue for additional therapy following polypectomy, three have been most consistent: (1) the presence of carcinoma at the resection line, (2) poorly differentiated (grade III of III) carcinoma, and (3) lymphatic or vascular invasion by malignant cells.

As indicated, one problem in reviewing published reports of malignant polyps is a lack of uniformity regarding definitions of histological criteria. While it is generally accepted that adenomas with carcinoma in situ lack metastatic potential, this term has been variably applied. In general histological terms, carcinoma in situ refers to the presence of cytologically malignant cells replacing normal cells within a given epithelium but restricted to the usual anatomic domain (above the basement membrane). In the colon and rectum, however, several studies apply the term carcinoma in situ to foci of malignant cells which have invaded through the basement membrane into lamina propria but have not reached the muscularis mucosa. Fenoglio and Pascal have offered alternative terms for these two situations: intraepithelial carcinoma for those lesions in which malignant cells are confined to the original crypts of Lieberkühn without involvement of the lamina propria, and intramucosal carcinoma for those lesions in which malignant cells invade into lamina propria but do not involve the muscularis mucosa.[1]

It is believed that both intraepithelial and intramucosal carcinoma have little or no metastatic potential due to the paucity of lymphatics in the colon and rectum superficial to the muscularis mucosa. While this lessens the significance of the confusion in terminology, a careful comparison of different studies is difficult nonetheless, especially in regard to the minority of cases where metastases accompanying these early lesions is claimed. Most studies have recognized the presence of "invasive carcinoma" when malignant cells invade into or through the muscularis mucosa. There has been less agreement as to the optimal method of classifying the level of invasion. Some studies have defined invasion relative to the morphological domains of the adenoma such as the head or stalk of pedunculated lesions, whereas others have not attempted such distinctions but have considered all invasive carcinomas together irrespective of degree of invasion. This further complicates study comparison. Uniform to all studies has been documentation of the presence or absence of carcinoma at the resection line, and most studies have concluded that the status of the margin is of paramount importance in assessing the risk of recurrence or residual tumor following polypectomy. Even here, however, there is not total uniformity, in that some studies assess only the cauterized margin itself, while others group lesions with malignant cells at or near this margin. Unfortunately, "near" has not been defined uniformly and in some studies it has not been defined at all. In spite of these difficulties, several published studies within the past few years have provided for consideration a growing number of patients who have undergone endoscopic removal of malignant polyps. Some of the larger studies will be reviewed.

In 1975 Wolff and Shinya reported 46 patients with malignant polyps representing a mixture of pedunculated and sessile lesions.[2] Invasion was defined as malignant cells penetrating into or through the muscularis mucosa. Twenty-five patients underwent subsequent colectomy for various reasons, whereas the remaining 21 were treated by polypectomy only. Of the resected specimens, only one contained metastatic carcinoma within regional lymph nodes and this followed incomplete excision of a malignant polyp. The authors defined three criteria that would indicate a need for further therapy after polypectomy: (1) malignant cells near the resection line, (2) lymphatic invasion by malignant cells, and (3) poorly differentiated carcinoma. No precise definition of inadequate margin was provided in this study. Nonetheless, the authors concluded that the absence of these three findings in a pedunculated adenoma indicated that the lesion could be treated safely by polypectomy only.

In 1981 Colacchio described 39 patients with pedunculated malignant polyps.[3] Invasion was defined as malignant cells invading up to or through the muscularis mucosa. Twenty-four patients underwent colonic resection, whereas 15 were treated by endoscopic polypectomy alone. Of the 24 patients undergoing colonic resection, 6 (25%) were found to have positive lymph nodes. The authors observed that such features as size, depth of invasion, histological differentiation, and involvement of lymphatics by malignant cells failed to predict these lesions which metastasized. Therefore, they concluded that all patients with polyps containing invasive carcinoma should undergo standard colonic resection. This study has the unusual feature that 12 of the 24 patients who underwent colectomy did not, in fact, undergo prior endoscopic resection of the malignant polyps. Instead, they had initial colectomy with subsequent polypectomy performed upon the pathological specimen. While it was the opinion of the authors that these lesions could have been excised totally by endoscopic excision, the comparability of this study is questionable.

In 1982 Rossini reported 31 patients with malignant polyps, 24 of whom were treated by polypectomy only and 7 of whom underwent subsequent colonic resection.[4] Twenty-two patients were available for follow-up, which ranged from 1 to 6 years in length, and no metastasis or recurrences were observed. Although the levels of invasion and the nature of an adequate margin were not clearly defined, the authors concluded that endoscopic polypectomy was adequate therapy in the absence of malignant cells near the resection margin, lymphatic invasion by malignant cells, and poorly differentiated carcinoma.

In 1983 Cooper described 56 patients with endoscopically removed malignant polyps, including a careful pathological description of the lesions.[5] Twenty-four patients underwent subsequent colonic resection, while the remaining 22 patients were treated by polypectomy only and were followed for a mean of 4.5 years. Five patients were found to have metastatic tumor within lymph nodes and 3 had metachronous liver metastases. To define adverse and favorable pathological features, Cooper recognized three categories of polyps: long-stalk (3 mm or more) pedunculated polyps, short-stalk (less than 3 mm) pedunculated polyps, and sessile lesions. No metastasis or recurrence was observed among 28 long-stalk polyps and 4 short-stalk polyps with tumor limited to the head of the lesion. In contrast, a 25% incidence of regional lymph node metastases or local recurrence was observed in short-stalk polyps with deeper tumor invasion and in sessile polyps. The author concluded that long-stalk malignant polyps and short-stalk polyps with cancer limited to the head could be treated by polypectomy alone in the absence of poorly differentiated carcinoma, lymphatic invasion, or tumor at or near the resection margin (here defined as within 0.8 mm). All other lesions should invoke consideration of subsequent resection. This rather cumbersome method of pathological analysis has not been duplicated by other studies.

Also in 1983, Lipper et al. reported 51 patients who had undergone endoscopic removal of 53 malignant polyps.[6] Four levels of invasion were recognized, with level 1 representing invasion not reaching the muscularis mucosa, levels 2 and 3 representing superficial and deeper invasion into the muscularis mucosa, and level 4 representing penetration through the muscularis mucosa into the submucosa. Twenty-three patients were treated by polypectomy only and were followed for a mean of 3.5 years. Only 1 patient developed recurrence, and this patient had a positive margin in the original polypectomy specimen. Twenty-three patients underwent subsequent colectomy, only one of which was considered justified by the authors. This one case demonstrated residual tumor in the colectomy specimen which was predicted by a positive resection line of the polyp. No other specimen demonstrated residual tumor. The authors found no clinical significance associated with the level of invasion within a malignant polyp and advocated a conservative approach to malignant polyps in the absence of a positive margin (defined as malignant cells at the resection line).

In 1984 Morson and colleagues from St. Marks Hospital in London described 60 patients with malignant polyps, all of whom had a least a 5-year period of follow-up.[7] In this study, invasion was defined as tumor penetrating through the muscularis mucosa. Forty-six patients were treated by polypectomy only, in that excision was judged to be complete and the invasive carcinoma was either well or moderately differentiated. No recurrence developed in these patients. Fourteen patients underwent subsequent surgical excision, with the findings of residual tumor in 2 patients and metastatic carcinoma in 1 patient who had poorly differentiated invasive cancer within the original polyp. The 2 patients with residual tumor had positive resection margins on the original polypectomy specimen. The authors advocated polypectomy as therapy of a malignant polyp in the absence of a positive resection margin or high-grade carcinoma.

Also in 1984, Christie described his experience with 83 consecutively encountered malignant polyps.[8] These occurred in 80 patients who were followed for a median time period of 36 months. Invasion was not precisely defined. Forty-nine pedunculated malignant polyps were removed colonoscopically. Eight patients in this group underwent subsequent colectomy due to the presence of malignant cells in the stalk region of the polyp. No residual tumor or positive lymph nodes were found in these specimens. The author considered colonoscopic polypectomy to be curative for pedunculated malignant polyps provided the stalk region of the lesion was not invaded by malignant cells, there was no lymphatic or vascular invasion, the carcinoma was well differentiated, and follow-up examination of the polypectomy site revealed no residual tumor. The absence of clear histological description in this study, especially regarding stalk invasion, makes comparison with other studies difficult.

In a careful clinical and pathological study in 1985, Haggitt et al. studied 129 malignant polyps in which invasion was no deeper than the submucosa of the underlying colonic wall.[9] Invasion in this study was defined as the penetration of malignant cells through the muscularis mucosa into the submucosa. Four levels of invasion were defined wherein invasion was limited to the head, the neck, the stalk, or the submucosa of the bowel wall below the stalk of the polyp. These regions were carefully defined descriptively and schematically. Sixty-three patients were treated by polypectomy alone and 66 by colectomy (with only 21 of the latter having antecedent polypectomy). Of 64 patients with invasive carcinoma, 8 had an adverse outcome (defined as death, recurrent carcinoma, or positive lymph nodes at the time of colectomy). Only level 4 invasion and rectal location proved to be statistically significant adverse prognostic factors. Level 4 invasion (defined as malignant cells extending into the submucosa below the level of the stalk of the polyp) predicted adverse outcome. It is important to recognize that this level of invasion could be determined only by a combined analysis of the endoscopic and pathological findings, and could not be determined by either evaluation alone. In an analysis of the literature, the authors concluded that the prognostic significance of lymphatic invasion and tumor grade could not be determined due to the limited number of cases available for study. They also questioned the significance of a positive margin independent of level of invasion in view of the limited number of cases. The authors concluded that there is no indication of significant risk of metastatic disease until an invasive carcinoma reaches the submucosa of the colonic wall below the insertion site of a malignant polyp. In an accompanying editorial analyzing this and earlier studies, Riddell concluded that pedunculated malignant polyps containing invasive carcinoma could be treated conservatively in the absence of four histological and clinical findings: (1) poorly differentiated carcinoma, (2) lymphatic invasion, (3) invasive carcinoma at the resection margin, and (4) invasive carcinoma at the level of the submucosa of the adjacent large bowel.[10]

In 1986 Cranley et al. reported 39 patients with 41 malignant polyps with a minimum 4-year follow-up.[11] Invasion was defined as the infiltration of malignant cells into the submucosa. In an analysis of their cases, the authors defined three favorable histological findings: (1) well- or moderately differentiated carcinoma, (2) a free margin of resection (defined as tumor more than 2 mm from the cautery artifact), and (3) the absence of lymphatic invasion. Fourteen patients had favorable histological features and none had residual or recurrent tumor, including 10 who were treated by polypectomy only. In contrast, of the 24 patients with unfavorable histological features, 42% either had residual tumor or metastatic carcinoma demonstrated subsequently. The high percentage of patients with histologically adverse lesions in this study is a marked contrast to most other studies. The authors concluded that endoscopic polypectomy alone is adequate therapy for colonic polyps provided that the aforementioned favorable histological features are present.

Also in 1986, Fucini reported 35 patients with invasive carcinoma within an adenoma, with invasion defined as infiltration into or through the muscularis mucosa.[12] Of 17 patients with malignant polyps treated by polypectomy only with negative resection margins, two experienced recurrent carcinomas. Both recurrent lesions were detected early and treated successfully. Eighteen patients underwent immediate colonic resection with the finding of residual carcinoma in two specimens but with no example of lymph node metastases demonstrated. The authors concluded that endoscopic polypectomy alone is adequate therapy for malignant polyps if the resection margins are free and if a plan of thorough follow-up is pursued, consisting in this study of endoscopic reexamination and biopsy 6 to 12 weeks later followed by a subsequent examination in 6 months if no recurrent lesion is detected. The absence of a careful description of the levels of invasion and a definition of a free margin in this study makes comparison difficult.

In 1987 Conte and colleagues described the clinical and pathological features of 87 patients with 89 malignant polyps removed endoscopically.[13] Upon pathological review, 54 lesions were found to have carcinoma in situ, defined as the presence of malignant cells in the mucosa but without penetration into the muscularis mucosa. Thirty lesions contained invasive carcinoma, defined as penetration beyond the muscularis mucosa. The authors observed that 4 of the 30 patients with a malignant polyp (14%) would have been treated inadequately by polypectomy alone, since 1 had residual disease at the polypectomy site, 1 had lymph node metastases, 1 had liver metastases at the time of colectomy, and 1 subsequently developed liver metastases. Three histological criteria correctly predicted all 4 cases in which residual or recurrent disease occurred: (1) the presence of malignant cells at the resection margin, (2) lymphatic invasion, and (3) poorly differentiated carcinoma. These authors concluded that polypectomy alone is adequate therapy for malignant polyps in the absence of these three histological findings.

Later in 1987, Richards et al. reported 80 patients with invasive carcinoma in malignant polyps defined as penetration beyond the muscularis mucosa.[14] Of these 80 patients, 44 underwent subsequent bowel resection, with the finding of residual tumor or metastatic carcinoma to lymph nodes in 10 patients. Each of the 10 had at least 1 of 5 indications of an inadequate resection: (1) incomplete excision, (2) poorly differentiated carcinoma, (3) invasion of the line of resection, (4) invasion of the stalk of the polyp, and (5) invasion of venous or lymphatic channels. The authors concluded that patients with a malignant polyp demonstrating any 1 of these 5 adverse findings should undergo colonic resection and regional lymphadenectomy. Patients with none of these risk factors should have endoscopic reexamination 3 months after the initial polypectomy to reevaluate the polypectomy site. The authors made the important observation that 3 of their patients had metastatic tumor to regional lymph nodes after colectomy in spite of having well-differentiated carcinomas and clear resection lines. Unfortunately, no description of the methods used was provided in this paper and there was no evidence of a primary review of the histology of the cases encountered during the 15-year interval studied retrospectively.

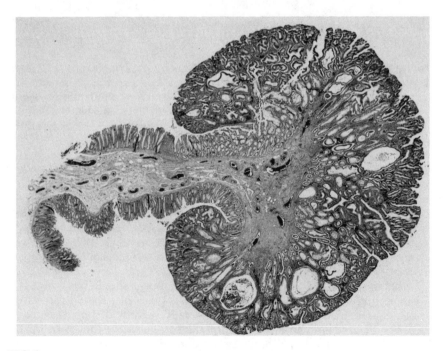

FIG 1.
Low-power magnification of a tubular adenoma (adenomatous polyp) which has been removed endoscopically in total and processed in optimal fashion. The plane of resection demonstrates the neoplastic head of the lesion, the stalk covered by normal colonic mucosa, and the excision line. No carcinoma is present in this specimen.

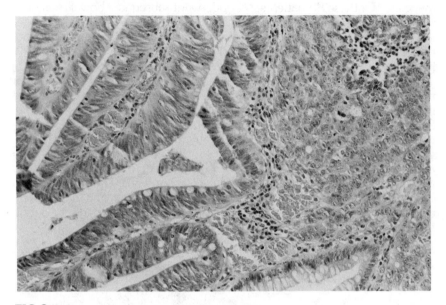

FIG 2.
High-power view of invasive carcinoma in a tubulovillous adenoma. The solid sheets of malignant cells in the right side of this field show marked pleomorphism and no attempt at gland formation and therefore are poorly differentiated (grade III of III). Most published series have found that only a small minority of cases of malignant polyps show grade III carcinoma.

What conclusions can be derived from these studies? It seems most evident that great care must be exercised in the procurement and handling of adenomas whenever they are encountered endoscopically. Standardized methods of examination and reporting must be employed and open communication between all involved persons must be fostered. It also can be concluded that cautious acceptance of the conservative management of malignant polyps is appropriate, provided certain clinical and pathological requirements are met.

What are some of these requirements? Any polyp should be removed as a single fragment whenever possible. The endoscopist should record the gross characteristics of the lesion, especially regarding the presence or absence of a stalk. The level of amputation relative to the plane of the mucosal surface should be noted and recorded. This information must be provided to the pathologist. In the laboratory, careful gross inspection of the lesion should be undertaken, and it is useful to locate and mark the amputation site with India ink. A recommended method of preserving orientation during fixation is to impale the lesion with a needle or pin through the amputation site along the axis which would be perpendicular to the mucosal plane. The adenoma should not be sectioned unfixed or partially fixed, as significant distortion will likely occur during processing. This mandates a fixation period of approximately 24 hours prior to sectioning. After complete fixation, the lesion should be sectioned in a manner which allows optimal microscopic evaluation. For smaller adenomas (less than 1 cm) hemisection through the amputation site perpendicular to the resection plane is advocated (Fig 1). For larger lesions, sections should be examined again through the amputation site perpendicular to the resection plane.

The pathologist has a number of obligations in interpreting colorectal polyps. The nature of the lesion (neoplastic or non-neoplastic) must be determined. The presence or absence of carcinoma must be specified. If carcinoma is present, the level of invasion should be specified, especially relative to the muscularis mucosa (which is critical to the definition of "invasive" in most studies). Ambiguous terms such as "superficial carcinoma" or "focal cancer" should be avoided. The histological grade and presence or absence of lymphatic invasion should be specified (Fig 2). The margin of resection should be evaluated and an indication of the distance from the carcinoma to the margin provided (Figs 3 and 4). Finally, it seems prudent

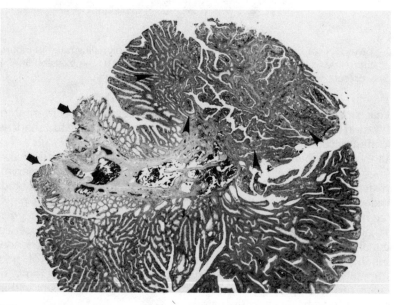

FIG 3.
Low-power magnification of invasive adenocarcinoma within the head of a pedunculated tubulovillous adenoma. The area of invasive carcinoma (outlined by *arrowheads*) invades through the muscularis mucosa but is confined within the bulbous head of the lesion. The distance to the excision line (indicated by *arrows*) can be readily assessed in this histological preparation.

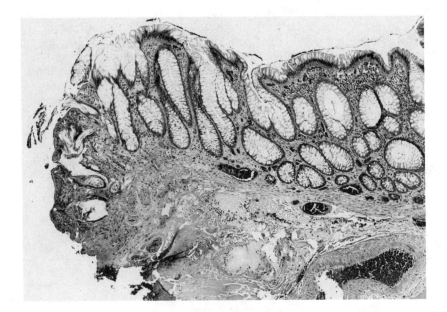

FIG 4.
High-power view of the excision line of the malignant polyp illustrated in Figure 3. The cautery line artifact of the tissue readily identifies this as the excision line. The mucosa present which coats the polyp stalk is non-neoplastic.

that each example of a malignant polyp should precipitate direct verbal communication between pathologist and endoscopist to minimize the chances of miscommunication.

Although an analysis of the existing literature is difficult for the reasons outlined previously, there does seem to be reasonable cause for conservative management of most malignant polyps. Such cause must be rooted in consideration of the greatest good versus the possible risk to the patient. Three histological criteria have been cited most frequently which suggest a minimal risk lower than that of surgery for many patients: (1) the absence of malignant cells at the cauterized margin of resection, (2) the absence of lymphatic invasion by malignant cells, and (3) the absence of poorly differentiated carcinoma. Careful surveillance following polypectomy, usually with repeat endoscopsy and biopsy of the polypectomy site within 6 weeks to 3 months, is also advocated.

Finally, it must be concluded that optimal management of malignant polyps is an issue not totally resolved. Resolution can only follow additional study applying rigorous and standardized clinical and pathological criteria.

References

1. Fenoglio CM, Pascal RR: Colorectal adenomas and cancer: Pathologic relationships. *Cancer* 1982; 50:2601–2608. *An excellent discussion of the pathological aspects and variance in nomenclature of adenomas with and without malignant foci.*

2. Wolff WI, Shinya H: Definitive treatment of "malignant" polyps of the colon. *Ann Surg* 1975; 182:516–524. *In a review of 46 patients with malignant polyps, the authors conclude that endoscopic polypectomy only is adequate therapy in the absence of poorly differentiated carcinoma, a positive resection line, and lymphatic invasion.*

3. Colacchio TA, Forde KA, Scantlebury VP: Endoscopic polypectomy: Inadequate treatment for invasive colorectal carcinoma. *Ann Surg* 1981; 194:704–707. *In an analysis of 24 patients with malignant polyps who underwent segmental colonic resection, the authors found that size, depth of invasion, differentiation, and involvement of lymphatics did not predict which cases would have lymph node metastases.*

4. Rossini RP, Ferrari A, Coverlizza S: Colonoscopic polypectomy in diagnosis and management of cancerous adenomas: An individual and multicentric experience. *Endoscopy* 1982; 14:124–127. *In a review of 31 patients with malignant polyps, the authors conclude that endoscopic polypectomy alone is adequate therapy in the absence of malignant cells near the resection margin, lymphatic invasion, and poorly differentiated carcinoma.*

5. Cooper HS: Surgical pathology of endoscopically removed malignant polyps of the colon and rectum. *Am J Surg Pathol* 1983; 7:613–623. *A detailed pathological analysis of 56 malignant polyps concludes that polyps with long stalks are more amenable to adequate therapy by polypectomy than are polyps with short stalks.*

6. Lipper S, Kahn LB, Ackerman LV: The significance of microscopic invasive cancer in endoscopically removed polyps of the large bowel. *Cancer* 1983; 52:1691–1699. *In a review of 51 patients with 53 malignant polyps, the authors advocate a conservative approach to malignant polyps in the absence of a positive resection margin.*

7. Morson BC, Whiteway JE, Jones EA, et al: Histopathology and prognosis of malignant colorectal polyps treated by endoscopic polypectomy. *Gut* 1984; 25:437–444. *Sixty patients with malignant polyps are studied with clinical follow-up; polypectomy only is advocated in the absence of a positive resection line and high-grade carcinoma.*

8. Christie JP: Malignant colon polyps — cure by colonoscopy or colectomy? *Am J Gastroenterol* 1984; 79:543–547. *In a personal experience with 83 consecutively encountered malignant polyps, the author concludes that colonoscopic polypectomy can be considered curative for malignant pedunculated polyps, provided the stalk portion of the lesion is totally uninvolved with carcinoma, there is no lymphatic or vascular invasion, the carcinoma is well differentiated, and follow-up endoscopic examination of the polypectomy site reveals no residual or recurrent tumor.*

9. Haggitt RC, Glotzbach RE, Soffer EE, et al: Prognostic factors in colorectal carcinomas arising in adenomas: Implications for lesions removed by endoscopic polypectomy. *Gastroenterology* 1985; 89:328–336. *A comprehensive clinical and pathological analysis of 129 patients with malignant polyps concludes that the level of invasion should be the major factor in determining prognosis for the management of carcinoma arising in an adenoma.*

10. Riddell RH: Hands off "cancerous" large bowel polyps. *Gastroenterology* 1985; 89:432–441. *An excellent editorial which accompanies reference 9 and which discusses the overall issue of therapy of malignant polyps.*

11. Cranley JP, Petras RE, Carey WD, et al: When is endoscopic polypectomy adequate therapy for colonic polyps containing invasive carcinoma? *Gastroenterology* 1986; 91:419–427. *The authors reviewed 39 patients with 41 malignant polyps and concluded that endoscopic polypectomy is adequate therapy for these lesions provided the following favorable histological features are present: free margin of resection, absence of poorly differentiated carcinoma, and absence of lymphatic invasion.*

12. Fucini C: An appraisal of endoscopic removal of malignant colonic polyps. *Mayo Clin Proc* 1986; 61:123–126. *In a review of 35 patietns with malignant polyps, the authors conclude that endoscopic polypectomy alone is adequate for malignant polyps if the resection margin is free and an adequate plan of follow-up is pursued.*

13. Conte CC, Welch JP, Tennant R, et al: Management of endoscopically removed malignant polyps. *J Surg Oncol* 1987; 36:116–121. *A study of 87 patients with 89 malignant polyps concludes that endoscopic polypectomy alone is adequate therapy for polyps with carcinoma in situ and for polyps with invasive carcinoma, provided the carcinoma was not poorly differentiated, did not involve the resection line, and did not invade lymphatics.*

14. Richards WO, Webb WA, Morris SJ, et al: Patient management after endoscopic removal of the cancerous colon adenoma. *Ann Surg* 1987; 205:665–672. *Five adverse features are identified which mandate segmental resection for malignant colorectal polyps: (1) incomplete excision, (2) poorly differentiated carcinoma, (3) postiive resection margin, (4) invasion of the stalk of the polyp, and (5) invasion of venous or lymphatic channels.*

Negative

Anton J. Bilchik, M.D.
Garth H. Ballantyne, M.D.

The colon is the second most common site of visceral cancer in the United States, exceeded only by the lung.[1] Unfortunately, the results of treating colorectal cancer have failed to improve during the last 40 years.[2] Indeed, crude 5-year survival in the United States and the United Kingdom for patients with colorectal cancer is only about 30%.[3] The results of treating early colorectal cancers, however, are excellent. Turnbull, for example, reported a 98% 5-year survival rate for 103 patients with Dukes' A lesions (i.e., lesions limited to the bowel wall without lymph node involvement).[4] These results would suggest that the best strategy for improving survival for patients with colorectal cancer is to discover these lesions while they remain limited to the bowel wall. Endoscopic examination of the colon and rectum has proven the best means of finding such early curable lesions.[5,6] The endoscopic identification of colorectal cancers while they remain confined to the submucosa or particularly limited to the body of a polyp offers the best possibility for implementing effective treatment.

The purpose of this paper is to demonstrate that invasive carcinoma contained within a colorectal polyp is a life-threatening malignancy. Specifically, we will review the factors that are associated with poor outcomes for patients with these lesions. Furthermore, we will demonstrate that the majority of these lesions are best treated by traditional surgical techniques. Unfortunately, we will show that the criteria which often are utilized in advocating colonoscopic polypectomy as adequate treatment for malignant polyps are found only in a small group of patients. Finally, we will question the ability of a pathological staging system to predict treatment outcome in individual patients.

Definitions

Invasive Carcinoma in a Colorectal Polyp

This review will examine the results of treating invasive carcinoma in colon and rectal polyps. A colorectal neoplasm is considered to be an invasive carcinoma when the lesion has penetrated through the muscularis mucosa.[7,8] The treatment of lesions which have not penetrated this layer will not be included in this discussion.[9] Also, the results of treating polypoid cancers have been excluded from this review.

Conservative Therapy

The *Oxford Universal English Dictionary* defines the word conservative as "characterized by a tendency to preserve or keep intact and unchanged; preservation."[10] Thus, conservative therapy would indicate the utilization of traditional techniques. Surgical resection has been the standard method of treating colorectal cancer throughout this century. Therefore, in this review, conservative therapy will represent traditional surgical techniques of resecting colorectal cancer. This includes colectomy and also techniques of locally resecting rectal cancers. The evolution of the surgical treatment of colorectal cancer has been discussed elsewhere.[11] The intent of this review, however, is not to discuss the relative merits of different surgical techniques.

Factors Contributing to Poor Outcome Following Endoscopic Polypectomy

The satisfactory treatment of invasive colorectal cancer requires complete excision of the lesion as well as any involved lymph nodes. Consequently, endoscopic polypectomy can be utilized only in treating patients in whom disease is limited to the confines of the polyp. Whenever the lesion is not limited to the excised tissue, a poor outcome for the patient follows. Unfortunately, the majority of invasive carcinomas in colorectal polyps have features which suggest that endoscopic polypectomy may not offer the best opportunity for a satisfactory treatment outcome (Table 1). Whenever these features are present, treatment success can be assured only by traditional, i.e., conservative, techniques of surgical resection.

Rate of Treatment Failures

The effectiveness of endoscopic treatment of invasive cancers in colorectal polyps can be judged only by end results. A number of studies have analyzed the outcome of patients treated for these lesions.[7,8,12-16] Treatment in these studies was not limited to endoscopic polypectomy. A patient was considered to have suffered a poor outcome when lymph nodes were found to have contained cancer, the patient was alive with recurrent disease, or the patient died of his disease. Deaths from unrelated conditions were not included in the category of poor outcome. Overall, more than 10% of 291 patients reported in seven series sustained poor outcomes following the treatment of invasive carcinomas in colorectal polyps (Table 2). These results indicate that invasive carcinoma, even when limited to a polyp, represents a life-threatening condition.

TABLE 1.
Characteristics of Malignant Polyps of the Colon and Rectum Which Tend to Favor Operative Resection for Treatment

Sessile
Villous
Poorly differentiated
Lymphatic invasion
Greater than 2 cm in diameter
Cancer near or at margin of resection
Right-sided lesion
Rectal lesion
Clinical features of malignancy
Found in patients at high risk for developing colorectal cancer
Not amenable to colonoscopic polypectomy

TABLE 2.
Number of Patients That Suffered Poor Outcomes Following Treatment of Malignant Polyps*

First Author	Year	Number of Patients With Poor Outcome	Total Number of Patients	Percent
Cooper HS[8]	1983	7	56	12.5%
Lipper S[12]	1983	0	39	0%
Fried GM[13]	1984	0	22	0%
Morson BC[7]	1984	1	51	2.0%
Haggitt RC[14]	1985	8	64	12.5%
Cranley JP[15]	1986	10	38	26.3%
Contee CC[16]	1987	4	21	19.0%
Totals		30	291	10.3%

*Poor outcome is defined as lymph nodes found to contain cancer, recurrence of cancer, or death from cancer.

Rate of Lymph Node Involvement

The selection of the best means for resecting a malignancy requires information regarding the likelihood that the lesion has already metastasized to the regional lymph nodes. Dukes believed that colorectal cancers rarely spread to regional lymph nodes until the lesion had penetrated through the full thickness of the bowel wall.[17] Unfortunately, even when confined to a polyp, colorectal cancer often metastasizes before the lesion reaches the muscular wall of the bowel.[18] Table 3 lists the number of patients treated for invasive carcinomas in colorectal polyps in whom carcinoma was found in lymph nodes. Among 401 patients compiled from 11 series, metastatic disease was found in the lymph nodes of 8.2% of the patients.[8,9,13–15,19–24] These reports illustrate the point that the complete excision of malignancy in patients with invasive carcinoma in a colorectal polyp often can be accomplished only by traditional surgical techniques in which the involved segment of bowel with its attached mesentery is resected. The presence of several features of individual polyps increases the likelihood that the lesion has spread to the regional lymph nodes.

TABLE 3.
Number of Patients With Malignant Polyps of the Colon and Rectum in Whom Cancer Was Found in Lymph Nodes

First Author	Year	Number of Patients With Postitive Lymph Nodes	Total Number of Patients	Percent
Grinnell RS[19]	1958	10	71	14.1%
Helwig EB[20]	1959	1	14	7.1%
Waye JD[21]	1974	0	10	0%
Wolff WI[9]	1975	1	46	2.2%
Colacchio TA[23]	1981	6	24	25.0%
Cooper HS[8]	1983	5	56	8.9%
Langer JC[24]	1984	0	19	0%
Fried GM[13]	1984	0	22	0%
Nivatvongs S[22]	1985	6	41	14.6%
Haggitt RC[14]	1985	4	64	6.3%
Cranley JP[15]	1986	0	34	0%
Totals		33	401	8.2%

Sessile Polyps

Several studies have indicated that sessile polyps containing invasive carcinomas are frequently associated with poor outcomes. Among 100 patients having sessile lesions compiled from the literature, 15 had lymph nodes containing cancer.[22] Furthermore, an additional 6% of these patients had residual disease found when they underwent colectomy. Thus, in this compiled series, 21% of patients with sessile lesions containing invasive carcinomas were treated inadequately by polypectomy. Cranley and colleagues reported that 40% of patients (2 of 5) with sessile lesions suffered poor treatment outcomes.[15]

Sessile polyps represent a substantial portion of the polyps that contain invasive carcinoma. Wolff and Shinya found invasive carcinomas in 10.2% of 127 sessile polyps which had been endoscopically excised.[9] Sessile polyps containing carcinoma represented 28% of the invasive carcinomas found in polyps by Wolff and Shinya and 41% of the malignant lesions found by Christie.[9,25] Based on these results, several reports have recommended that all sessile polyps with invasive carcinomas be treated with colectomy.[9,23,25] This one criterion by itself suggests that between 28% and 41% of all polyps containing carcinoma should be treated by traditional techniques of operative resection.

Villous Adenomas

Several studies have reported a high rate of poor treatment outcomes in patients in whom invasive carcinomas were found in villous polyps.[15,23,26] At The Cleveland Clinic, lymph nodes containing cancer were found in 21% of these lesions (16 of 75).[26] Cranley reported poor outcomes in 3 of 7 patients with this type of lesion.[15] In contrast, at Thomas Jefferson University Hospital only 1 of 20 villous polyps containing invasive carcinoma was associated with lymph nodes positive for carcinoma.[8] Similarly, at St. Mark's Hospital in London, no poor outcomes ensued in ten patients with villous polyps containing invasive carcinoma.[7] This wide range of results may reflect differences in design among these several studies. The Cleveland Clinic study included all villous polyps with invasive carcinoma treated in their institution, whereas the reports from Thomas Jefferson University Hospital and St. Mark's Hospital presented only those patients who were treated endoscopically.[7,8,26]

Invasive carcinomas are found more commonly in villous polyps than in tubular or villotubular polyps. Table 4 lists the histological types of polyps in which 301 invasive cancers were found.[7,9,12,13,23,26,27] Among these lesions, 39% were found in villous polyps. Thus, utilizing the villous polyp as a criteria for colectomy by itself would indicate the need for operative resection in more than one third of patients.

TABLE 4.
Distribution by Histological Type of 301 Polyps in Which
Invasive Carcinoma Was Discovered

First Author	Year	Tubular	Villotubular	Villous	Total
Wolff WI[9]	1975	17	10	14	41
Coutsoftides T[26]	1979	17	20	75	112
Lipper S[12]	1983	9	18	12	39
Morson BC[7]	1984	25	17	10	52
Fried GM[13]	1984	15	5	2	22
Fucini C[27]	1986	26	5	4	35
Totals		109	75	117	301
Percent		36.0%	25.0%	38.9%	100%

Lymphatic Invasion

Invasion of the lymphatics by colorectal cancers is associated with frequent treatment failures.[28] Fortunately, the invasion of submucosal lymphatics is rarely observed in cancers contained within polyps. Nonetheless, when such lymphatic invasion is observed in polyps, a poor treatment outcome is likely. Metastatic spread to regional lymph nodes was found to be present in 5 of 17 patients with lymphatic invasion within the polyp reported in five series.[8,12,14,15,23] Patients in whom lymphatic invasion is observed should be treated with operative resection.

Poorly Differentiated Carcinoma

Patients who develop poorly differentiated colorectal carcinomas fare poorly with their disease.[29] This appears to be true also for poorly differentiated carcinomas found within polyps. In six series, poorly differentiated lesions were found in the polyps of 17 patients.[7,8,14,15,23,30] Lymph nodes containing carcinoma or poor treatment outcomes were reported in 65% of these patients. Poorly differentiated carcinoma in a colorectal polyp is best treated by operative resection.

Cancer at or Near the Margin of Resection

The histological identification of residual tumor at or near the margin of resection is associated with both a high rate of local recurrence of disease and lymph node involvement with tumor. At the University of Toronto, residual cancer was found in 80% of patients (4 of 5) who underwent colectomy because of tumor at or near the margin of resection.[24] Similarly, at The Cleveland Clinic, 10 patients suffered adverse outcomes among 22 who had tumor at or near the margin.[15] The rate of lymph node involvement with cancer is high among these patients; 24% of patients (23 of 97) reported in seven series who had tumor at or near the margins of resection had cancer found in lymph nodes.[8,9,15,23,26,30,31] Unfortunately, the discovery of cancer near the margin of resection is common. Indeed, in some series tumor is found near the margin of resection in 33% to 58% of lesions.[15,24] Some authors consider this finding the most important indication for treating patients with colectomy.[15,32] This criterion by itself suggests the need for operative resection for treating one third to one half of patients with invasive carcinoma in a polyp.

Size Greater Than 2 cm

The risk of a polyp containing invasive cancer increases with the size of the polyp. At St. Mark's Hospital, for example, invasive carcinoma was found in 1.3% of polyps less than 1 cm in diameter, in 9.5% of polyps 1 to 2 cm in diameter, and in 17% of polyps greater than 2 cm in diameter.[33] Furthermore, 73% of all polyps containing invasive carcinoma were greater than 2 cm in diameter. The risk of perforation during endoscopic polypectomy increases with increasing size of the polyp.[34] Consequently, the lesions most likely to contain invasive carcinoma, i.e., polyps greater than 2 cm, are the ones which are the most difficult to remove endoscopically. Although the overall risk of perforation during colonoscopic polypectomy generally is stated at about 1%,[34] the rate of perforation in relation to the size of the polyp generally is not stated. Consequently, it is difficult to estimate the relative risk of polypectomy for large polyps.

The difficulty of endoscopically excising large polyps is reflected in the low number of large polyps included in series of endoscopically excised malignant polyps. Among 41 polyps containing invasive cancer excised by Wolff and Shinya, 66% were under 2 cm in diameter.[9] Similarly, Cranley and coworkers reported that 45% of endoscopically excised polyps containing invasive cancer were less than 2 cm in size, while Richards and colleagues reported 53% less than 2 cm.[15,35] This is about double the percentage that we would expect based on the aforementioned data from St. Mark's.[33] This indicates that a significant proportion of polyps containing invasive carcinoma have not been included in endoscopic polypectomy series because these lesions were never treated by this technique. Many polyps greater than 2 cm in diameter are not suitable for colonoscopic polypectomy.

Lesions Proximal to the Splenic Flexure

Polyps containing invasive carcinoma which are located proximal to the splenic flexure have not often been treated by endoscopic polypectomy. Among 210 malignant polyps reported in five series, only 9% were found in the right colon or transverse colon.[13,15,24,25,35] In any case, this is many fewer lesions than would be expected based on the generally reported distribution of colorectal cancers.[36] No explanation for this observation has been presented. Perhaps colon carcinomas of the midgut are less often amenable to endoscopic polypectomy. Additionally, because of the few reported cases, little information about treatment outcome is available for patients with right-sided lesions.

Rectal Lesions

The rectum offers specific advantages for surgical resection of neoplastic lesions. Surgical approaches for local complete excision of rectal polyps and cancers have been practiced commonly since the late 19th century.[11] In addition, long-term results utilizing these procedures in patients with early rectal cancers are well documented.[37] When large polyps or ones likely to contain malignancy are encountered in the rectum, surgical excision is the preferred method of resection.

Clinical Features of Malignancy

An experienced endoscopist often can identify colorectal polyps which contain invasive carcinoma by their gross appearance.[38] Shinya has described several characteristics associated with invasive carcinoma.[1] Deep ulcerations, a concave surface with an irregular nodular appearance, a granular and friable surface, discoloration, and disproportion in size between the head and the stalk all are features which suggest the presence of malignancy. Polyps which have these characteristics often should be treated by endoscopic biopsy followed by traditional surgical resection.[38]

Malignant polyps that are treated initially by surgical resection often are excluded from published series which consider the treatment of these lesions.[8,12,15,24,27,35] This group represents a significant portion of all malignant polyps. In the report by Haggitt and colleagues, 35% of polyps containing carcinoma were treated initially by colectomy.[14] Only 64 of these 129 polyps had invasion through the muscularis mucosa. Thus, the surgically treated polyps may represent an even greater proportion in this series. In the report of Fried and coworkers, 10 of 22 patients (45%) with malignant polyps were treated initially by surgical resection, 4 were treated by colectomy, and 6 were treated by operative local excision.[13] These data suggest that many published series excluded as many as one half of colorectal polyps that contained invasive carcinoma because these lesions were not treated by endoscopic polypectomy.

High-Risk Patients

Several groups of patients have an extremely high risk of dying from colorectal cancer (Table 5).[3,39,40,41] When invasive carcinoma is found within a polyp in patients in one of these groups, total abdominal colectomy with ileorectostomy or total proctocolectomy is often the best treatment. Patients from these high-risk groups generally are excluded from studies which examine treatment outcome for malignant polyps.

Inadequate Histological Information

Invasive colorectal carcinoma, even when limited to a polyp, is a life-threatening condition. Several features outlined above increase the likelihood that endoscopic polypectomy may not provide adequate therapy. A number of authors have emphasized the importance of meticulous pathological examination of the polyp in order to discover these features.[7,8,14,15,22] Whenever adequate histological assessment is not available, traditional surgical techniques should be used in treating these patients.

Predicting Treatment Outcome

Several groups have advocated that the treatment of individual patients in whom colorectal polyps containing invasive carcinoma have been found should be determined by histological criteria.[13–15,42] The ability to predict which patients will be adequately treated by low-risk therapeutic modalities is, of course, very desirable. Unfortunately, no pathological staging system for colorectal cancer has even proven to be completely accurate in predicting outcome for individual patients.[18] Thus, the utilization of pathological criteria for determining treatment must be done cautiously.

Treatment results for colorectal cancer generally are reported after follow-up information is available for more than 5 years for all patients. This seems

---

TABLE 5.
Diseases in Which Malignant Polyps Generally Should Be Treated by Abdominal Colectomy or Total Proctocolectomy*

Familial polyposis
Chronic ulcerative colitis
Crohn's colitis
Hereditary nonpolyposis colon cancer (Lynch Syndromes I and II)
Multiple synchronous colorectal cancers
Multiple synchronous polyps

*Data from references 3 and 39–41.

---

particularly important in reporting treatment outcomes for malignant polyps. As we have seen earlier, patient populations included within studies concerning colorectal polyps containing invasive carcinoma represent highly preselected groups. Furthermore, many of these patients were identified at a time when their lesions were asymptomatic and were treated by a method not previously available. Consequently, it may be difficult to compare these patient groups to historical groups. An element of lead time bias may be present in patient groups treated with endoscopic polypectomy. The natural history of these lesions may have been different than, for example, the Dukes' A lesions reported by Turnbull.[4] Unfortunately, 5-year follow-up for all patients in individual studies has been reported only on several occasions.[7,14,15,27] For the present, therefore, we must agree with the following statement of Dr. Kenneth Barwick of Yale University: "At the current time there are insufficient data to determine the exact risk and indicated management for patients after the complete endoscopic removal of a polyp with superficially invasive carcinoma."[43]

References

1. Shinya H, Hsu M, Cwern M: Colonoscopy. *Probl Gen Surg* 1985; 2:211–218.
2. Ballantyne GH, Modlin IM: Postoperative follow-up for colorectal cancer: Who are we kidding? *J Clin Gastroenterol* 1988; 10:359–364. *Improvement in treatment outcome can be realized only with earlier identification of colorectal cancer. Endoscopic screening by primary care physicians trained in the techniques of flexible endoscopy is the author's solution to this problem.*
3. Goligher J: *Surgery of the Anus, Rectum and Colon.* London, Bailliere Tindall, 1984.
4. Turnbull RB Jr: The no-touch isolation technique of resection. *JAMA* 1975; 231:1181–1182.
5. Gilbertsen VA, Nelms JM: The prevention of invasive cancer of the rectum. *Cancer* 1978; 41:1137–1139.
6. Longo WE, Ballantyne GH, Modlin IM: Colonoscopic detection of early colorectal cancers: Impact of a surgical endoscopy service. *Ann Surg* 1988; 207:174–178. *The establishment of a surgical endoscopy service with more aggressive use of flexible sigmoidoscopy led to a fourfold increase in the number of early cancers (Dukes' A and B). Occult blood testing and patients symptoms were late indicators of colonic cancer.*
7. Morson BC, Whiteway JE, Lones EA, et al: Histopathology and prognosis of malignant colorectal polyps treated by endoscopic polypectomy. *Gut* 1984; 25:437–444.
8. Cooper HS: Surgical pathology of endoscopically removed malignant polyps of the colon and rectum. *Am J Surg Pathol* 1983; 7:613–623.
9. Wolff WI, Shinya H: Definitive treatment of "malignant" polyps of the colon. *Ann Surg* 1975; 182:516–525. *Endoscopic resection appears to be adequate therapy for pedunculated polyps with invasive cancer in the head*

unless (1) the cancer is close to the site of resection, (2) the cancer is found in the lymphatics, or (3) the tumor is highly undifferentiated. Recommendations are made based on a review of 892 polypectomies.

10. *Oxford Universal English Dictionary.* Oxford, Oxford University Press, 1937.

11. Ballantyne GH: Theories of carcinogenesis and their impact on surgical treatment of colorectal cancer: An historical review. *Dis Colon Rectum* 1988; 31:513–517.

12. Lipper S, Kahn LB, Ackerman LV: The significance of microscopic invasive cancer in endoscopically removed polyps of the large bowel: A clinicopathologic study of 51 cases. *Cancer* 1983; 52:1691–1699. *The presence of cancer at the resection line is the only absolute finding capable of predicting residual disease. Skillful removal of the polyps to permit successful evaluation of the specimens by the pathologist is essential.*

13. Fried GM, Hreno A, Duguid WP, et al: Rational management of malignant colon polyps based on long-term follow-up. *Surgery* 1984; 96:815–820.

14. Haggitt RC, Glotzbach RE, Soffer EE, et al: Prognostic factors in colorectal carcinomas arising in adenomas: Implications for lesions removed by endoscopic polypectomy. *Gastroenterology* 1985; 89:328–336. *The level of invasion is the major factor in determining prognosis for the management of carcinoma arising in an adenoma. The worst prognosis is associated with invasion of the submucosa of the colonic wall; the significance of a positive stalk margin is controversial.*

15. Cranley JP, Petras RE, Carey WD, et al: When is endoscopic polypectomy adequate therapy for colonic polyps containing invasive carcinoma? *Gastroenterology* 1986; 91:419–427.

16. Contee CC: Management of endoscopically removed malignant colon polyps. *J Surg Oncol* 1987; 36:116–121.

17. Dukes CE: The classification of cancer of the rectum. *J Pathol Bacteriol* 1943; 35:323–332.

18. Phillips RKS, Hittinger R, Blesovsky L, et al: Large bowel cancer: Surgical pathology and its relationship to survival. *Br J Surg* 1984; 71:604–610.

19. Grinnell RS, Lane N: Benign and malignant adenomatous polyps and papillary adenomas of the colon and rectum. An analysis of 1856 tumors in 1335 patients. *Int Abst Surg* 1958; 106:519–525.

20. Helwig EB: Adenomas and the pathogenesis of cancer of the colon and rectum. *Dis Colon Rectum* 1959; 2:5–17.

21. Waye JD, Frankel A: Treatment of early colon cancer (abstract). *Gastroenterology* 1974; 66:796.

22. Nivatvongs S: Management of polyps containing invasive carcinoma, in Kodner IJ, Fry RD, Roe JP (eds): *Colon, Rectal and Anal Surgery. Current Techniques and Controversies.* St Louis, CV Mosby, 1985; pp 173–180.

23. Colacchio TA, Forde KA, Scantlebury VP: Endoscopic polypectomy. Inadequate treatment for invasive carcinoma. *Ann Surg* 1981; 194:704–707. *The surgical authors use their experience (729 patients) to conclude that all patients with polyps containing invasive carcinoma should undergo standard colon resection. They believe it is impossible to predict which lesions have lymph node metastases at the time of resection.*

24. Langer JC, Cohen Z, Taylor BR, et al: Management of patients with polyps

containing malignancy removed by colonoscopic polypectomy. *Dis Colon Rectum* 1984; 27:6–9.

25. Christie JP: Malignant colon polyps —cure by colonoscopy or colectomy. *Am J Gastroenterol* 1984; 79:543–547. *The author believes that colonoscopic polypectomy is curative for malignant pedunculated polyps provided the stalk portion of the lesion is totally uninvolved with the malignant process, there is no lymphatic or vascular invasion, the malignancy is well differentiated, and follow-up endoscopy reveals no residua or recurrence.*

26. Coutsoftides T, Lavery I, Benjamin SP, et al: Malignant polyps of the colon and rectum: A clinicopathologic study. *Dis Colon Rectum* 1979; 22:82–86.

27. Fucini C, Wolff BG, Spencer RJ: An apraisal of endoscopic removal of malignant colonic polyps. *Mayo Clin Proc* 1986; 61:123–126. *The authors conclude on the basis of a study group of 65 patients that colonic polyps with carcinoma in situ can be treated safely with complete endoscopic removal; such management incurs the responsibiity of thorough follow-up studies.*

28. Fielding LP, Ballantyne GH: Classification systems for staging colorectal cancer: Past, present, and future. *Probl Gen Surg* 1987; 4:39–53.

29. Rankin FW, Broders AC: Factors influencing prognosis in carcinoma of the rectum. *Surg Gynecol Obstet* 1928; 46:660–667.

30. Lockhart-Mummery HE, Dukes CE: The surgical treatment of malignant rectal polyps. *Lancet* 1952; 2:751–755.

31. Nivatvongs S, Goldberg SM: Management of patients who have polyps containing invasive carcinoma removed via colonoscope. *Dis Colon Rectum* 1978; 21:8–11.

32. Pearl RK: Management of malignant polyps. *Probl Gen Surg* 1987; 4:54–60.

33. Muto T, Bussey HJR, Morson BC: The evolution of cancer of the colon and rectum. *Cancer* 1975; 36:2251–2270.

34. Katon RM, Keeffe EB, Melnyk CS: *Flexible Sigmoidoscopy.* New York, Grune & Stratton, Inc. 1985.

35. Richards WO, Webb WA, Morris SJ, et al: Patient management after endoscopic removal of the cancerous colon adenoma. *Ann Surg* 1987; 205:665–672. *Colon resection after endoscopic polypectomy is reserved for the following: (1) incomplete excision, (2) poorly differentiated tumor, (3) invasion of the line of resection, (4) invasion of the polyp stalk, and (5) invasion of venous or lymphatic channels.*

36. Greene FL: Distribution of colorectal neoplasma: A left to right shift of polyps and cancer. *Am Surg* 1983; 43:62–65.

37. Lock MR, Cairns DW, Ritchie JK, et al: The treatment of early colorectal cancer by local excision. *Br J Surg* 1978; 65:346–349.

38. Schrock T: Discussion, in Richards WO, Webb WA, Morris SJ, et al: Patient management after endoscopic removal of the cancerous colon adenoma. *Ann Surg* 1987; 205:670.

39. Ballantyne GH: Risk of colorectal cancer in patients with chronic ulcerative colitis and Crohn's disease. *Probl Gen Surg* 1987; 4:154–167.

40. Greenstein AJ, Heimann TM, Sachar DB, et al: A comparison of multiple synchronous colorectal cancer in ulcerative colitis, familial polyposis coli, and de novo cancer. *Ann Surg* 1986; 203:123–128.

41. Fitzgibbons RJ Jr, Lynch HT, Stanislav GV, et al: Recognition and treatment

of patients with hereditary nonpolyposis colon cancer (Lynch Syndromes I and II). *Ann Surg* 1987; 206:289–295.

42. Riddell RH: Hands off "cancerous" large bowel polyps. *Gastroenterology* 1985; 89:432–441.

43. Barwick KW: The use of endoscopic biopsy in evaluation of polypoid lesions of the colon. *Yale J Biol Med* 1986; 59:33–40. *The author discusses the limitation of endoscopic biopsies due to sampling errors and the inability to reach the deep submucosal cores of polyps where malignant invasion may occur.*

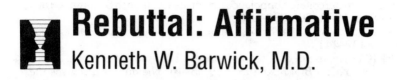

Rebuttal: Affirmative
Kenneth W. Barwick, M.D.

Changes come slowly in the practice of medicine, as well they should. Any departure from standardized, accepted practice should follow only upon careful analysis of the potential gain in clinical outcome vs. the potential risk to the patients involved. However, there invariably is tension in such evolution as the necessary data are accrued, because any such transition is characterized by an interval during which relative uncertainty prevails while a bridge from the accepted to the proposed is constructed. A number of such efforts currently are being undertaken in medicine and especially in the field of surgery. Examples include narrowing the resection margins in the surgical treatment of cutaneous malignant melanoma, utilizing more limited forms of resection in the surgical therapy of breast carcinoma, and consideration of polypectomy alone as therapy for selected malignant colorectal polyps.

Drs. Bilchik and Ballantyne have offered a very fine argument for retaining the standard surgical approach to malignant polyps. Surgeons are generally conservative by nature, as indeed they should be. The same is true of my own discipline, which may be in part why I find much of their argument compelling and convincing. I am also intrigued by their application of the word "conservative." This is backed by no less an authority than the *Oxford Universal English Dictionary*. However, any linguist knows that difficult decisions must be made in defining a word. Conservative is also defined as "characterized by moderation, tending to preserve." There is conflict between the time-honored usage of a word and the usage that evolves over time in the community which it serves that is, ultimately, a conflict between form and function. So it is with medicine and with the medical literature which we use to record our progress and our experience and thus to guide us.

Regarding malignant colorectal polyps, we must ask, what is our experience and how should our practice be impacted? It is here that I have some differences with Drs. Bilchik and Ballantyne. The question is, what does the literature say and are we being directed to bridge to a modified form of therapy? In my review of the literature provided earlier in this chapter, it seems that most authors believe this bridge is indicated, that is, that carefully selected malignant colorectal polyps can be treated safely by endoscopic polypectomy alone. My colleagues have a number of reservations about this, including the following: (1) more than 10% of patients with polyps containing invasive carcinoma have poor treatment outcome; (2) many polyps are not amenable to polypectomy only, due to morphology, size, or other considerations; (3) identifying polyps with favorable histology remains problematic;

and (4) the published series of individuals with malignant polyps may not well reflect the population at large.

These are all worthwhile reservations that cannot be totally refuted. Nonetheless, the references which I have quoted earlier provide good evidence that the "more than 10% who will have adverse outcome" can be predicted. The overwhelming majority of such patients have one or more of the three major adverse histological guidelines which have been defined as: (1) a positive resection margin, (2) poorly differentiated carcinoma, or (3) lymphatic invasion by malignant cells. Virtually all would agree that these patients should be treated by standard segmental colonic resection. One quarrel I have with the position of Drs. Bilchik and Ballantyne is that much of the literature they review addresses this group of patients and not the group with favorable histology.

Whether most malignant polyps will not be amenable to polypectomy alone (that is, will have unfavorable histology or morphology) is unclear. Again, in the published series to date, a variable but substantial percentage of patients with malignant polyps have favorable histology. Moreover, if we succeed in what we must do to combat colorectal cancer (i.e., create effective surveillance programs for early detection) then we will encounter greater numbers of small polyps with superficially invasive carcinoma and the question will only become more relevant.

It is true that accurately and reproducibly identifying patients with favorable histology remains problematic. Much of the available literature stresses the necessity of removing and examining colorectal polyps in such a way as to allow optimal diagnostic information to be derived. It is essential that endoscopists and pathologists follow the guidelines which are now well defined. I have reviewed these guidelines and the problems which persist with the nomenclature of malignant polyps previously.

The concern which I most share with my colleagues is whether the published studies accurately reflect experience with the population at large relative to recurrence, survival, and compliance with follow-up regimens. A new study published since the submission of our original manuscripts addresses some of these concerns.[1] This study is of a large population of individuals with colorectal adenomas followed at a gastrointestinal institute in West Germany. It was undertaken by a group of clinicians, pathologists, and statisticians. During a 10-year interval, 1,769 polyps were endoscopically removed from 1,219 patients. The authors indicate that their study differs from several earlier studies in that it was performed at a large group practice which serves urban and rural areas. The follow-up of such patients more accurately reflects the outcome of patients seen in a physician's office.

Areas of invasive adenocarcinoma infiltrating the muscularis mucosa were demonstrated in adenomas from 61 patients (5.0%). Another 97 patients (8.0%) had areas of severe atypia without invasion. The same three criteria which have been used in several earlier studies to determine favorable histology (negative resection margin, absence of poorly differentiated carcinoma, and absence of lymphatic invasion) were employed. Of the patients with malignant polyps, 25 (41%) had favorable histology and were treated by polypectomy only.

Patients with malignant polyps and those with polyps containing areas of severe atypia were asked to have follow-up examinations at 3-month intervals for 1 year, at 6-month intervals for a second year, and at 3-year intervals beginning with the third year. Compliance in these groups was poor during the first year when follow-up intervals were short, but improved during the second and following years to a rate which was superior to that of patients with benign adenomas. Of the patients with malignant polyps, 80% returned for surveillance examinations. The 5-year survival rate of patients with malignant polyps was 84.3%, not different from that of patients with severe atypia only (79.0%), but superior to that of patients who underwent colectomy following endoscopic polypectomy (55.4%). The latter figure undoubtedly reflects the more aggressive biology of these lesions as predicted by the unfavorable histology criteria. No recurrences of tumor were observed in the patients with endoscopically removed malignant polyps. The authors concluded that endoscopic polypectomy alone is acceptable therapy for patients with malignant polyps having favorable histology. This paper, combined with others, suggests that a significant number of malignant polyps will have favorable histology, and that those which will behave aggressively can be predicted.

Finally, I am flattered that my colleagues chose to close their article by quoting my reservations regarding conservative (or liberal?) therapy of malignant polyps. Since I wrote those words in 1985 for submission, five additional major articles have been published (referenced earlier) which support endoscopic polypectomy only for malignant polyps with favorable histology. In my opinion, it is time to embrace this cautiously as an option in the therapy of colorectal neoplasia.

Reference

1. Eckardt VF, Fuchs M, Kanzler G, et al: Follow-up of patients with colonic polyps containing severe atypia and invasive carcinoma. Compliance, recurrence, and survival. *Cancer* 1988; 61:2552–2557.

Rebuttal: Negative

Anton J. Bilchik, M.D.
Garth H. Ballantyne, M.D.

The purpose of this rebuttal is to demonstrate how our approach to the management of malignant polyps differs from that of Dr. Barwick. Also, we hope to highlight several assumptions that are implicit in Dr. Barwick's argument which are left unstated. Furthermore, we hope to emphasize that the ideal management of individual patients can be selected only based upon an integration of both clinical and morphological data. Finally, we must reiterate that 50 years of clinical experience with various staging systems for colorectal cancer strongly suggest that simplified pathological staging systems are unable to reliably predict treatment outcome for individual patients.

Statement of the Controversy

We disagree with the statement made earlier by Dr. Barwick that "...there does seem to be reasonable cause for conservative management of *most* malignant polyps." We believe that we have demonstrated that the majority of polyps containing invasive carcinoma require resection by traditional surgical techniques. We agree, however, that there is a small group of patients for whom endoscopic polypectomy may accomplish curative therapy. This group of patients represents a *minority* of all patients with invasive carcinoma in a polyp. In order to fall within this group, the lesion in these patients must not contain any of the characteristics listed in Table 1. Unfortunately, whether endoscopic polypectomy provides adequate treatment for even this highly preselected group of patients remains unproven.

Critique

Dr. Barwick has offered a superb synopsis of the available literature which records the results of endoscopically treating patients with polyps containing invasive carcinoma. He has described in detail the results published in 12 original articles spanning the period from 1975 to 1987. Furthermore, he has critically analyzed the techniques utilized in these studies and has attempted to compare their results. He pointed out that the numbers of patients in the quoted studies is small and highly preselected, and that the follow-up on these patients is poor. He has noted rightly that the varying techniques and definitions of invasive carcinoma found in these publications often make comparisons between studies elusive or tenuous. Because of the small number and short follow-up of patients in most of these studies, Dr. Barwick concludes that the determination of optimal management will require "additional study."

The most significant element of Dr. Barwick's discusion is his description of the role of the pathologist in evaluating polyps containing invasive carcinoma. He describes the best means of preparing endoscopically excised polyps for pathological evaluation. He further emphasizes the need for communication between the clinician and the pathologist. With all of these points, we agree.

Dr. Barwick has approached the topic of debate somewhat differently than we addressed it. Although the management of "malignant polyps of the colon and rectum" is the issue of concern, Dr. Barwick has limited his discussion to only "endoscopically removed malignant polyps." Unfortunately, as pointed out above, this excludes almost one half of all malignant polyps from discussion. Also, Dr. Barwick limits his discussion of treatment to only those patients for whom "certain clinical and pathological requirements are met." The criteria that are emphasized are (1) the removal of the polyp as a single fragment, (2) the absence of malignant cells at the cauterized margin of resection, (3) the absence of lymphatic invasion by malignant cells, and (4) the absence of poorly differentiated carcinoma. Each of these items, of course, further limits the number of patients included for consideration. Thus, Dr. Barwick does not address the management of the majority of patients with invasive carcinoma in a polyp but rather limits his discussion to a small, heavily preselected group of patients. In contrast, we attempted to address the factors influencing treatment decision for the entire group of patients with malignant polyps.

The definition of "conservative managment" utilized by Dr. Barwick apparently differs from ours. Although this term is not characterized, he seems to equate endoscopic polypectomy with conservative management. We feel that this is an unfortunate use of the term, since it might imply that endoscopic excision is a long-established and generally accepted treatment for invasive carcinoma of the colon and rectum. It might also imply that the primary physician should resort to "radical" therapy such as operative exicision of invasive colorectal cancer only under unusual circumstances. We believe that we have demonstrated that endoscopic polypectomy may be adequate therapy for only a small group of patients and, therefore, that operative excision continues to represent the well-established and generally accepted treatment of invasive colorectal cancer for the majority of patients with invasive carcinoma in a polyp.

Dr. Barwick appears to assume that endoscopic polypectomy is a safer procedure than operative excision of malignant polyps. This is oversimplification. Rectal lesions, for example, often can be excised more easily and safely by transanal or transperineal approaches than by endoscopic polypectomy. Similarly, right colectomy is often a less morbid procedure than endoscopic excision of a sessile cecal lesion. Thus, the selection of the safest therapeutic modality for a particular patient requires an analysis of a variety of clinical issues. These include, but are not limited to, the condition of the patient, the presence of associated diseases such as ulcerative colitis, the gross morphological features of the polyp, the location of the polyp, the number of lesions, the difficulty of accomplishing endoscopic polypectomy, and the potential morbidity of various surgical approaches. The ideal therapy for individual patients can be selected only by an experienced clinician after weighing all mitigating variables.

We disagree with one additional assumption that is implicit in Dr. Barwick's argument. He assumes that a purely histological classification of a colorectal cancer can predict treatment outcome for an individual patient. As we have discussed earlier, no previous pathological staging system for colorectal cancer has succeeded in this task. Consequently, reliance upon histological criteria for predicting treatment outcome would seem premature, at best.

Summary

The results of treating colorectal cancer have not improved in the last 30 years. The crude 5-year survival rate for this disease is only about 30%. Furthermore, no successful treatment of metastatic carcinoma has been identified. Even when limited to a polyp, invasive carcinoma is a life-threatening disease. Indeed, more than 10% of patients with polyps containing carcinoma suffer poor outcomes. Consequently, clinicians managing patients with polyps containing invasive cancer must select a treatment which offers the best chance of a satisfactory outcome. This, of course, requires balancing the morbidity of the treatment against the potential of curative resection of the lesion.

We have summarized the data available which indicate that the majority of patients with malignant polyps are best treated by the traditional surgical techniques of resection. The reasons for poor outcome if the patient is treated only by endoscopic polypectomy may reflect features of the polyp, associated disease, or practical considerations. Several characteristics of malignant polyps augur a poor outcome if the lesion is treated only by endoscopic polypectomy. These include a sessile polyp, a villous adenoma, a poorly differentiated carcinoma, invasion of the lesion into lymphatics, a polyp greater than 2 cm in diameter, and cancer at or near the margin of resection. Patients with associated conditions such as familial polyposis, chronic ulcerative colitis, Lynch syndromes, multiple synchronous polyps, or multiple synchronous carcinomas generally are best treated by abdominal colectomy or total proctocolectomy. Sometimes practical considerations mitigate against treatment by endoscopic polypectomy. The lesion may not be amenable to endoscopic polypectomy because of inaccessibility, location, or size. On occasion, adequate histological information is not available because of piecemeal excision or inappropriate sectioning of the lesion. Unfortunately, the *majority* of patients with malignant polyps fall into one of these categories. Consequently, the *majority* of patients with polyps containing invasive carcinoma are best treated by traditional operative techniques.

The concept of identifying a small group of patients for whom endoscopic polypectomy will offer adequate therapy for patients with malignant polyps is attractive. At best, this will prove adequate therapy for only a small *minority* of such patients. It must be stressed, however, that although this is an attractive hypothesis, little substantial data exist at present for its support.

Editor's Comments
Thomas P. Duffy, M.D.

This debate constitutes a healthy and lively engagement wherein the surgical pathologist, Dr. Kenneth Barwick, ably meets the etymologic and scientific thrusts of Dr. Ballantyne's sallies. The conservative (traditional), aggressive (nonconservative) surgical resection of malignant colorectal polyps may now give way to endoscopic removal of such polyps in specific, selected circumstances. Both parties agree that certain characteristics of the resected specimen (tumor differentiation, lymphatic invasion, and tumor involvement of the resection margin) demand aggressive intervention. Dr. Barwick argues convincingly (and provides a more recent and larger series of studies to buttress his arguments) that a definite group of patients with these lesions can be identified and spared the burden of bowel resection. But the eventual outcome in this gray area depends not only upon the initial pathology of the tumor but also upon the adequacy of follow-up and the patient's compliance with that follow-up. Endoscopic polypectomy creates a shared responsibility to maximally guarantee that the critical "conservative" management has cured the lesion.

The debate highlights another dimension in managing this problem which is central to all of the controversies in medicine. That dimension is the patient's choice from the various options presented by his or her physician. The different perspectives of the surgeon and internist must be recognized as influencing the recommendations that they make. Confrontations such as the one which is contained in this debate are not simple academic exercises but the content of the common clinical discussions between doctors and their patients. Where uncertainty exists as to a therapeutic recommendation, the patient's informed consent and choice from these options often will best solve the debate surrounding the gray areas. The physician and his or her community continue to assume their appropriate responsibility for scholarship in gathering data to narrow and ultimately eliminate the gray areas.

Should Surgeons Perform Gastrointestinal Endoscopy?

Chapter Editor: Thomas P. Duffy, M.D.

Affirmative: William H. Marks, M.D., Ph.D.
Associate Professor of Surgery, Director,
Endoscopy-Surgical Service, Department of
Surgery, Yale University School of
Medicine, Yale-New Haven Hospital, New
Haven, Connecticut

Negative: John Dobbins, M.D.
Professor of Medicine, Director, GI
Procedure Center, Department of Medicine,
Yale University School of Medicine, New
Haven, Connecticut

Editor's Introduction

Endoscopy traditionally has been the means by which a gastroenterologist examined the gut in order to identify and biopsy any pathologic features. Today, advances in technology and application have made it possible for this nonsurgical technique to be used to correct lesions that previously required laparotomy. Thus, the "viewing" endoscopist has now become the "interventional" endoscopist; placing stents to relieve obstruction, performing papillotomies, and crushing stones are only a few newfound capabilities. In addition, sclerotherapy of bleeding esophageal lesions is now used in some cases as a substitute for portal decompression procedures.

Not unexpectedly, this incursion of the gastroenterologist into the field of the surgeon has led to the appropriation of endoscopy as a tool to be used by both practitioners. This development has created the following debate in which a medical gastroenterologist and a surgeon-endoscopist defend their opposing positions regarding who should perform endoscopy.

Thomas P. Duffy, M.D.

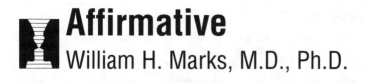

Affirmative
William H. Marks, M.D., Ph.D.

The surgeon should endoscopically view the lesion which he or she is going to treat prior to the operation. Whether "lesion" refers to a neoplasm or to a site of bleeding, this seems to be a straightforward and benign statement regarding surgical disease — or is it? Not all general surgeons are qualified endoscopists and, in fact, the majority of preoperative endoscopic evaluations are performed by medical endoscopists. In our current medical system, internists are the endoscopists. This situation has evolved for many reasons, not the least of which is that surgeons chose to neglect endoscopy during the procedure's developmental years. Be that as it may, the fundamental question we must address is whether the system is acceptable in its current form, and why?

For the surgeon/endoscopist, the need to view endoscopically the lesion to be treated surgically is straightforward. Any system that does not afford the surgeon this ability is inadequate. "After all," my endoscopy mentor, Tom Dent, used to admonish his residents at the University of Michigan, "the endoscopic examination is part of the complete physical examination of the gastrointestinal tract." When the surgeon is not the endoscopist, he or she must rely on a colleague for evaluation of the patient. In other words, the surgeon must be dependent on someone else to complete part of the patient's physical examination. It is undesirable and potentially detrimental to patient care for the surgeon to rely on secondhand information in this regard.

The history and physical examination are the cornerstones of clinical practice and the physical examination is a "contact sport." For each medical or surgical discipline, the physical examination becomes a unique synthesis of tactile sensation and instinctual awareness. The latter results from both the examiner's experience and, of course, his or her "point of view." The physical examination is a subjective experience with the potential for remarkably enhancing subtle signs of a disease process which may prove important for the diagnosis and management of a given problem. The unique perspective of the general surgeon with regard to anatomy and a "feel" for the tissues is an important addition to the standard physical examination of the gastrointestinal tract, and one which the internist cannot provide.

In the course of a patient's work-up, the surgeon/endoscopist will endoscope any patient being evaluated as a potential surgical candidate with three goals in mind: (1) to see the nature of the lesion (usually obtaining biopsy proof of a malignant process in the case of a neoplasm or assessing therapeutic strategies in the case of a bleeding site), (2) to clear the gastrointestinal tract of simultaneously occurring lesions, and (3) to aid in planning the operation. If the surgeon cannot perform the examination directly, then a weak link is introduced into the chain of decision-making concerning the patient. The surgeon will be obliged to base his or her decisions on the results of a physical examination performed by someone else, and his or her interpretation may be limited to some extent by the endoscopist's ability to communicate relevant findings.

It is likely that the amount of misinformation transmitted to the surgeon will be related inversely to the reporting endoscopist's level of experience. The observations of the endoscopist are colored with a point of view that is critical for establishing a preoperative plan for the patient. "Point of view" can be equated with "orientation" and is the product of training and prior experience in this case. The internist/endoscopist approaches the gastrointestinal lesion from a medical point of view with a static view of anatomy and a limited "feel" for tissues. The internist follows a series of maneuvers designed to answer specific questions relating to the disease process at hand, but not necessarily to address fundamental surgical questions. Surgical intervention is requested only when the internist believes that a problem needs to be addressed by a surgeon and any request is limited to a specific lesion. Information about the lesion is passed along from the endoscopist to the surgeon. It is at this point that responsibility for patient care is also likely to shift from the internist to the surgeon, making it an easy place for a breakdown in physician communication to occur which can result in patient injury.

Since the impression that the internist/endoscopist passes on to the surgeon is a major component of the data base used to determine the operative approach to the patient, and since there is a clear danger in miscommunication, why cannot this problem simply be avoided by having the surgeon attend the patient's endoscopy? The answer to this question is all too obvious. Time and economic constraints prevent dual attending coverage by both an endoscopist and a surgeon from becoming standard practice at every endoscopic procedure concerning a potential surgical lesion. Alternatively then, given the current availability of electronic equipment and computers, why not record a video of the case for review by the surgeon? Certainly we make excellent use of such technology for coronary angiography and contrast gastrointestinal radiology. Again, the answer boils down to time and fiscal constraints. As a practical matter, both viewing an unedited videotape and editing one into a concise and informative record are cumbersome and expensive procedures. In addition, such technology requires an institutional investment in hardware as well as personnel to operate it. Even if a real-time visual record were always available, it clearly cannot accurately relay a "feel" for the examination. Therefore, most endoscopy/surgery teams depend on interpersonal communication.

Interpersonal communication may consist of either verbal or written reports. However, the human inability to relate unedited information accurately is well know and has become engrained as part of the conventional wisdom. Therefore, the descriptive notes the surgeon will receive will contain secondhand information which is subject to the interpretation, skills, and point of view of the endoscopist. Even if the information is passed on by direct communication, interpretive descriptions and static photos do not always tell the surgeon the whole story. Acting solely on this information is akin to accepting someone else's physical examination of a patient suspected of having an acute abdomen as the basis for operation. The surgeon taking responsibility for the case must examine the patient in order to reach a valid surgical decision. Performing this examination through an endoscope is no less important in forming a surgical opinion. Descriptive phrases such as "mild," "moderate," "severe deep tenderness," or "exquisitely tender" are not different than "superficial," "partially circumferential," "angry," "mild diverticular disease," "no bleeding beyond this point," "distensible wall," or "deep ulcer." Without a "laying on" of hands, the surgeon is prevented from gathering the most complete information available about the lesion being addressed.

Do patients suffer under the current system or is our concern just a smoke screen designed to hide some underlying territorial dispute? Under our current system of practice in which the endoscopist is separate from the surgeon, two outcomes are regularly predictable for any case. Either the lesion will be properly identified and described by the endoscopist and the proper surgical procedure will be performed, or the lesion will not be properly identified and/or described and the case will be handled incorrectly. In the latter case, the patient may be forced to suffer a second procedure or, worse, the consequences of inadequately treated disease. I am aware of at least two currently pending lawsuits which have resulted from exactly this situation. In both cases, inaccurate endoscopic evaluation of the lesion led to the need for a second procedure.

A variant of this problem derives from the surgeon's need to make adequate preoperative plans and to inform the patient and family of the anticipated procedure(s) and statistical chances that alternative procedures may be necessary. For instance, consider a patient having a "rectal" carcinoma identified by colonoscopy who also has had his colon cleared of synchronous lesion by colonoscopy. Both he and the surgeon are told that the lesion is in a position which makes resection easy. After he and his concerned family members have been informed that a simple, one-stage colon resection will be performed, it is discovered at operation that the lesion is actually much lower than expected, making resection remarkably difficult or impossible. The patient and his family may be upset to find that he now has a colostomy. It would have served them best to inform them from the outset that a colostomy may be necessary.

What makes the endoscopic examination any different than any other "diagnopeutic" technique (diagnostic techniques with direct therapeutic potential and/or applications such as angiography or interventional radiology)? Unlike many other techniques, endoscopy lends itself to daily surgical practice. A detailed knowledge of complicated equipment is not required and interpretation of the findings is not dependent on a set of clinical skills which are outside the training of a surgeon, as might be the case with radiology. The techniques are easily learned and complement other mechanical skills which the surgeon is already accustomed to using in daily practice. Finally, it cannot be overemphasized that endoscopy provides timely and direct sensory input which the surgeon needs to complete his or her evaluation of the patient.

A nonsurgeon performing an endoscopic examination is unlikely to approach it as part of the routine work-up for a potential surgical disease process, a difference in approach that can be frustrating to a surgeon. However, if the surgeon is not an endoscopist, the usual politics of referral patterns and reputation can force him or her to accept the "medical approach" to a patient with a surgical problem. A patient presenting with a potential surgical lesion will require either elective or urgent/emergent endoscopy. The elective case is easy to address; performing the endoscopy tonight, today, tomorrow, or 7 days from now is adequate to suit the needs of both surgeon and patient. However, when the case has an urgent/ emergent status, the picture often becomes cloudy. Obviously, there are straightforward emergencies that require immediate treatment, either endo-scopic or open surgical. However, there is a large group of patients who fall into a medical gray zone. What is a "now" case for the surgeon is often a "happy to do first thing in the morning" case for his gastroenterology colleague.

Is this a fair argument? Is the care of the patient seriously affected by these minor conflicts? Is it not really just for the surgeon's convenience that the now-stable 2-unit gastrointestinal bleeder in the cardiac intensive care unit be endoscoped at 2 A.M.? The importance of point of view cannot be overemphasized! Endoscopy in this situation offers both diagnosis and potential treatment. Most importantly, it allows the surgeon to formulate a plan. The typical question asked of the surgeon requesting immediate endoscopy at odd hours is "will you operate if I find X, Y, or Z?" It is asked because a "maybe" or "no" answer apparently will justify a delay in the service. However, the surgical point of view is that the planning which the endoscopy will allow is an important part of the treatment algorithm for the patient. Delay in future steps can be avoided, for example, if the lesion and the anatomy are known, as well as any unusual features such as concurrent gastric and duodenal erosions. Often, this knowledge results in more efficient delivery of care to the patient; occasionally, it provides lifesaving information. For instance, consider a patient with pyloric stenosis due to peptic ulcer disease who has now stopped bleeding. Rapid rebleeding from a duodenal ulcer is best served by immediate operation rather than by an attempt to endoscope an area which is not accessible to the scope. A delay in endoscopy will translate into a delay in operation or into an operation performed with less information than might otherwise be available to the operating surgeon.

However, as noted previously, most surgeons today are not qualified endoscopists. Skills in diagnostic and minor therapeutic endoscopy must await the next generation of surgeons — residents currently in training who, by mandate of the Board of Surgery, will be trained in these techniques in order to qualify for Board certification.

What then does one do when the surgeon performing the operation is not an endoscopist? There appear to be only two alternatives: (1) have a qualified internist perform the endoscopy, or (2) have another surgeon qualified in endoscopy perform the procedure. How does one make such a choice? In many areas of the United States, the question is moot. Small towns, rural communities, and "undesirable" areas within larger communities often lack access to a qualified specialist such as a gastroenterologist. The general surgeon may be the only physician in such an area with the necessary mechanical skills to adopt endoscopic techniques. On the other hand, it is possible that a gastroenterologist may be the only other "game in town." In either case, it is clear that the clinician offering the skill in such an area will receive the referral and perform the procedure. Whether or not this is a good situation is not relevant to this discussion. Rather, what must be considered in this forum is the situation in which both a medical and a surgical service are available. For the sake of this argument, I will assume that both persons offering the service are well qualified in gastrointestinal endoscopy. Which endoscopist then, should perform the endoscopy?

I believe that on a cold and pragmatic level it can be stated that in today's fiscally aware medical community the entire health care system is best served by having a surgeon perform an endoscopic procedure for a potential surgical lesion. Each patient must be approached as a potential operative candidate. The operating room needs to be informed in order to plan instruments, personnel, anesthesiology coverage, and reservations. Blood bank and laboratory facilities need to be informed, and the recovery room, intensive care units, and/or surgical floors may need to be more actively mobilized. The proper timing of a proposed procedure is critical, in relation to both the urgency of the procedure for the care of the patient and the way in which the case will impact on the operating room schedule. The surgeon performing his own endoscopy does so with an understanding of the complicated logistics associated with any operation.

Preoperative work-ups and orders require time to implement. Booking cases and obtaining other tests requires time and is dependent on available manpower. The urgency in evaluating a patient may be determined by far more than simply the status of the lesion. A late afternoon endoscopy that is postponed until the next day instead of being performed in the evening may result in a patient being unable to proceed through a necessary work-up for several days because of delays in scheduling or an intervening weekend. A poorly timed report or observation by the endoscopist may have consequences extending far beyond the doctor/patient relationship.

An equally important consideration is that endoscopic procedures have become increasingly invasive, and even relatively benign procedures are not without complications. Medical endoscopists have not simultaneously developed the skills necessary to deal with these complications. Once a complication occurs, it must be dealt with in a forthright manner. Complications of endoscopy are largely surgical in nature, involving aspiration, perforation, bleeding, or a complication of anesthesia. Since a surgeon is trained to handle these problems, if he or she performs the endoscopy, no time will be lost in evaluating and/or preparing the patient for the operating theater. The surgeon/endoscopist is trained in a surgical point of view and a "feel" for surgical disease, making him or her the best alternative when the attending surgeon is not an endoscopist.

Whatever reasons surgeons offer for believing that either they should perform their own endoscopies or another surgeon should do so for patients having surgical problems, their motives are open to suspicion. After all, until recently, endoscopy has been a surgical orphan. For whatever reason, this technique has not been considered a technical tour de force by the surgical community. So why is it now? What motives are powering this mounting enthusiasm? Surgeons clearly have discovered that endoscopy is an important tool for physical diagnosis, treatment planning, and therapy. As discussed above, peforming their own endoscopies allows surgeons to manage surgical problems in surgical terms and to exercise greater control than if they are dependent on medical endoscopists. In addition, improved equipment and innovative techniques now make endoscopy technically interesting. Performing endoscopy today requires excellent eye-hand coordination, instrumentation, and three-dimensional thinking, basic skills that are part of general surgical training. The general surgery residency is set at 5 years in length in order to hone both the intellectual and the mechanical skills of the resident. Thus, endoscopy has become an attractive skill for the surgeon.

But is there really something else at play here? Of course there is. Both surgeons and internists want to perform endoscopy for two reasons which are all too obvious: endoscopic procedures are lucrative and provide a source of power. Why is gastrointestinal endoscopy considered to be lucrative to the internist? Technical procedures have always been the most lucrative part of medical practice. Traditionally, these procedures have been surgical. As technology has advanced in numerous areas, both diagnostic and therapeutic, skill in performing specialized and increasingly invasive procedures has been developed in most specialties. The substantial costs associated with these procedures are justified by the extra training, time, and skill they require; the information they provide; and the treatment they facilitate. It would be naive to ignore the lucrative nature of endoscopy, since it is the most profitable portion of a gastroenterology practice. One colonoscopy alone can provide in real income the equivalent of seven to ten office visits with one-tenth the time investment.

But why is this important to the surgeon? After all, the surgeon performs major invasive procedures that carry large price tags. Surely he or she is not concerned that the only alternative income will be derived from the office. The reason is related to the fact that gastrointestinal endoscopic procedures are charge-intensive. Since they are relatively brief (at least when compared to major surgical operations), numerous procedures can be performed within a short time span. Importantly, patients require little follow-up care or other investment of time once the procedure is complete. The procedures provide quick answers to important diagnostic questions and can be potentially therapeutic. Therefore, a constant source of patients is available once referral patterns are established. Gastrointestinal endoscopy is a skill that provides an important and necessary service but does little to interfere with the physician's "schedule." To ignore the importance of financial considerations in this argument would be both naive and callous.

What type of power can endoscopy hold within an institution? Control over a budget, space, and personnel are all necessary to run an endoscopy unit. These are also the administrative components from which power is derived within any institution. The individual(s) and department who control these areas accrue a degree of "say-so" about the way the institution operates. For the endoscopist or group, the controlling department also gains high visibility within the institution and automatically becomes a part of the referral network that is a clinician's lifeblood.

In summary, I believe that both the medical and surgical communities have legitimate interests in performing gastrointestinal endoscopy. The reasons are numerous and range from power and money to concerns over patient care. However, it is my contention that both the patient and the medical system are best served in the case of a surgical lesion if the endoscopy is performed by either the surgeon responsible for the case or by another qualified surgeon.

References

1. Dent TL: The surgeon and fiberoptic endoscopy. *Surg Gynecol Obstet* 1973; 137:278. *This article offers important insights from the surgical point of view.*
2. Dent TL: Surgeons, gastroenterologist, endoscopists (editorial). *Surg Gynecol Obstet* 1981; 153:733. *This editorial offers key aspects of the debate.*
3. Donahue PE, Abcarian H, Nyhus LM: Surgeons as endoscopists. *Surg Gastroenterol* 1982; 1:73–76. *This classic report is required reading.*
4. Kukora JS, Clericuzio CP, Dent TL: The case for surgical training in gastrointestinal endoscopy. *Am J Gastroenterol* 1984; 79:907–909. *The surgeon's case is substantiated by this report.*
5. Dent TL, Leibrandt TJ: Teaching surgical endoscopy of the gastrointestinal tract, in Dent TL, Strodel WE, Turcotte JG (eds): *Surgical Endoscopy.* Chicago, Year Book Medical Publishers, Inc, 1985. *This is an important and comprehensive assessment of surgical endoscopy.*

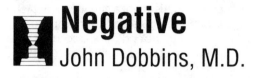

Negative
John Dobbins, M.D.

Until recently, who should perform gastrointestinal endoscopy has not been an issue at most institutions. Gastroenterologists have predominantly performed this procedure since the modern era of gastrointestinal endoscopy was ushered in with the development of fiberoptic instruments. Relatively few surgeons performed endoscopy and training in this area was not a requirement in most surgical residency programs. However, in 1983, the American Board of Surgery decreed that surgical residency programs would include training in gastrointestinal endoscopy. The result has been the establishment of "surgical gastrointestinal endoscopy" units and programs around the country and an increase in the number of surgeons who perform this procedure. These "surgical" endoscopists perform the same procedures as do "medical" endoscopists (gastroenterologists), placing the two groups in direct competition and leading to the inevitable question of who should perform the procedures.

The two major pioneers in gastrointestinal endoscopy were gastroenterologists themselves. Rudolf Schindler developed the first practical gastroscope to receive worldwide usage in 1932.[1] This instrument used prisms and lenses to convey light through a semiflexible tube. Although this was the first practical endoscope, its deficiencies limited widespread application of its use. The modern era of endoscopy was ushered in by the development of the flexible fiberoptic endoscope by Basil Hirschowitz and his colleagues at the University of Michigan in 1957.[2]

Fiberoptic endoscopy was limited to the esophagus initially, but an instrument long enough to visualize the stomach and duodenum as well soon became available. Development of the equipment and techniques necessary to perform colonoscopy and endoscopic retrograde cholangiopancreatography (ERCP) was quick to follow. In the 1970s, refinements in instrumentation made the technique easier and more informative for both the endoscopist and the patient. The advent of therapeutic procedures such as polypectomy, papillotomy, sclerotherapy, and laser therapy has further increased the usefulness of endoscopy, and the Japanese have contributed mightily to these technological advances.

This remarkable explosion in the utilization of endoscopic procedures has resulted in endoscopy almost replacing barium contrast examination (upper gastrointestinal series, barium enema) of the gastrointestinal tract as the primary diagnostic procedure in the initial evaluation of abnormalities in this area. As stated previously, the rapid expansion in the use of endoscopy occurred at a time when gastroenterologists were by far and away the primary group performing these procedures. This is not a situation in which the procedure was introduced by gastroenterologists and then applied by surgeons. The surgeons have been latecomers to the endoscopic scene. Only in 1983 did the American Board of Surgery state that surgical residents should have "exposure" to gastrointestinal endoscopy.

Why have surgeons decided to get into the endoscopy business? Is it only because this experience will result in the training of better surgeons? Is it because traditional surgical procedures have been eroded or eliminated by endoscopic procedures? Endoscopic polypectomy, papillotomy, dilatation, stents, electrocautery, heat therapy, and laser therapy clearly have decreased the utilization of such surgical procedures as colonic and gastric resections for polyps, common bile duct explorations for stones, choledochoduodenostomy, choledochojejunostomy, resection of strictures, and various surgical techniques utilized to treat gastrointestinal bleeding. Is it because surgeons realize how lucrative the performance of endoscopy can be?

Whatever the reason, surgeons have decided to perform gastrointestinal endoscopy and, in doing so, have entered into direct competition with internist-gastroenterologists. Is this competition good for medicine? Should gastroenterologists give up this "procedural" skill to the surgeon and hone the "cognitive" skills traditionally associated with internists? I believe that the internist-gastroenterologist should continue to perform endoscopy and, indeed, should be the primary specialist performing these procedures.

My first argument is relatively simple. What have gastroenterologists done wrong or poorly that they should relinquish this responsibility to the surgeon? Gastroenterologists have initiated and presided over the rapid and extensive advances made in gastrointestinal endoscopy. As a group, they should be proud of these accomplishments. The diagnostic and therapeutic advances resulting from endoscopy can be compared favorably to those afforded by other new technologies such as ultrasonography and computed tomography. Would the surgeons have done better? Would they have done as well? Would endoscopy be less expensive if controlled by surgeons?

Would surgeons be as skeptical and critical as internist-gastroenterologists? There have been at least seven controlled (some double-blind) trials on the efficacy of endoscopy in acute upper gastrointestinal bleeding.[3] All of these studies concluded that endoscopy did not influence the hospital course of these patients. In fairness, therapeutic techniques were not utilized in these studies, but this is beside the point. If surgeons were controlling endoscopy, would there have been seven studies saying that endoscopy did not affect the outcome of upper gastrointestinal bleeding? Endoscopic sclerotherapy for variceal bleeding is another example. After an initial flurry of primarily uncontrolled, poorly controlled, or small trials suggesting its efficacy, more recently performed, better controlled, and larger trials are questioning the efficacy of this procedure. I submit that internists are more likely to perform the painstaking, frequently tedious task of designing and rigorously adhering to these protocols and collecting the data. Gastroenterologist-endoscopists have been viewed critically by their colleagues in internal medicine. Will surgical endoscopists be examined as critically by their colleagues?

Internist-gastroenterologists not only perform endoscopy, but are also involved in the long-term care of many of their patients. In general, surgeons have relatively short-term encounters with their patients. When a patient only has colonic polyps that need to be removed, it does not matter whether it is done by a surgical endoscopist, a gastrointestinal endoscopist, or, for that matter, a dermatological endoscopist. When a patient has ulcerative colitis or Crohn's disease, however, firsthand knowledge of endoscopy can only help in management. Stated differently, when a patient has ulcerative colitis, who should perform the endoscopy — the gastroenterologist with whom the patient has or will have a long-term relationship or the surgeon that the patient will see only if medical management fails or a malignancy develops? The same could be asked for patients with other chronic intestinal diseases, such as severe reflux esophagitis, other peptic disease, or cirrhosis.

What about the patient who presents with abdominal pain or other symptoms suggestive of gastrointestinal disease? Except in cases of acute abdominal processes requiring emergent or semiemergent surgery, these patients are usually evaluted by internists and gastroenterologists. Should surgeons now be brought onto the scene just to perform the endoscopy? I think not. A patient complaining of abdominal pain was recently referred to me by a surgical resident who saw the patient in the emergency room. An acute abdomen was excluded and the patient was referred to the gastrointestinal clinic for further evaluation, a common procedure. The patient was also scheduled for a colonoscopy in the recently established surgical endoscopy clinic. By the time I saw the patient, the colonoscopy had been performed, the results were negative, and no further evaluation was being performed by the surgeons. Our evaluation revealed peptic ulcer disease and the patient was rendered asymptomatic on standard therapy.

Because he referred the patient to the gastrointestinal clinic, the surgical resident in the emergency room clearly thought medical evaluation was necessary. However, he also apparently wanted to support the newly created surgical endoscopy service. I doubt that this fragmentation of the work-up is good for the patient. It could be argued that the emergency room resident's scheduling of the colonoscopy is little different from scheduling a barium enema to precede the patient's appointment in the gastrointestinal clinic. Firsthand knowledge of a procedure, however, whether it is a barium enema or a colonoscopy, is always better than a written report. Of course, we cannot be trained in all diagnostic procedures and must rely on the expertise of others, but this is not the case here. The gastroenterologist to whom the patient was referred is trained in performing colonoscopy. Should he not perform the indicated procedure rather than relying on the report of a surgical endoscopist?

Stated another way, the physician expected to diagnose and manage the problem should either perform or be involved in the work-up of the patient as much as possible, simply because it gives him or her a more intimate knowledge of the disease process. No one disputes the enormous value of a good history and physical examination in the evaluation of symptoms that are not specific to one disorder. In this regard, endoscopy is simply an extension of the physical examination. To the extent that the internist-gastroenterologist is serving as the primary diagnostician, as in the preceding case, he or she should perform the endoscopy.

There are a number of important questions that need to be answered in regard to gastrointestinal endoscopy. For instance, how frequently should follow-up colonoscopy be performed for surveillance after a colonic polyp has been removed? How often should endoscopic surveillance be performed for dysplasia in cases of Barrett's esophagus or ulcerative colitis? What is the evolution or natural history of inflammation that can proceed to dysplasia and then to malignancy? Is endoscopic sclerotherapy for bleeding esophageal varices any good? These and other questions are being addressed at a number of institutions through studies being conducted primarily by gastro-enterologists, epidemiologists, and pathologists.

If surgeons were controlling endoscopy, would these questions be answered? Though the trend is clearly changing, as all of medicine is, surgeons are still less apt to answer these kinds of questions. This may be because of their heavy clinical burden, their apprenticeship type of training system which still relies to a certain extent on dogma, or their interest in other areas. Whatever the reason, internists are more research-oriented and more likely to propose, properly design, and execute the studies needed to answer questions such as those raised in the previous paragraph. Even today, much of the surgical literature is in the form of extended care reports or chart-review types of studies. Indeed, in gastroenterology, it could be argued that surgeons played much more of an investigative role 20 to 30 years ago than they do today.

Another issue is the training of surgical residents in endoscopy. Internists receive endoscopy training after entering a gastroenterology fellowship are commiting themselves to that subspecialty. Since, as far as I am aware, there is no similar subspecialty pathway for gastrointestinal surgeons, the real possibility exists that a surgical resident trained in endoscopy could end up in another surgical subspeciality and never utilize this training. In the current era of great emphasis on cost-containment in medicine, can we afford such luxury?

Also at issue is the extent to which surgical residents will be trained in endoscopy. Gastroenterology fellows receive at least 1 and usually up to 2 years of very extensive endoscopy training. Considering the increasing complexity of endoscopic procedures, this extensive training seems quite justified. Indeed, many gastroenterologists require postgraduate training to become adept at more difficult procedures, such as endoscopic papillotomy and stent placement. For surgical residents to become equally trained, they would have to undertake a training program like that of gastrointestinal fellows. To my knowledge, few if any such programs currently exist and one could certainly question such duplication of effort within a university medical school were they to be proposed, since both programs could be seriously diluted. Are there enough cases of biliary tract disease requiring endoscopic papillotomy at most centers to justify training both gastrointestinal fellows and surgical residents in this technique? If the intent is to "expose" surgical residents to endoscopy without training them to the level of competence, then is a separate training program really needed? Could they not be incorporated into the existing endoscopy program? With the rapidly growing popularity of video endoscopy which allows both multiple viewing and videotaping of procedures for use in classrooms, it has become possible to teach indication, findings, complications, and therapeutic techniques in depth without providing time-consuming "hands-on" experience to each surgical resident.

It could be argued that competition between gastroenterologists and surgeons over endoscopy is good, because competition usually drives prices down and we are all aware of the national concern about the cost of health care. However, this does not appear to be happening. Recently, a well-trained surgical endoscopist joined the surgical faculty at Yale University. Given the fact that he was the first full-time surgical endoscopist on staff, it would not have been surprising if he had charged fees below or at least equal to those of the gastroenterologists performing the same procedures. Instead, his prices are $100 to $200 higher. In fairness, these are the same prices he was charging when he came from the Midwest; however, it does not indicate that this competition is going to result in any savings for the consumer.

Having argued that internists-gastroenterologists should continue to be the main group performing endoscopy, as was my task in this article, let me conclude by saying that I do not think that surgeons should be totally excluded from performing endoscopy. Direct information obtained at endoscopy certainly helps surgeons to decide when to operate and what operation to perform. Surgeons can reasonably argue that they should be able to perform surveillance colonoscopy on their own patients with colonic polyps or malignancy. If a surgeon can perform an operative sphincteroplasty, why not an endoscopic papillotomy? At issue is which surgeons to train and how extensively to train them.

Medicine and surgery are changing rapidly and many of the classical distinctions that have separated these specialties are disappearing as a result of rapid technological advances. The same can also be said of radiology, which has evolved into "diagnostic imaging" as a result of the relatively recent development of nonradiological techniques such as ultrasonography, magnetic resonance imaging, and computed tomography. It is not clear into which department some of the newer technologies will fall. For instance, extracorporeal shock wave lithotripsy for gallstones which is now becoming established in this country on an experimental basis is under the primary control of either radiology, surgery, or gastroenterology at different institutions. Clearly, these three disciplines must work together for the successful application of this new technology.

Changing technology has resulted in new alliances. The gastroenterologist today has much more contact with gastrointestinal surgeons and "diagnostic imagers" than with members of his own department such as cardiologists and hematologists. At Yale University, a "Hepato-Biliary-Pancreatic Clinic" is being established which will be attended by surgeons, gastroenterologists, hepatologists, and radiologists specializing in disorders of these organs. The same is occurring in gastrointestinal oncology. I would not be surprised to see training become oriented more around disease entities or organ systems than around medical or surgical treatment. In such a system, the "digestive disease specialist" may receive training in gastroenterology, endoscopy, gastrointestinal surgery, and gastrointestinal imaging procedures after a suitable period of training in basic medical and surgical skills.

References

1. Schindler R: Ein vollig ungefahrliches flexibles Gastroskop. *Munchen Med Wochenschr* 1932; 79:1268–1269. *This article is the classic basis of gastrointestinal endoscopy.*
2. Hirschowitz BI, Curtiss LE, Peters CW, et al: Demonstration of a new gastroscope, the "fiberscope." *Gastroenterology* 1958; 35:50–53. *This is an important article in the history of endoscopy.*
3. Peterson WL: Gastrointestinal bleeding, in Sleisenger ML, Fordtran JS (eds): *Gastrointestinal Disease.* 3rd ed. Philadelphia, WB Saunders, 1983, p 186. *This important chapter establishes the role of endoscopy in the management of gastrointestinal bleeding.*

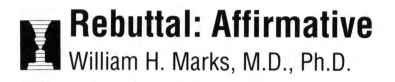

Rebuttal: Affirmative
William H. Marks, M.D., Ph.D.

I read with great interest the arguments of my medical colleague regarding the current conflict between surgeons and internists who perform gastrointestinal endoscopy. My colleague is indeed correct when he notes that endoscopy is a mechanical skill, and that developments in this technique have been furthered by the input of numerous internists. However, internists have not been solely responsible for all development in this field. I am sure that he is well aware that many legitimate contributions such as snare polypectomy, pecutaneous gastrostomy, and peritonoscopy have been made by surgical investigators with interest in this field. I initially orchestrated a rebuttal centered on my opponent's concern that surgeons and surgical thought would in some manner corrupt the practice of endoscopy. In the end, I concluded that an argument which attempts to associate unethical medical practices and conflict of interest was beyond the scope of this article. The emergence of the *Journal of Surgical Endoscopy* and the Society of American Gastrointestinal Endoscopic Surgeons (SAGES), illustrate the serious and committed interest of surgeons to this field as both investigators and clinicians.

I heartily agree with my colleague's concern over the economic issues on which this sort of debate focuses. I believe that economics is the overwhelming point on which most arguments between surgical and medical endoscopists pivot, be they members of community or academic institutions. In the final analysis, my opponent's point is that there is room for the practice of gastrointestinal endoscopy by internists and surgeons alike. In fact, I wholeheartedly agree. It is up to all of us as endoscopists to devise a system that will benefit our patients most. I believe that patients can be "divided" on the basis of the discipline (medicine or surgery) that cares for them. Rarely is there a need for confusing overlap. Lesions which come to the surgeon's attention or those that require chronic monitoring by medical specialists, are generally well-defined and agreed upon by the conventional wisdom of those who practice gastrointestinal endoscopy. Divorced from economic considerations, decisions regarding diagnostic or therapeutic intervention by endoscopists having either a surgical or a medical background become much easier to sort out. I hope, as my opponent indicated in his arguments, that we will soon reach that time when the skill of the operators and the collegiality of the specialty will allow for the distribution of patient cases based on the diagnosis and projected needs of each patient.

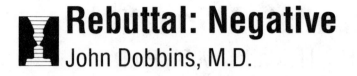

Rebuttal: Negative
John Dobbins, M.D.

Dr. Marks argues that the surgeon who is going to operate on a patient should be the person who performs the endoscopy. I certainly cannot argue with this, since I rely on similar logic in advocating that the internist should endoscope the patient with a chronic problem such as ulcerative colitis. Only in malignancy, however, is endoscopy routinely followed by surgery. In cases of gastrointestinal bleeding, the other example that Dr. Marks uses, 85% of these patients will stop bleeding spontaneously or with conservative management, and only a portion of the 15% who do not will require surgery. Many of these will be variceal bleeders, in which case I doubt that observing blood pouring from a varix will enable the surgeon to do a better job in the operating room.

Should we be training all general surgeons to perform endoscopy so that they can "see" the tumors and occasional gastrointestinal bleeding sites that they will subsequently treat surgically? The answer would be yes if there were evidence that patients did better when endoscopy and surgery were performed by the same individual. But there is no such evidence in the literature. Indeed, as mentioend previously, there are many studies which indicate that diagnostic endoscopy has no effect on the outcome of gastrointestinal bleeding. Dr. Marks even makes a big point that "early" endoscopy (2 A.M., the presumption being that surgeons are more willing to perform endoscopy at this hour) in gastrointestinal bleeders will result in better, more efficient patient care, a surgical "point of view" that clearly is not supported by the seven or more controlled trials reported in the literature.[1] Thus, before we begin the expensive, duplicative, time-consuming task of training surgeons to be good endoscopists as well as good surgeons, it would not be unreasonable to obtain a few controlled trials to support such an effort. After all, many vaunted surgical procedures (i.e., the Vinberg procedure) have wilted when scrutinized by controlled trials.

Dr. Marks goes on to argue that when the attending surgeon is not a trained endoscopist, he should select a surgical rather than a medical colleague to perform the procedure. He argues again that the surgical endoscopist will be more aware of the urgency (presumably in the case of a gastrointestinal bleed) and will expedite the procedure to the benefit of the patient, despite evidence to the contrary in the literature. He then goes on to argue that the surgical endoscopist can deal with complications such as perforation better than can the medical endoscopist. Why this would matter to a surgeon calling in an endoscopist is unclear to me, since the surgeon himself presumably could handle any surgical complications.

In summary, Dr. Marks talks a lot about the surgical point of view and "feel" that presumably makes the surgeon a better endoscopist and/or physician better able to incorporate endoscopic data into the total management of the surgical patient. He may be right, but I doubt it. However, Dr. Marks' views can be tested by the performance of controlled clinical trials comparing surgical endoscopists to medical endoscopists. As a scientist as well as a surgeon and endoscopist, I am sure that Dr. Marks would agree that we should end the current controversy by performing these necessary studies.

Reference

1. Peterson WL: Gastrointestinal bleeding, in Sleisenger ML, Fordtran JS (eds): *Gastrointestinal Disease,* 3rd ed. Philadelphia, WB Saunders, 1983, p 186.

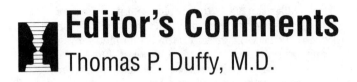

Editor's Comments
Thomas P. Duffy, M.D.

One must be sympathetic to the historical antecedents of endoscopy and its origins in gastroenterology as outlined by Dr. Dobbins, but such claims of precedence and tradition are weak obstacles to the commandeering of these skills by others. In the same vein, one cannot be very sympathetic to the opposing claim of Dr. Marks that endoscopy represents an access to power and control in an institution, especially when one considers the impact and excitement that a creative surgeon can provide. The territorial rights to endoscopy should be determined in the same fashion as are so many other disputes in medicine and surgery, that is, by deciding how this technology and its practitioners can best be mobilized in the best interest of patients.

There is little question that patients with clinical syndromes suggestive of medical illness should be endoscoped by gastroenterologists, the physicians who will medicate and care for these problems, as is well argued by Dr. Dobbins. However, it seems just as appropriate for the surgeon to examine and view a lesion which he or she will be called upon to resect. It would seem feasible that a cooperative, concomitant endoscopy with both gastroenterologist and surgeon present is possible, although the two discussants have doubts regarding such a collaboration. Until then, it would appear that referral patterns will determine the outcome of this debate. Medical endoscopists will continue to retain major control of this technology with infrequent incursions of surgeons into the territory.

Is *Campylobacter pylori* a Significant Etiological Agent in Peptic Ulcer Disease?

Chapter Editor: Gary Gitnick, M.D.

Affirmative: James S. Barthel, M.D.
Assistant Director, Gastrointestinal
Endoscopy, Department of
Gastroenterology, The Cleveland Clinic
Foundation, Cleveland, Ohio

Negative: William E. Karnes, M.D.
Assistant Professor of Medicine, UCLA
School of Medicine, Associate Investigator,
Center for Ulcer Research and Education,
Veterans Administration Medical Center,
West Los Angeles, Los Angeles, California

Paul Guth, M.D.
Key Investigator, Center for Ulcer Research
and Education, Professor of Medicine,
University of California, Los Angeles, UCLA
School of Medicine; Assistant Chief of
Gastroenterology, Veteran's Administration
Medical Center, West Los Angeles, Los
Angeles, California

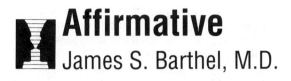

Affirmative
James S. Barthel, M.D.

To argue that *Campylobacter pylori* is a significant etiological agent in peptic ulcer disease is, in essence, to propose a totally new theory of ulcer pathogenesis. Merely presenting the data will serve this endeavor poorly. Data can be interpreted in many different ways. Inevitably, unexpected data, such as the discovery of *C. pylori,* is initially interpreted as representing an exception to existing theory and not evidence against it. To determine whether unexpected new data warrant a new theory or nothing more than a footnote to existing theory, it is necessary to look beyond the data and examine the scientific history of the phenomenon in question.[1] Henry Margenau[2] suggested that the ultimate test of a valid theory is its ability to simply, elegantly, and logically explain both new and old observations. What is the situation with peptic ulcer disease? Does etiological heterogeneity simply, elegantly, and logically explain all observations old and new? Or is it time for a new theory of ulcerogenesis based on the concept of chronic infection?

Virchow, the 19th century German pathologist, was probably the first to suggest that microorganisms might play a role in peptic ulcer disease. Virchow was troubled by Rokitansky's hypothesis[3] that duodenal ulcer was caused by vagally mediated gastric hyperacidity. Virchow pointed out that Rokitansky's theory could not account for the focal nature of ulcers[4] and he postulated that a second local factor was necessary to produce them. He proposed ischemia, infection, and toxins as possible local factors necessary for the production of peptic ulcer disease.

Early in the 20th century, the theory that an infectious process was the immediate cause of peptic ulcer disease enjoyed brief popularity. Between 1913 and 1915, Rosenow[5] attempted to demonstrate that streptococci played an etiological role in peptic ulcer disease. In 1917, Dragstedt[6] reported that the healing of silver nitrate–induced duodenal ulcers was not affected by the presence or absence of gastric juice. He observed that the ulcers frequently were infected and concluded that infection was the important factor in chronic peptic ulcer. Dragstedt later abandoned these opinions in favor of vagally mediated hyperacidity as the cause of peptic ulcer.[7] In 1922, Warthin[8] reported three cases of peptic ulcer which he attributed to syphilitic arteritis. Subsequent attempts to report cases of syphilitic gastritis and ulcer disease were criticized because the large numbers, location, and morphology of the spirochetes seen were not typical for syphilitic lesions and the Wassermann reactions were sometimes negative.[9]

These attempts to link an infectious process to peptic ulcer disease were abandoned as an improved understanding of gastric secretory physiology evolved. During the 1890s Heidenhain's pupil, Pavlov, modified the experimental gastric pouch such that it remained innervated and thus was able to demonstrate that gastric secretion in response to the sight, smell, and chewing of food was vagally mediated. This supported Rokitansky's concept of ulcerogenesis. In 1903, Popielski advanced the view that histamine, long recognized as a gastric secretogogue, was the substance responsible for the ability of organ extracts to stimulate gastric secretion. Popielski also proposed the theory of local reflex mechanisms, observing that the ability of certain foods to stimulate gastric secretion when introduced directly into the Heidenhain (denervated) pouch must be a locally mediated phenomenon.[10] In 1906, Edkins[11,12] postulated the existence of a gastric secretogogue produced in the pyloric gland mass which, after transportation via the blood to the oxyntic gland area, stimulated gastric secretion. With the articulation of Karl Schwartz' famous dictum "no acid, no ulcer,"[13] the gap between physiology and pathophysiology was bridged and the reign of acid began.

In 1914, technological innovations made the routine study of human acid secretion feasible. In that year, Rehfuss[14] described the weighted rubber gastric sampling tube and the technique of fractional gastric analysis. Rehfuss et al.[15] studied nine medical students and described isosecretory, hypersecretory, and hyposecretory states in response to an Ewald test meal. The idea rapidly evolved that the hypersecretory state was associated with peptic ulceration. Numerous "tube studies" were performed subsequently in an attempt to prove this hypothesis. Recently, the technology of acid secretion tube studies has neared perfection with the advent of the ingestible continuous pH monitoring probe. Despite this technological progress, a consistent association between duodenal ulcer disease and acid hypersecretion has not been demonstrated.

The Zollinger-Ellison syndrome[16] was described in 1956. Five years later Gregory and Tracy[17] reported the isolation of gastrin, thereby conclusively proving Edkins' gastrin hypothesis. These discoveries further intensified interest in abnormalities of acid secretory physiology as the cause of peptic ulcer disease. In 1952, Cox reported that the parietal cell mass was greater in ulcer patients than in normal individuals.[18] This finding was amplified by the report of Card and Marks[19] which related histamine-stimulated maximal acid output to parietal cell mass. In 1963, Baron[20] suggested that patients with peptic ulcer disease possessed an increased drive to secrete acid manifest by greater basal or resting gastric acid secretion. The year 1975 was a good year for reports of acid secretory abnormalities in patients with peptic ulcer disease. Isenberg reported that lower doses of exogenous gastrin were required to stimulate one-half maximal gastric output[21] and concluded that patients with peptic ulcer disease possessed an increased parietal cell sensitivity to gastrin and its analogues. These findings were expanded later by Lam,[22] who described an increased sensitivity to endogenous gastrin in patients with peptic ulcer disease. Walsh[23] reported experiments which suggested that peptic ulcer patients had defective acid-induced inhibition of gastric acid secretion. Cano and Isenberg[24] reported an increase in duodenal acid load in duodenal ulcer patients, possibly related to rapid emptying of gastric contents.[25] However, the rate at which the stomach empties in peptic ulcer disease is not a settled issue and contradictory evidence exists.[26,27] An alternative explanation for increased duodenal acid load was provided by Fiddian-Green and Hosley,[28] who reported impaired duodenal bicarbonate release in patients with peptic ulcer disease. Holt and Isenberg observed that none of these abnormalities occur in all patients with duodenal ulcers. Individual defects occur in 20% to 50% of peptic ulcer patients and some patients possess no abnormalities of acid secretion.[29] This inability to demonstrate excess acid production consistently or to identify a commonly occurring, acid-related pathophysiological mechanism in peptic ulcer patients led theorists to look elsewhere for explanations.

With the recognition that the putative aberrations of acid secretory physiology would not produce a simple acid aggression theory of peptic ulcer pathogenesis, attention turned to mucosal defenses. In 1954, Hollander[30] proposed a two-component system for gastric mucosal acid protection consisting of alkaline mucus overlying a rapidly regenerating epithelial cell layer. In 1959, Heatly[31] refined Hollander's concept by proposing that the gastric mucus served as an unstirred layer which allowed H^+ diffusing from the lumen to be neutralized by HCO_3 secreted by the gastric surface epithelial cells. The intensity with which these theories were ignored is notable. At the time, acid resistance was thought to occur at the level of the epithelial lining and not the mucus. Robert's macroscopic observations that prostaglandins protect the gastric mucosa from noxious substances[32] reinforced the idea that acid resistance occurred at the level of the epithelial lining. Robert did not attempt to demonstrate prostaglandin-mediated microscopic cytoprotection. Subsequently, other workers using Robert's rat model demonstrated that microscopic epithelial protection did not exist.[33] In 1981, investigators using antimony microelectrodes reported the demonstration of a pH gradient across rat[34] and rabbit[35] gastric mucus. These findings gave new support to the idea that mucus played an important role in mucosal protection.

The multitude of alleged acid secretory aberrations and mucosal defense defects led to abandonment of the idea that a simple pathophysiological theory could explain peptic ulcer disease. In 1973, Cowan[36] proposed the theory of the polygenetic inheritance of peptic ulcer disease to explain the apparent presence of genetic markers in some patients with peptic ulcer disease. He proposed that the hereditary component of peptic ulcer disease reflects the combined contribution of many genes which act in consort with environmental factors to create a threshold beyond which the disease is manifest. In 1977, Rotter and Rimoin proposed the theory of etiological heterogeneity as an alternative to the theory of polygenetic inheritance[37]: "Peptic ulcer is the final common manifestation of a variety of distinct diseases with different etiologies (genetic and nongenetic) and pathophysiologic mechanisms." The acid secretory and mucosal defense physiologists were particularly enamored with the theory of etiological heterogeneity because it allowed for the description of an infinite number of acid secretory and mucosal defense aberrations[38] without having to account for their significance with respect to the peptic ulcer disease which they allegedly caused.

Unfortunately, the theory of etiological heterogeneity is nothing more than an articulation of the fact that laboratory observations defy coherent, logical explanation by medical scientists. Wormsley's criticism[39] aptly describes the problem and undoubtedly will soon be recognized as marking the twilight of etiological heterogeneity:

This hypothesis proposes that ulcer disease reflects pathophysiological heterogeneity — in other words, whatever apparent disturbance of function one happens to find, that particular dysfunction is somehow implicated in the genesis of the ulcer disease and if one does not find anything, then (presumably) lack of defensive factors — which are unmeasurable, like mucus synthesis or secretion — must be responsible.

I think that it is time to call a halt. Pathophysiological disturbances, like the gastric hypersecretion which occurs in one sixth to one third of patients with duodenal ulcer, are changes from the usual physiological situation and that is all they are. There is no evidence whatsoever that these variant reactions are anything other than that, or that they are in any way ulcerogenic. Indeed, these pathophysiological disturbances may be merely a consequence of the disease and it is not impossible to conceive that some even reflect a defensive reaction associated with the development of a duodenal mucosal lesion. To take the argument further, there is really no evidence that there are any endogenous aggressive factors or that gastric juice is ever aggressive towards normal alimentary mucosa. That being so, there are normally no defensive factors, either.

Despite the uncertainty concerning ulcer pathogenesis, successful therapies for healing ulcers evolved. Approaches to acid neutralization were refined.[40,41] Anticholinergic agents were combined with antacids to attenuate vagally mediated acid secretion and slow gastric emptying. H_2 receptor antagonists (cimetidine, ranitidine, famotidine, nizatidine) were developed to block histamine-mediated acid secretion pharmacologically. Various prostaglandins administered in antisecretory doses were demonstrated to heal peptic ulcers.[42] Omeprazole, a cellular proton pump inhibitor with the unique ability to completely paralyze acid secretion, was developed.[43] The clinical use of these various acid inhibitory agents inevitably produced an ulcer healing rate of approximately 80% at 1 month and an ulcer recurrence rate of 40% to 60% within 1 year after therapy was stopped.[44,45] Colloidal bismuth compounds and sucralfate are considered mucosal protective agents; however, their true mechanisms of action are not fully understood. Some evidence suggests that the ulcer recurrence rate after therapy with these agents is lower.[46–50] Any credible theory of ulcer pathogenesis must account for the success of these therapies.

The most recent significant finding with respect to the pathogenesis of peptic ulcer disease fits better with Virchow's theory of acid acting in consort with a second local factor to produce peptic ulcer than with the theory of etiological heterogeneity. In 1983, Warren and Marshall[51] reported the isolation of a gram-negative, spiraled, microaerophilic *Campylobacter*-like organism from antral mucosal biopsies in patients with histological gastritis. The organisms ultimately were given the name *Campylobacter pylori*. The association between *C. pylori* and histological gastritis in both symptomatic and asymptomatic[52] patients was observed throughout the world. When a microaerophilic technique was used, the organism could be cultured from up to 90% of the biopsies in which it was observed histologically. Reports of *C. pylori* serum antibody responses detected by complement fixation assay[53] and enzyme-linked immunosorbent assay[54] in patients with *C. pylori* and gastritis strongly suggested a pathogenetic role for the organism. Proof of *C. pylori* pathogenicity was provided by two human ingestion experiments[55,56] conducted in such a manner as to fulfill Koch's third and fourth postulates.

The association between *C. pylori* histological gastritis and duodenal ulcer disease was reported also by Marshall and Warren.[57] Others[58–61] soon confirmed the report. In some studies, the association between *C. pylori* gastritis and duodenal ulcer disease approached 100%. This association was particularly puzzling with respect to an etiological link between *C. pylori* and duodenal ulcer disease, because *C. pylori* could not be found in duodenal mucosa. Then Phillips et al.[62] reported that *C. pylori* could be found in the duodenum, but only in foci of gastric metaplasia.

It seems reasonable to postulate that *C. pylori*–infected foci of duodenal gastric metaplasia represent foci of diminished acid resistance where peptic ulceration begins. Duodenal gastric metaplasia occurs in 30% to 64% of healthy volunteers[63,64] and in 45% to 100% of patients with duodenal ulcer.[65,66] *C. pylori* appears to damage the mucosal barrier directly. Marshall and coworkers[57] have published photomicrographs demonstrating thinning of the mucus layer in the presence of *C. pylori* infection with the return of normal mucus thickness upon eradication of the organism. Slomiany et al.[67] have reported that *C. pylori* secretes a protease capable of degrading gastric mucus. Evidence that *C. pylori* produces a large molecular weight toxin with an in vitro cytopathic effect has been presented.[68] The effects of the inflammatory response induced by *C. pylori* on the mucosal barrier have not been investigated, but it seems likely that such effects would only serve to weaken the mucosal barrier further.

The hypothesis that *C. pylori* plays a primary etiological role in duodenal ulcer disease is intellectually appealing because it can explain a number of perplexing aspects of duodenal ulcer disease which are not readily explained by competing theories of ulcerogenesis. The phenomenon of duodenal ulcer location can be explained readily if a focus of inflamed, *C. pylori*–infected antral metaplasia is recognized as the point where an ulcer begins. The problem of ulcer recurrence after the cessation of acid suppression therapy can be explained when one realizes that acid suppression therapy has little or no effect on *C. pylori* and its associated inflammation. The persistent observation that less than one half of duodenal ulcer patients actually have hyperacidity or abnormalities of acid secretory physiology can be explained by the fact that acid only plays a role in ulcer pathogenesis when the mucosa is infected and inflamed, and its defenses are malfunctioning. Under such conditions any acid, not just excess acid, will likely result in mucosal damage. Of course, this fits nicely with Schwartz' dictum and the fact that acid suppression therapy obviously works when administered to ulcer patients who do not hypersecrete acid.

Despite the success of an ulcerogenesis theory based on *C. pylori* infection in explaining the problematic areas of idiopathic peptic ulcer disease, it remains absolutely true that not all ulcers are linked to *C. pylori*. Diseases such as Zollinger-Ellison syndrome produce ulcers independent of *C. pylori*. Likewise, ulcerogenic drugs produce ulcers by a different mechanism. In this sense, etiological heterogeneity is a concept with applicability at the margins of the peptic ulcer phenomenon. However, this is not the situation which the theory was created to explain. Etiological heterogeneity exists at the margins of any phenomenon, and when applied in such a manner is nothing more than a simplistic truism. It becomes an argument lacking interconnection with other biological theories and devoid of logical fertility.

In conclusion, a theory of ulcerogenesis based on the concept that idiopathic peptic ulcer disease is an infectious process (Fig 1) simply,

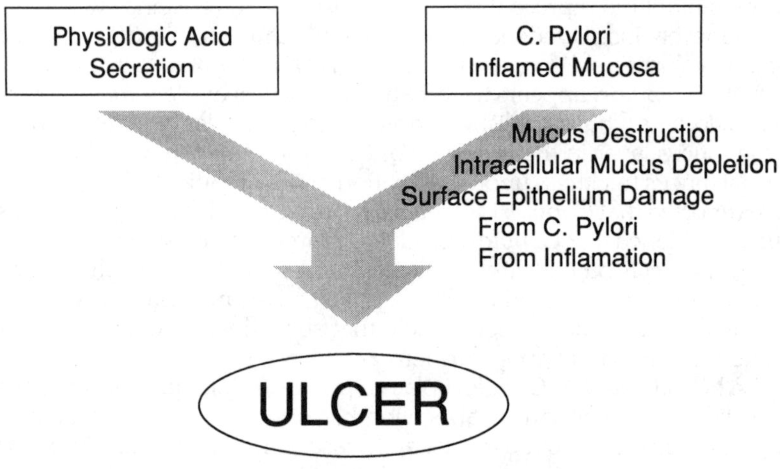

FIG 1.
Schematic representation of acid acting in conjunction with *C. pylori* to produce peptic ulcer disease.

elegantly, and logically accounts for both old and new observations concerning the peptic ulcer phenomenon. The multitude of "aggressive" and "defensive" factor aberrations observed in peptic ulcer disease which gave rise to the theory of etiological heterogeneity are simply epiphenomena representing the effect of the causative agent at various times throughout the course of its natural history, rather than the cause itself.

References

1. Kuhn TS: *The Structure of Scientific Revolutions,* 1st ed. Chicago, The University of Chicago Press, 1968, pp 52–65. *This monograph is a classic philosophy of science work which describes the impact of nonscientific forces upon the acceptance of new scientific theories.*

2. Margenau H: *The Nature of Physical Reality,* 1st ed. Woodbridge, Ox Bow Press, 1977, pp 75–102. *This work offers a discussion of the nonempirical aspects of scientific theory creation and verification.*

3. Rokitansky C: *Manual of Pathological Anatomy,* vol 2. London, 1849. *This is the original description of the hypothesis that duodenal ulcer disease is caused by vagally mediated hyperacidity. This theory has been referred to as the central theory of ulcerogenesis.*

4. Virchow R: Einfaches chronisches Magengeschwur. *Virchows Arch [A]* 1853; 5:362–64. *The original description of the local factors theory is presented. This theory fell into disrepute in the early 20th century because of the inability of medical scientists of the time to demonstrate convincingly that local factors, particularly microorganisms, played an important role in ulcerogenesis.*

5. Rosenow EC: Elective localization of streptococci. *JAMA* 1915; 65:1687–1691. *Rosenow is credited with demonstrating that streptococci produce pharyngitis. He believed that bacteria isolated from a lesion in a diseased host, when injected into the bloodstream of a healthy host, would travel to the same anatomic location and produce the same lesion. He attempted unconvincingly to demonstrate this for peptic ulcer disease with various streptococci which he isolated from ulcer tissue. Unfortunately, the microbiology techniques of the early 20th century did not permit the isolation of C. pylori.*

6. Dragstedt LR: Contributions to the physiology of the stomach: Gastric juice in duodenal and gastric ulcers. *JAMA* 1917; 68:330–333. *Ironically, Dragstedt's early work in peptic ulcer disease was in keeping with the popularity of the local factors/infection theories of the time.*

7. Dragstedt LR: Pathogenesis of gastroduodenal ulcer. *Arch Surg* 1942; 44:438–451. *In this paper, Dragstedt presents his views concerning the importance of vagally mediated acid secretion in the production of ulcers.*

8. Warthin AS: Syphilis of the medium and smaller arteries. *N Y Med J* 1922; 115:69–73. *In this paper Warthin described three cases of syphilitic ulcer disease. He believed that peptic ulcers frequently were the result of acid corrosion of syphilitic gumma.*

9. Singer HA: Syphilis of the stomach with special reference to the significance

of spirochetes. *Arch Intern Med* 1932; 46:754–770. *This is a criticism of Warthin's hypothesis.*

10. Carlson AJ: The secretion of gastric juice in health and disease. *Physiol Rev* 1923; 3:1–40. *This review article describes Popielski's theory concerning the local reflex mechanism of acid secretion. Popielski's work provided the foundation for modern concepts of paracrine-mediated acid secretion.*

11. Edkins JS: The chemical mechanisms of gastric secretion. *J Physiol* 1909; 34:133–144. *This paper describes Edkins' work, which demonstrated the presence of endocrine-mediated acid secretion.*

12. Edkins JS, Tweedy M: The natural channel of absorption evoking the chemical mechanism of gastric secretion. *J Physiol* 1909; 38:263–267. *As above.*

13. Schwartz K: Uber penetricrende magen und jejunalgeschwur. *Beitr Klin Chir* 1910; 67:96–128. *This is the paper in which Schwartz pedantically concludes that ulcers do not occur in the absence of acid. His thoughts on the matter were later distilled into the dictum "No acid, no ulcer" by others.*

14. Rehfuss ME: A new method of gastric testing with a description of a method for the fractional testing of the gastric juice. *Am J Med Sci* 1914; 147:878–955. *The method of fractional sampling of gastric juice described in this paper is the origin of modern techniques for studying gastric acid secretion.*

15. Rehfuss ME, Bergeim O, Hawk PB: Gastrointestinal studies. I. The question of the residuum found in the empty stomach. *JAMA* 1914; 63:11–13. *This paper represents the first attempt to quantitatively define hyper- and hyposecretion of gastric acid. Acceptable methods of comparative statistical analysis were not applied to the data.*

16. Zollinger RM, Ellison EH: Primary peptic ulcerations of the jejunum associated with islet cell tumours of the pancreas. *Ann Surg* 1955; 142:709–728. *This paper is the original description of the Zollinger-Ellison syndrome. The description of this syndrome provided additional evidence for an endocrine-mediated mechanism of acid secretion as originally proposed by Edkins.*

17. Gregory RA, Tracy HJ: The preparation and properties of gastrin. *J Physiol* 1961; 156:523–43. *This paper describes the isolation of the secretory peptide gastrin, thus proving the existence of an endocrine-mediated mechanism of acid secretion.*

18. Cox AJ: Stomach size and its relation to chronic peptic ulcer. *Arch Pathol* 1952; 54:407–422. *This article proposes that patients with peptic ulcer disease have increased parietal cell masses. Acceptable methods of comparative statistical analysis were not applied to the data.*

19. Card WI, Marks NI: The relationship between the acid output of the stomach following "maximal" histamine stimulation and the parietal cell mass. *Clin Sci* 1960; 19:147–163. *As above.*

20. Baron JH: Studies of basal and peak acid output with an augmented histamine test. *Gut* 1963; 4:136. *This paper describes variations in acid secretion observed in some ulcer patients.*

21. Isenberg JI, Grossman MI, Maxwell V, et al: Increased sensitivity to stimulation of acid secretion by pentagastrin in duodenal ulcer. *J Clin Invest* 1975; 55:330–337. *As above.*

22. Lam SK: Gastric acid secretion (GAS) is more sensitive to endogenous gastrin

in duodenal ulcer (DU) than in normals (N) (abstract). *Gastroenterology* 1979; 76:1178. *As above.*

23. Walsh JH, Richardson CT, Fordtran JS: pH dependence of acid secretion and gastrin release in normal and ulcer subjects. *J Clin Invest* 1975; 55:462–468. *As above.*

24. Cano R, Isenberg JI: Demonstration of increased duodenal acid load in duodenal ulcer patients. *Clin Res* 1975; 23:97A. *This article describes the presence of variations in acid disposal in some duodenal ulcer patients.*

25. Hurst AF: New views on the pathology, diagnosis, and treatment of gastric and duodenal ulcer. *Br Med J* 1920; 55:559–563. *As above.*

26. Bromster D: Gastric emptying rate in gastric and duodenal ulceration. *Scand J Gastroenterol* 1969; 4:193. *This paper presents data suggesting that acid disposal is not abnormal in ulcer patients.*

27. Hunt JN: Influence of hydrochloric acid on gastric secretion and emptying in patients with duodenal ulcer. *Br Med J* 1957; 1:681. *As above.*

28. Fiddian-Green RG, Hosley M: Defective bicarbonate secretion in response to duodenal acidification in patients with chronic gastric or duodenal ulceration. *S Afr Med J* 1976; 50:479–481. *These authors present evidence that duodenal bicarbonate secretion may be defective in peptic ulcer disease.*

29. Holt KM, Isenberg JI: Peptic ulcer disease; Physiology and pathophysiology. *Hosp Pract (Off)* 1985; 20:89–106. *This is a review of gastric acid physiology and its relationship to peptic ulcer disease with an acknowledgement that the majority of patients with peptic ulcer disease do not have demonstrable abnormalities of acid secretion.*

30. Hollander F: The two component mucus barrier. *Arch Intern Med* 1954; 93:107–120. *This is an original article suggesting that mucus plays an important role in the protection of the gastric mucosa from the effects of gastric acid.*

31. Heatly NG: Mucosubstance as a barrier to diffusion. *Gastroenterology* 1959; 37:313–317. *This is an original article suggesting that mucus represents an unstirred layer over the gastric mucosa which retards the diffusion of hydrogen ions.*

32. Robert A, Nezamis JE, Lancaster C, et al: Cytoprotection by prostaglandins in rats: Prevention of gastric necrosis produced by alcohol, HCl, NaOH, hypertonic NaCl, and thermal injury. *Gastroenterology* 1979; 77:433–443. *This is an original article suggesting that prostaglandins possess gastric mucosal cytoprotective properties.*

33. Lacy ER, Ito S: Microscopic analysis of ethanol damage to rat gastric mucosa after treatment with a prostaglandin. *Gastroenterology* 1982; 83:619–625. *This article suggests that prostaglandins do not prevent microscopic epithelial damage and thus may not possess true cytoprotective effects. A current area of controversy is the exact level within the mucosa at which prostaglandin-mediated cytoprotection occurs.*

34. Ross IN, Bahari HMM, Turnberg LA: The pH gradient across mucus adherent to rat fundic mucosa in vivo and the effect of potential damaging agents. *Gastroenterology* 1981; 81:713–718. *This paper presents evidence which supports Heatly's theory that gastric mucus plays an important role in protecting the gastric epithelial surface from destruction by acid.*

35. Williams SE, Turnberg LA: Demonstration of a pH gradient across mucus adherent to rabbit gastric mucosa: Evidence for a 'mucus-bicarbonate' barrier. *Gut* 1981; 22:94–96. *As above.*

36. Cowan WK: Genetics of duodenal and gastric ulcer. *Clin Gastroenterol* 1973; 2:539–545. *This original article proposes the theory of polygenetic inheritance as an explanation for the etiology of peptic ulcer disease.*

37. Rotter JI, Rimoin DL: Peptic ulcer disease — a heterogeneous group of disorders? *Gastroenterology* 1977; 73:604–607. *This is the original article proposing the theory of etiological heterogeneity as an explanation for the etiology of peptic ulcer disease.*

38. Grossman MI, Kurata JH, Rotter JI, et al: Peptic ulcer: New therapies, new diseases. *Ann Intern Med* 1981; 95:609–627. *This is a good review article which neatly catalogues the myriad acid secretory, acid disposal, and mucosal defense aberrations which comprise the substance of the theory of etiological heterogeneity.*

39. Wormsley KG: Duodenal ulcer: Does pathophysiology equal aetiology. *Gut* 1983; 24:775–780. *An extremely well-articulated criticism of the theory of etiological heterogeneity.*

40. Peterson WL, Sturdevant RAL, Frankl HD, et al: Healing of duodenal ulcer with an antacid regimen. *N Engl J Med* 1977; 297:341–345. *This is an investigation concerning the efficacy of antacids in healing duodenal ulcer.*

41. Kumar N, Vij JC, Karol A, et al: Controlled therapeutic trial to determine the optimum dose of antacids in duodenal ulcer. *Gut* 1984; 25:1199–1202. *As above.*

42. Hawkey CJ, Walt RP: Prostaglandins for peptic ulcer: A promise unfulfilled. *Lancet* 1986; ii:1084–1086. *Prostaglandin agents are capable of healing ulcers only when administered in doses large enough to inhibit acid secretion. Lower doses which allegedly produce cytoprotection do not heal ulcers.*

43. Friedman G: Omeprazole. *Am J Gastroenterol* 1987; 82:188–191. *Friedman discusses the ultimate pharmacological weapon in acid inhibition.*

44. Strum WB: Prevention of duodenal ulcer recurence. *Ann Intern Med* 1986; 105:757–761. *This paper discusses the strikingly high ulcer recurrence rate after a course of ulcer-healing acid inhibition.*

45. Ippoliti A, Elashoff J, Valenzuela J, et al: Recurrent ulcer after successful treatment with cimetidine or antacid. *Gastroenterology* 1983; 85:875–880. *As above.*

46. Martin DF, May SJ, Tweedle DEF, et al: Difference in relapse rates of duodenal ulcer after healing with cimetidine or tripotassium dicitrato bismuthate. *Lancet* 1981; i:7–10. *This article presents evidence that agents which allegedly heal ulcers by mucosal protective mechanisms produce lower ulcer recurrence rates than do those which heal ulcers by acid reduction.*

47. Vantrappen G, Schuurmans P, Retgeerts P, et al: A comparative study of colloidal bismuth subcitrate and cimetidine on the healing and recurrence of duodenal ulcer. *Scand J Gastroenterol* 1982; 17(suppl 80):23–30. *As above.*

48. Miller PJ, Faragher EB: Relapse of duodenal ulcer: Does it matter which drug is used in initial treatment? *Br Med J* 1986; 293:1117–1118. *As above.*

49. Hamilton I, O'Connor HJ, Wood NC, et al: Healing and recurrence of

duodenal ulcer after treatment with tripotassium dicitrato bismuthate (TDB) tablets or cimetidine. *Gut* 1986; 27:106–110. *As above.*

50. Marks IN, Wright JP, Lucke W, et al: Relapse rates following initial ulcer healing with sucralfate and cimetidine. *Scand J Gastroenterol* 1983; 18(suppl 83):53–56. *As above.*

51. Warren TR, Marshall B: Unidentified curved bacilli on gastric epithelium in active chronic gastritis (letter). *Lancet* 1983; ii:1273–1275. *This is the original report of Warren and Marshall describing the histological identification of a unique curved bacterium in gastritis patients and its isolation in pure culture.*

52. Barthel JS, Westblom TU, Havey AD, et al: Gastritis and *Campylobacter pylori* in healthy asymptomatic volunteers. *Arch Intern Med* 1988; 148:1149–1151.

53. Jones DM, Lessells AM, Eldridge J: *Campylobacter*-like organisms on the gastric mucosa: Culture, histological, and serological studies. *J Clin Pathol* 1984; 37:1002–1006. *This is one of the initial reports concerning the presence of an antibody response to C. pylori.*

54. Jones DM, Eldridge J, Fox AJ, et al: Antibody to the gastric *Campylobacter*-like organism ("*Campylobacter pyloridis*")—clinical correlations and distribution in the normal population. *J Med Microbiol* 1986; 22:57–62. *As above.*

55. Marshall BJ, Armstrong JA, Mcgechie DB, et al: Attempt to fulfill Koch's postulates for pyloric *Campylobacter*. *Med J Aust* 1985; 142:436–439. *This reference describes human ingestion experiments performed to fulfill Koch's third and fourth postulates. Dr. Marshall succeeded in fulfilling Koch's third postulate, but not the fourth. Dr. Morris fulfilled both the third and fourth postulates. Unfortunately, he now has chronic symptomatic C. pylori gastritis.*

56. Morris A, Nicholson G: Ingestion of *Campylobacter pyloridis* causes gastritis and raised fasting gastric pH. *Am J Gastroenterol* 1987; 82:192–199. *As above.*

57. Marshall BJ, Warren JR: Unidentified curved bacilli in the stomach of patients with gastritis and peptic ulceration. *Lancet* 1984; i:1311–15. *This report represents a more comprehensive description of the findings described in reference 51.*

58. Marshall BJ, McGechie DB, Rogers PA, et al: Pyloric *Campylobacter* infection and gastroduodenal disease. *Med J Aust* 1985; 142:439–444. *This paper represents an initial report confirming the association between antral gastritis and C. pylori.*

59. Lambert JR, Dunn KL, Eaves ER, et al: Pyloric CLO in the human stomach. *Med J Aust* 1985; 143:174. *As above.*

60. Tytgat GNJ, Lagenberg ML, Rauws E, et al: *Campylobacter*-like organisms (CLO) in the human stomach (abstract). *Gastroenterology* 1985; 88:1620. *As above.*

61. Price AB, Levi J, Dolby JM, et al: *Campylobacter pyloridis* in peptic ulcer disease: Microbiology, pathology, and scanning electron microscopy. *Gut* 1985; 26:1183–1188. *As above.*

62. Phillips AD, Hine KR, Holmes GKT, et al: Gastric spiral bacteria. *Lancet* 1984; ii:100–101. *This is the first report of C. pylori in the duodenum.*

63. Kreuning J, Bosman FT, Kuiper G, et al: Gastric and duodenal mucosa in 'healthy' individuals; an endoscopic and histopathological study of 50 volunteers. *J Clin Pathol* 1978; 31:69–77. *This paper discusses the prevalence of duodenal metaplasia in healthy individuals.*

64. Greenlaw R, Sheahan DG, Deluca V, et al: Gastroduodenitis: A broader concept of peptic ulcer disease. *Dig Dis Sci* 1980; 25:660–672. *As above.*

65. Kang JY, Nasiry R, Guan R, et al: Influence of the site of a duodenal ulcer on its mode of presentation. *Gastroenterology* 1986; 90:1874–1876. *This article presents data on the prevalence of antral metaplastic foci in the duodenum of patients with duodenal ulcer disease.*

66. Shousha S, Barrison IG, El-Sayeed W, et al: A study of incidence and relationship of intestinal metaplasia of gastric antrum and gastric metaplasia of duodenum in patients with nonulcer dyspepsia. *Dig Dis Sci* 1984; 29:311–316. *As above.*

67. Slomiany BL, Bilski J, Sarosiek J, et al: *Campylobacter pyloridis* degrades mucin and undermines gastric mucosal integrity. *Biochem Biophys Res Commun* 1987; 144:307–314. *This paper was the first report of the mucus-degrading activity of C. pylori.*

68. Morgan DR, Leunk RD, Kraft WG: Identification of a toxin produced by strains of *Campylobacter pylori*. Presented at *Campylobacter pylori* — A Multidisciplinary Workshop, Keystone, Colorado, 1987.

Negative

William E. Karnes, M.D.
Paul Guth, M.D.

Duodenal ulcer disease remains an important and costly medical problem despite the development of potent antisecretory drugs. While existing therapies accelerate ulcer healing, they do little to affect the natural history of duodenal ulcers; ulcers recur.[1] Increased acid secretion does not explain the occurrence of duodenal ulcer disease in many individuals.[2] Additional aggressive and/or defective defensive factors must be involved in the pathogenesis and maintenance of chronic duodenal ulcer disease. Until the "soil" from which ulcers develop is understood, duodenal ulcer disease will remain an incurable source of suffering and expense.

The discovery of an association between *Campylobacter pylori* and duodenal ulcer disease has stirred considerable excitement. Duodenal ulcer disease is rarely found in the absence of gastric colonization with *C. pylori*. Colonization is accompanied by mucosal infiltration of polymorphonuclear cells, mucus depletion, and ultrastructural changes in surface epithelial cells. These histological findings have been interpreted as evidence that *C. pylori* induces a defect in the mucosal defense which could precipitate the development of duodenal ulcer disease. Numerous epidemiological and therapeutic studies have added support to the belief that *C. pylori* is ulcerogenic. A century after first being observed,[3,4] this previously ignored gastric colonist has emerged as a potential explanation for many, if not most, of the mysteries of chronic duodenal ulcer disease. The excitement has led some investigators to adopt a new dogma of duodenal ulcer disease: "no bug, no ulcer."

However, acceptance of this concept is unwarranted. Important gaps in our understanding persist largely due to the fact that the full spectrum of clinical disease seen in association with *C. pylori* is unique to humans. Animal models with gastric *Campylobacter*-like organisms have not been reported to develop ulcer.[5,6] In an attempt to fulfill Koch's hypothesis, two cases of self-inoculation resulted in acute gastritis but not ulcers.[7,8] Larger human inoculation studies are not possible because the organism may be difficult (or impossible) to eradicate.[9,10] The remaining indirect pathways toward defining the relationship between *C. pylori* and duodenal ulcer disease must be pursued with a degree of skepticism.

Overview

C. pylori colonizes gastric-type epithelium wherever it is found, including the stomach, duodenum, esophagus,[11] and rectum.[12] Histological evidence that *C. pylori* causes gastric mucosal disease is compelling and includes rarely observed adherence pedestals between *C. pylori* and epithelial cells, depletion of mucin granules from gastric epithelium in proximity to organisms, intercellular invasion of bacteria with separation of intercellular tight junctions, and recruitment of polymorphonuclear cells into the underlying mucosa.[13-16]

Superficial antral gastritis is found in essentially all cases of active colonization and the prevalence of colonization is significantly higher in individuals with biopsy-proven superficial antral gastritis than in age-matched controls.[17-21] Follow-up studies indicate that superficial gastritis and *C. pylori* colonization are chronic conditions.[22-24] The only direct evidence that *C. pylori* causes superficial antral gastritis is derived from self-inoculation and acute acquisition case reports in which acute upper gastrointestinal symptoms, acute superficial antral gastritis, and hypochlorhydria have been observed.[7,8] Several small studies have reported histological improvement in gastritis when *C. pylori* is cleared from the stomach with antibiotics and bismuth-containing compounds.[25-27] Most individuals with *C. pylori* colonization, however, are asymptomatic and have normal endoscopic exams.[28-30] In summary, *C. pylori* chronically colonizes human stomachs and probably causes acute and chronic microscopic superficial antral gastritis of unknown clinical significance.

C. pylori is found in practically all patients with duodenal ulcers.[31,32] Unlike *C. pylori*–associated gastritis, however, ulcers are found in only a minority of those who are colonized with *C. pylori*. Studies which predate the discovery of *C. pylori* demonstrated that duodenal ulcer is nearly always associated with superficial antral gastritis.[33] Based on what we know presently, these cases of superficial antral gastritis likely were *C. pylori*–associated. One could have predicted, therefore, that *C. pylori* would be associated with duodenal ulcer.

Only a small fraction of individuals who are colonized with *C. pylori* develop ulcers. Also, highly selective vagotomy reduces ulcer recurrence without affecting *C. pylori* colonization.[34] These observations indicate the *C. pylori* is not independently involved in duodenal ulcer pathogenesis. However, the rarity with which ulcers occur in the absence of *C. pylori* is evidence that *C. pylori* is involved in ulcerogenesis. These discrepant observations could be explained in several ways: (1) the environment which predisposes to ulcer disease may be particularly well-suited for colonization by *C. pylori,* with the two events occurring independently; (2) there may be rare ulcerogenic and common nonulcerogenic forms of *C. pylori,* all of which are capable of inducing gastritis; and (3) *C. pylori* may be necessary for ulcer formation but dependent on the presence of other predisposing condition(s).

Three investigative strategies have been utilized to define the relationship between *C. pylori* and duodenal ulcer disease. Retrospective and short-term prospective epidemiological approaches have defined a clear association between *C. pylori* colonization and duodenal ulcer, but have failed to determine "which came first." Recent attempts to identify potential ulcerogenic mechanisms by *C. pylori* have yielded interesting but inconclusive results. A third tactic has been to study healing and recurrence rates of duodenal ulcer after treatment with antibiotics and bismuth-containing agents which have in vitro inhibitory activities against *C. pylori* but no known effects on acid secretion. This chapter critically summarizes the information available on *C. pylori* as it relates to duodenal ulcer disease. Alternative interpretations of the literature and suggestions for new approaches are presented.

Method of Detection

Endoscopic techniques for detecting *C. pylori* colonization require biopsy and include culture, staining, and the rapid urease test. Studies utilizing endoscopy have significant selection bias because normal controls are difficult to recruit. Serological screening methods utilizing the enzyme-linked immunosorbent assay (ELISA) have been used to study the prevalence of *C. pylori* in populations. First-generation ELISAs utilizing crude extracts of *C. pylori* have good sensitivity but relatively poor specificity, due to the inclusion of antigens which cross-react with circulating antibodies to other organisms.[35,36] When sera are diluted to 1:800, these crude antigen preparations have better specificity.[37] Purified antigens which are specific to *C. pylori* may improve specificity and sensitivity even further. Breath tests which measure carbon dioxide liberated by the action of *C. pylori* urease on carbon isotopes of ingested urea have been reported to have high sensitivity and specificity.[38] A third method for detecting gastric urease activity by measuring ammonia in gastric secretion after urea ingestion has been introduced.[39] The utilization of breath tests and second-generation serological tests is now underway. Most available data are based on first-generation serological tests and endoscopic evaluations. Any interpretation of the results of these tests must take into account the intrinsic error and selection bias, respectively.

Epidemiology of *Campylobacter pylori* Colonization

The prevalence of seropositivity for *C. pylori* varies between population groups. In Western societies including the United States, Great Britain, and Australia, seropositivity is rare in children and increases with age at a rate of approximately 1% per year.[40-43] In less developed societies, as many as 80% of individuals become seropositive by the age of 20 years.[44,45] The rates of acquisition of *C. pylori* appear to parallel the acquisition rates of superficial antral gastritis.[46] A similar parallel between *C. pylori* and duodenal ulcer disease is not universal. Whereas *C. pylori* seropositivity and duodenal ulcer disease are rare in Australian aborigines,[47] *C. pylori* seropositivity is ubiquitous and duodenal ulcer disease is rare in Peru.[48]

Epidemiological studies which probe the relationship between *C. pylori* and duodenal ulcer disease are lacking. For example, longitudinal serological studies which examine the relationship between the onset of seropositivity and the development of duodenal ulcer have not been performed. Family epidemiological studies could provide clues regarding potential sources of infection, factors involved in the acquisition of infection, and genetic factors which may affect the relationship between *C. pylori* and duodenal ulcer disease. Two small series have been published which examine seropositivity in families,[49,50] but the number of families examined has been too small to enable meaningful conclusions to be drawn.

Potential Pathogenic Factors

If *C. pylori* is important in the pathogenesis of duodenal ulcer disease, the mechanism must explain the relatively low number of colonized individuals who develop duodenal ulcer. Host-dependent and/or *C. pylori*–dependent variables may account for this phenomenon. Two broad approaches have been taken, one based on immunological and mucosal responses of the host to the organism and the other based on potential pathogenic factors produced by the organism. A key requirement missing in these investigations has been the identification of the way in which the hosts (or *C. pylori* strains) differ between cases of ulcer and nonulcer.

Host Factors

The host mounts an immune response as evidenced by circulating antibodies to a variety of *C. pylori* antigens and an inflammatory cell infiltration of the gastroduodenal mucosa. The antibody response to a battery of *C. pylori* antigens by Western blotting has been analyzed, with subtle differences between individuals noted. However, no differences in immunoblot profiles between ulcer and nonulcer patients have been identified yet.[37,51] If differences are present, the distinguishing antigens involved could prove to be important pathogenic factors.

Polymorphonuclear cells containing phagocytosed *C. pylori* have been observed in the gastric submucosal layers of infected individual and in vitro complement–dependent phagocytosis, and killing has been demonstrated by isolated human macrophages. Again, ulcer and nonulcer conditions have not been compared. Spontaneous clearance of *C. pylori* has been reported in isolated cases, suggesting that some individuals who are *C. pylori*–negative may share an ability to clear the organism.[7,52] The mechanism(s) that allows chronic colonization in the face of an immune response in many individuals, particularly members of older age groups, remains a mystery. A comparison of the effects of *C. pylori* on a variety of immune mechanisms in *C. pylori*–positive and *C. pylori*–negative individuals would help to define the apparent paralysis of effective immune-mediated clearance of the organism and to explore the hypothesis that mucosal structural changes associated with *C. pylori* infection are the result of inflammatory mediators rather than *C. pylori*–elaborated cytotoxins.

An histological analysis of *C. pylori*–associated fundal vs. body gastritis has shown that ulcer patients have less body gastritis than do nonulcer patients.[53] This observation suggests that healthy parietal and/or chief cell mass in the presence of *C. pylori* colonization could be a factor in ulcer development.

Gastric-type mucosa of the duodenum is commonly found in association with duodenal ulcer, and *C. pylori* is "only" found in the duodenum in association with gastric-type mucosa.[54–56] Gastric-type mucosa in the duodenum may occur primarily as heterotopic gastric mucosa or secondarily as gastric metaplasia in reponse to prior injury to the duodenum (such as excessive acid).[57] Whether gastric metaplasia-heterotopia in the duodenum and *C. pylori* colonization of the duodenum are interdependent factors in ulcerogenesis has not been determined.

Virulent Factors

Investigations into potential ulcerogenic substances elaborated by *C. pylori* have discovered weak mucolytic activity of *C. pylori* supernatants,[58] potential endotoxins,[59] lipolytic enzymes,[60] potential adhesion-colonization factors,[61,62] and cytopathic effects of filtrates of some isolates of broth-grown *C. pylori*.[63] Cytotoxic activity observed in the latter was seen more frequently in filtrates from ulcer-associated isolates compared to filtrates of isolates from nonulcer patients. The importance of these potential pathogenic factors has not been tested in vivo. The release of ammonia by the action of *C. pylori* urease on urea has been implicated as potentially toxic to gastric mucosa. Cytopathic effects of urea-supplemented supernatants or NH_4Cl alone have been demonstrated in cell culture and in animal models.[64–66] With the one noted exception, these investigations have not compared the activity of these potential pathogenic factors in isolates from ulcer and nonulcer patients.

Assuming the *C. pylori* proves to be an important pathogen, the search for potential pathogenic mechanisms could lead to specific therapies designed to interfere with pathogenesis without the need to eradicate the organism. Attachment factors and "ulcerogenic" toxins could be neutralized pharmacologically, "ulcerogenic" strains could be replaced with commensal nonulcerogenic strains, or ulcers could be prevented by immunization with attenuated "ulcerogenic" factors.

Therapeutic Trials

When duodenal ulcers are treated with antibiotic/bismuth combinations which have in vitro inhibitory activities against *C. pylori,* healing rates parallel clearance of the organism.[67] When bismuth compounds are compared side-by-side with H_2 blockers, ulcer healing rates are approximately equivalent.[68] H_2 blockers induce rapid healing without affecting the density of *C. pylori* or the degree of gastritis in the antrum.[69,70] Prior to the discovery of *C. pylori,* tripotassium dicitrato bismuthate had been shown to reduce the duodenal ulcer recurrence rate compared to cimetidine.[71] Several subsequent small trials have reported apparent reductions in recurrence rates in those who are initially cleared of *C. pylori* after the completion of treatment with bismuth/antibiotic combinations compared to H_2 blocker therapy.[72-76] Ulcer recurrence is associated with *C. pylori* reemergence, but some recurrences occur in patients who remain *C. pylori*–free.

Several problems arise in the design of these studies. First, treatments which include bismuth cannot be truly blinded because bismuth compounds produce black stools and darkening of the tongue. Knowledge by the subject that he or she is being treated with an agent effective against *C. pylori* may be significant (ulcer recurrence has been reported to be reduced by hypnotherapy at a rate very similar to that reported for bismuth treatment[77]). A second problem is the lack of a control group with duodenal ulcers that are not colonized with *C. pylori*. Bismuth compounds likely have "cytoprotective" effects in addition to bacteriosuppressant effects.[78] Trials which lack *C. pylori*–negative duodenal ulcer controls cannot differentiate *C. pylori*–suppressing activities from the potential "cytoprotective" activities of treatments.

The eradication of *C. pylori* has proven difficult; a very large percentage of those cleared of *C. pylori* become recolonized,[79] and a significant proportion of the reemergent bacteria are drug resistant.[80] Recolonization after clearance is usually by the same genetic strain, even when clearance has persisted up to a year off therapy.[9,81] Clearance often represents occult colonization. True eradication is rare and appears to require several weeks of bismuth-containing compounds used in conjunction with one or more antibiotics.[10] Long-term follow-up studies are needed to differentiate clearance from eradication.[76] Finally, the potential for significant toxicity with chronic bismuth administration should be defined before widespread use of this agent is advocated.

More information is needed concerning the biology of *C. pylori* within the human host. The worldwide prevalence of this organism indicates that it is among the most common chronic infections in man. Its ecological role in man needs to be fully elucidated before eradication can be considered. It is premature to assume that this organism is purely opportunistic; it may play a mutually beneficial commensal role by protecting its human host from the development of significant disease.

In summary, clinical studies have not yet shown a clear causal relationship between the presence of gastric *C. pylori* and duodenal ulcer, nor have they shown *C. pylori*–specific therapies to be superior to the established and proven safe acute and maintenance therapies. Additional evidence clearly is needed before considering a new approach to the treatment of duodenal ulcer disease. The definitive therapy for chronic duodenal ulcer disease will heal ulcers effectively and safely, prevent recurrence, and reduce the morbidity and mortality of duodenal ulcer disease. The first hurdle is to develop an effective and safe means of effecting the true eradication of *C. pylori*. The second challenge is to validly compare this therapy to established therapies for the treatment of recurrent duodenal ulcer in a large group of *C. pylori*–positive and –negative cases. Finally, the long-term effects of eradication will need to be explored to ensure that we are not eradicating a commensal organism that may be serving an unrecognized benefit to its host.

Conclusion

C. pylori possesses the capacity to colonize human gastric-type mucosa wherever it is found. It likely causes an acute and chronic active gastritis of unknown clinical significance. Its relationship to the pathogenesis of duodenal ulcer disease remains obscure. *C. pylori* is not independently involved in ulcer pathogenesis. Available evidence is inconclusive as to whether *C. pylori* interacts with other factors to cause duodenal ulcer, and a passive role has not been excluded. Additional work is needed to characterize the epidemiology of *C. pylori* colonization, including the sources, means of acquisition, time course of acquistion as it relates to onset of disease, and interaction of *C. pylori* colonization with other risk factors of duodenal ulcer disease. Investigations into potential pathogenic mechanisms should be accelerated; they may uncover important treatable pathogenic factors in duodenal ulcer disease which may or may not be directly related to *C. pylori*. Future investigations should be directed toward testing the following hypotheses: (1) the environment which predisposes to ulcer disease may be particularly well suited for colonization by *C. pylori*, with two events occurring independently; (2) there may be rare ulcerogenic and common nonulcerogenic forms of *C. pylori*, all of which are capable of inducing gastritis; and (3) *C. pylori* may be necessary for ulcer formation but dependent on the presence of other predisposing condition(s). Until these questions are answered, *Campylobacter pylori* cannot be implicated unequivocally in the pathogenesis of duodenal ulcer disease.

References

1. Van DeVenter GM: Approaches to the long-term treatment of duodenal ulcer disease. *Am J Med* 1984; 77(suppl 5B):15–22. *This article reviews the basis for the concept, "once an ulcer, always an ulcer."*
2. Wormsley KG, Grossman MI: Maximal histalog test in control subjects and patients with peptic ulcer. *Gut* 1965; 6:427. *This article indicates that many patients with duodenal ulcer disease have normal acid secretory function.*
3. Bottcher: *Dorpater Medicinische Zeitchrift* 1874; 5:148. *This is the first known observation of curved bacilli colonizing human gastric mucosa.*
4. Doenges L: Spirochetes in the gasric glands of macacus rhesus and of man without related disease. *Arch Pathol* 1939; 27:469–477. *This a commonly cited article indicating the presence of spirochetes in the stomachs of humans and monkeys. Rhesus monkeys have served as an animal model for C. pylori colonization (see reference 5).*
5. Baskerville A, Newell DG: Naturally occurring chronic gastritis and *C. pylori* infection in the Rhesus monkey: A potential model for gastritis in man. *Gut* 1988; 29:465–472. *This is a representative example of an animal model of C. pylori gastric colonization. Gastritis but not duodenal ulcers accompanies C. pylori colonization in this model.*
6. Krakowka S, Morgan DR, Kraft WG, et al: Establishment of gastric *Campylobacter pylori* infection in the neonatal gnotobiotic piglet. *Infect Immun* 1987; 55:2789–2796. *As above.*
7. Marshall BJ, Armstrong JA, McGechie DB, et al: Attempt to fulfill Koch's postulates for pyloric *Campylobacter*. *Med J Aust* 1985; 142:436–439. *Dr. Marshall reports a mild upper gastrointestinal illness and histological gastritis following self-ingestion of C. pylori. The infection and gastritis resolved spontaneously.*
8. Morris A, Nicholson G: Ingestion of *Campylobacter pyloridis* causes gastritis and raised fasting gastric pH. *Am J Gastroenterol* 1987; 82:192–199. *Morris was not as lucky as Marshall. He developed a more severe upper gastrointestinal illness with gasritis. While he is now asymptomatic, he continues to be chronically infected with C. pylori despite aggressive antibiotic/bismuth therapies.*
9. Langenberg W, Rauws EAJ, Widjojokusumo A, et al: Identification of *Campylobacter pyloridis* isolates by restriction endonuclease DNA analysis. *J Clin Microbiol* 1986; 24:414–417. *Utilizing restriction endonuclease profiles of the DNA of cultured C. pylori, these authors demonstrated recrudescence of colonization (with the same organism) after apparent eradication with antibiotics and bismuth.*
10. McNulty CAM: The treatment of *Campylobacter*-associated gastritis. *Am J Gastroenterol* 1987; 82:245–247. *McNulty reinforces the concept that C. pylori is difficult or impossible to eradicate with available antimicrobial agents and bismuth.*
11. Hazell SL, Carrick J, Lee A: *Campylobacter pylori* can infect the oesophagus when gastric tissue is present. *Gasroenterology* 1988; 94:A178. *These authors found histological evidence of C. pylori colonization of gastric metaplastic tissues in Barrett's esophagus.*

12. Pambianco DJ, Dye KR, Marshall BJ, et al: Gastritis in the rectum: *Campylobacter*-like organisms in heterotopic inflamed gastric mucosa. *Gastroenterology* 1988; 94:A340. *This group found an island of gastric metaplasia in the rectum with histological evidence of C. pylori colonization.*

13. Wyatt JI, Rathbone BJ: Immune response of the gastric mucosa to *Campylobacter pylori*. *Scand J Gastroenterol* 1988; 23(suppl 142):44–49. *This represents one of the important publications which describe the ultrastructural features of gastric mucosa and the accompanying mucosal inflammation in areas of C. pylori infestation.*

14. Pruul H, Lee PC, Goodwin CS, et al: Interaction of *Campylobacter pyloridis* with human immune defense mechanisms. *J Med Microbiol* 1987; 23:233–238. *As above.*

15. Goodwin CS, Armstrong JA, Marshall BJ: *Campylobacter pyloridis,* gastritis and peptic ulceration. *J Clin Pathol* 1986; 39:353–365. *As above.*

16. Bode G, Malfertheiner P, Ditschuneit H: Pathogenic implications of ultrastructural findings in *Campylobacter pylori* related gastroduodenal disease. *Scand J Gasroenterol* 1988; 23(suppl 142):25–39. *As above.*

17. Dwyer B, Nanxiong S, Kaldor J, et al: Antibody response to *Campylobacter pylori* in an ethnic group lacking peptic ulceration. *Scand J Infect Dis* 1988; 20:63–68. *This is one of the important articles which reveal the strong associations between C. pylori colonization and superficial gastritis.*

18. Booth L, Holdstock G, MacBride H, et al: Clinical importance of *Campylobacter pyloridis* and associated IgG and IgA antibody responses in patients undergoing upper gastrointestinal endoscopy. *J Clin Pathol* 1986; 39:215–219. *As above.*

19. Goodwin CS, Blincow E, Peterson G, et al: Enzyme-linked immunosorbent assay for *"Campylobacter pyloridis"* correlation with the presence of C. *pyloridis* in the gastric mucosa. *J Infect Dis* 1987; 155:488–493. *As above.*

20. Hazell SL, Hennessy SB, Borody TJ, et al: *Campylobacter pyloridis* gastritis II: Distribution of bacteria and associated inflammation in the gastroduodenal environment. *Am J Gastroenterol* 1987; 82:297–301. *As above.*

21. Jones DM, Eldridge J, Fox AJ, et al: Antibody to the gastric *Campylobacter*-like organism (*"Campylobacter pyloridis"*) — clinical correlations and distribution in the normal population. *J Med Microbiol* 1986; 22:57–62. *As above.*

22. Langenberg W, Rauws EAJ, Houthoff HJ, et al: Follow-up study of individuals with untreated *Campylobacter pylori*–associated gastritis and of noninfected persons with non-ulcer dyspepsia. *J Infect Dis* 1988; 157:1245–1249. *This is one of the important articles which examine the chronicity of superficial gastritis and C. pylori colonization.*

23. Rosch W, Demling L, Elster K: Is chronic gastritis a reversible process? Follow-up study of gastritis with step-wise biopsy. *Acta Hepato-Gastroenterol* 1975; 22:252–255. *As above.*

24. Siurala M, Sipponen P, Kekki M: Chronic gastritis: Dynamic and clinical aspects. *Scand J Gastroenterol* 1985; 20(suppl 109):69–76. *As above.*

25. McNulty CAM, Gearty JC, Crump B, et al: *Campylobacter pyloridis* and associated gastritis: Investigator blind, placebo controlled trial of bismuth salicylate and erythromycin ethylsuccinate. *Br Med J* 1986; 293:675–679. *This is one of the key articles which show that therapies directed toward*

the clearance of C. pylori administered in a double-blind placebo-controlled fashion result in the healing of gastritis.

26. Glupczynski Y, Burnette A, Labbe M, et al: *Campylobacter pylori*–associated gastritis: A double-blind placebo-controlled trial with amoxicillin. *Am J Gastroenterol* 1988; 83:365–372. *As above.*

27. Malfertheiner P, Stanescu A, Baczako K, et al: Chronic erosive gastritis — a therapeutic approach with bismuth. *Scand J Gastroenterol* 1988; 23(suppl 142):87–92. *As above.*

28. Rokkas T, Pursey C, Uzoechina E, et al: *Campylobacter pylori* and non-ulcer dyspepsia. *Am J Gastroenterol* 1987; 82:1149–1151. *This paper indicates that a significant proportion of patients colonized with C. pylori are asymptomatic and that the endoscopic appearance of the mucosa usually is normal in patients with C. pylori–associated gastritis.*

29. Barthel JS, Westblom TU, Havey AD, et al: Gastritis and *Campylobacter pylori* in healthy, asymptomatic volunteers. *Arch Intern Med* 1988; 148:1149–1151. *As above.*

30. Langenberg ML, Tytgat GNJ, Schipper MEI, et al: *Campylobacter*-like organisms in the stomach of patients and healthy individuals. *Lancet* 1984; 1:1348. *As above.*

31. Hornick RB: Peptic ulcer disease: A bacterial infections? *N Engl J Med* 1987; 316:1598–1600. *This is one of the key articles which show the high proportion of C. pylori colonization in patients with duodenal ulcer disease.*

32. Price AB, Levi J, Dolby JM, et al: *Campylobacter pyloridis* in peptic ulcer disease: Microbiology, pathology, and scanning electron microscopy. *Gut* 1985; 26:1183–1188. *As above.*

33. Tatsuta M, Iishi H, Okuda S: Location of peptic ulcers in relation to antral and fundal gastritis by chromoendoscopic follow-up examination. *Dig Dis Sci* 1986; 31:7–11. *This study, which predates the isolation of C. pylori, revealed the high incidence of antral gastritis in patients with duodenal ulcer disease.*

34. Graham DY, Jordan PH, Opekun AR, et al: *Campylobacter pylori* is not the cause of duodenal ulcers. *Gastroenterology* 1988; 94:A152. *Dr. Graham finds that patients who have undergone highly selective vagotomy for duodenal ulcer disease continue to have C. pylori colonization despite the low recurrence rates of duodenal ulcer disease in these individuals.*

35. Newell DG: Identification of the outer membrane proteins of *Campylobacter pyloridis* and antigenic cross-reactivity between *C. pyloridis* and *C. jejuni*. *J Gen Microbiol* 1987; 133:163–170. *This is one of the representative articles which address the sensitivity and specificity of ELISA for detecting C. pylori colonization using sonicated or acid-extracted antigen.*

36. Mills SD, Kurjanczyk LA, Penner JL: Identification of an antigen common to different species of the genus *Campylobacter*. *J Clin Microbiol* 1988; 26:1411–1413. *As above.*

37. Perez-Perez GI, Blaser MJ: Conservation and diversity of *Campylobacter pyloridis* major antigens. *Infect Immun* 1987; 55:1256–1263. *These investigators have shown that ELISA utilizing sonicated C. pylori has high sensitivity and specificity if patient sera are diluted to 1:800.*

38. Graham DY, Klien PD, Evans J, et al: *Campylobacter pyloridis* detected

noninvasively by the 13C-urea breath test. *Lancet* 1984; 1:1174–1177. *This is the first report of using nonradioactive carbon isotope–labeled urea to detect gastric urease activity. Dr. Graham shows that this test is quite accurate for the detection of C. pylori.*

39. Weber J, Astheimer W, Riemann JF: Ammonia production in the stomach by *Campylobacter pylori. Gastroenterology* 1988; 94:A489. *These investigators measured intragastric ammonia production following urea ingestion in a small series of patients. Their results suggest that this also may prove to be a sensitive and specific means of detecting C. pylori colonization.*

40. Czunn SJ, Lahms BB, Jacobs GH, et al: *Campylobacter*-like organisms in association with symptomatic gastritis in children. *J Pediatr* 1986; 109:80–83. *This article reveals the very low incidence of C. pylori colonization in children. The association of C. pylori and gastritis remains signficant in this group.*

41. Gnarpe H, Unge P, Klomqvist C, et al: *Campylobacter pylori* in Swedish patients referred for gastroscopy. *APMIS* 1988; 96:128–132. *This is an example of the epidemiological studies performed in developed countries which show a positive relationship between C. pylori colonization and age.*

42. Morris A, Nicholson G, Lloyd G, et al: Seroepidemiology of *Campylobacter pyloridis. N Z Med J* 1986; 99:657–659. *As above.*

43. Schaub N, Staler GA, Marbet UA, et al: *Campylobacter pylori,* gastritis and ulkuskrankheit, *Schweiz Med Wschenschr* 1988; 118:293–301. *As above.*

44. Graham DY, Klein PD, Opekun AR: Epidemiology of *Campylobacter pylori* infection: Ethnic considerations. *Scand J Gastroenterol* 1988; 23(suppl 142):9–12. *This is an epidemiological study in a developing country. The relationship of C. pylori positivity with age persists but is shifted dramatically toward younger ages.*

45. Gutierrez O, Sierra F, Gomez MC, et al: *Campylobacter pylori* in chornic environmental gastritis and duodenal ulcer patients (abstract). *Gastroenterology* 1988; 94:A163. *As above.*

46. Graham Y, Klein PD, Opekun AR, et al: Effect of age on the frequency of active *Campylobacter pylori* infection diagnosed by the [13C]urea breath test in normal subjects and patients with peptic ulcer disease. *J Infect Dis* 1988; 157:777–780. *These authors verify the age-related increase in C. pylori colonization and observe that the acquisition rate of C. pylori parallels that of superficial antral gastritis.*

47. Dwyer B, Nanxiong S, Kaldor J, et al: Antibody response to *Campylobacter pylori* in an ethnic group lacking peptic ulceration. *Scand J Infect Dis* 1988; 20:63–68. *This paper reveals that C. pylori seropositivity is rare in a group of Australian aborigines who essentially never get ulcers.*

48. Graham DY, personal communications, 1989.

49. Mitchell HM, Bohane TD, Berkowicz J, et al: Antibody to *Campylobacter pylori* in families of index children with gastrointestinal illness due to C. pylori. *Lancet* 1987; II:681–682. *This is one of only two articles published thus far which attempt to analyze the occurrence of C. pylori colonization within famiies. Mitchell et al found that family contacts of a C. pylori-positive index case were more likely to be seropositive than was the general population.*

50. Jones DM, Eldridge J, Whorwell PJ: Antibodies to *Campylobacter pyloridis*

in household contacts of infected patients. *Br Med J* 1987; 294:615. As above.

51. von Wulffen H, Grote HJ, Gatermann S, et al: Immunoblot analysis of immune response to *Campylobacter pylori* and its clinical associations. *J Clin Pathol* 1988; 41:653–659. *These authors were unable to identify unique bands in immunoblots which were predictive of duodenal ulcer disease.*

52. Hill ID, Sinclair-Smith C, Lastovica AJ, et al: Transient protein losing enteropathy associated with acute gastritis and *Campylobacter pylori*. *Arch Dis Child* 1987; 62:1215–1219. *This case report suggests the spontaneous clearance of C. pylori in a child who developed protein-losing enteropy.*

53. Mendes EN, Queiroz MM, Rocha GA, et al: *Campylobacter* colonization, duodenal ulceration, and changes in gastric mucosa. *J Clin Pathol* 1988; 41:1027. *These authors made the interesting observation that C. pylori–positive patients with duodenal ulcers had less body gastritis than C. pylori–positive individuals without ulcers.*

54. Steer HW: Surface morphology of the gastroduodenal mucosa in duodenal ulceration. *Gut* 1984; 25:1203. *This article addresses the issue of gastric metaplasia of the duodenum and C. pylori colonization of the duodenum. The consensus is that C. pylori colonizes the duodenum only in areas of gastric metaplasia.*

55. Wyatt JI, Rathbone BJ, Dixon MF, et al: *Campylobacter pyloridis* and acid induced gastric metaplasia in the pathogenesis of duodenitis. *J Clin Pathol* 1987; 40:841–848. *As above.*

56. Johnston BJ, Reed PI, Ali MH: Prevalence of *Campylobacter pylori* in duodenal and gastric mucosa—relationship to inflammation. *Scand J Gastroenterol* 1988; 23(suppl 142):69–75. *As above.*

57. Rhodes J: Experimental production of gastric epithelium in the duodenum. *Gut* 1964; 5:454–458. *Using animal models, these authors were able to induce gastric metaplasia of the duodenum with excessive acid.*

58. Saroseik J, Slomiany A, Slomiany BL: Evidence for weakening of gastric mucus integrity by *Campylobacter pylori*. *Scand J Gastroenterol* 1988; 23:585–590. *this is one of the key articles which investigate substances produced by C. pylori in vitro which may have pathogenic effects in vivo.*

59. Rathbone BJ, Wyatt JI, Heatley RV: Possible pathogenic pathways of *Campylobacter pylori* in gastro-duodenal disease. *Scand J Gastroenterol* 1988; 23(suppl 142):40–43. *As above.*

60. Sarosiek J, Slomiany A, VanHorn K, et al: Lipolytic activity of *Campylobacter pylori*: Effects of sofalcone (abstract). *Gastroenterology* 1988; 94:A399. *As above.*

61. Evans DG, Evans DJ, Moulds JJ, et al: N-acetylneuraminyllactose-binding fibrillar hemagglutinin of *Campylobacter pylori*: A putative colonization factor antigen. *Infect Immun,* 1988; 56:2896–2906. *As above.*

62. Levente E, Carlsson A, Ljungh A, et al: Mannose-resistant haemagglutination by *Campylobacter pylori*. *Scand J Infect Dis* 1988; 20:353–354. *As above.*

63. Figura N, Guglielmetti P, Rossolini A, et al: Cytotoxin production by *Campylobacter pylori* strains isolated from patients with peptic ulcer disease and from patients with chronic gastritis only. *J Clin Microbiol* 1989; 27:225–226. *As above.*

64. Tsujii M, Kawano S, Sato N, et al: *Campylobacter pylori* and gastric ulceration

(abstract). *Gastroenterology* 1988; 94:A467. *This article deals with the potential role of C. pylori urease as a pathogenic factor in the development of gastroduodenal disease.*

65. Murakami M, Yoo JK, Mizuno M, et al: Effects of ammonia, urea, and urease on the rat gastric mucosa (abstract). *Gastroenterology* 1987; 92:1544. *As above.*

66. Barer MR, Elliott TSJ, Berkley D, et al: Cytopathic effects of *C. pylori* urease. *J Clin Pathol* 1988; 41:597. *As above.*

67. Bayerdörffer E, Ottenjann R: The role of antibiotics in *Campylobacter pylori* associated peptic ulcer disease. *Scand J Gastroenterol* 1988; 23(suppl 142):93–100. *This paper describes a representative therapeutic trial directed toward the clearance of C. pylori which investigated the effects of various combinations of bismuth and antibiotics on duodenal ulcer healing and C. pylori clearance from the gastroduodenum.*

68. Lee FI, Samloff IM, Harman M: Comparison of tripotassium dicitrobismuthate tablets with ranitidine in healing and relapse of duodenal ulcers. *Lancet* 1985; 1:1299. *As above.*

69. Hui WM, Ho J, Lam SK: Persistence of *Campylobacter pylori* (CP) during remission and subsequent relapse in duodenal ulcer (DU) (abstract). *Gastroenterology* 1988; 94:A196. *As above.*

70. Hui W-M, Lam S-K, Chau P-Y, et al: Persistence of *Campylobacter pyloridis* despite healing of duodenal ulcer and improvement of accompanying duodenitis and gastritis. *Dig Dis Sci* 1987; 32:1255–1260. *As above.*

71. Martin DF, Hollanders D, May SJ, et al: Difference in relapse rates of duodenal ulcer after healing with cimetidine or tripotassium dicitrato bismuthate. *Lancet* 1981; 1:7–10. *As above.*

72. Coghlan JG, Gilligan D, Humphries H, et al: *Campylobacter pylori* and recurrence of duodenal ulcers — a 12 month follow-up study. *Lancet* 1987; 2:1109–1111. *As above.*

73. Marshall BJ, Goodwin CS, Warren JR, et al: Long-term healing of gastritis and low duodenal ulcer relapse after eradication of *Campylobacter pyloridis:* A prospective double-blind study (abstract). *Gastroenterology* 1987; 92:1518. *As above.*

74. Rauws EAJ, Langenberg W, Houthoff HJ, et al: *Campylobacter pyloridis*–associated chronic active antral gastritis: A prospective study of its prevalence and the effects of antibacterial and antiulcer treatment. *Gastroenterology* 1988; 94:33–40. *As above.*

75. Marshall BJ, Armstrong JA, Francis GJ, et al: Antibacterial action of bismuth in relation to *Campylobacter pyloridis* colonization and gastritis. *Digestion* 1987; 37(suppl 2):16–30. *As above.*

76. Borody T, Cole P, Noinan S, et al: Long-term *Campylobacter pylori* recurrence post-eradication (abstract). *Gastroenterology* 1988; 94:A43. *As above.*

77. Colgan SM, Faragher EB, Whorwell PJ: Controlled trial of hypnotherapy in relapse prevention of duodenal ulceration. *Lancet* 1988; 1:1299–1300. *This interesting investigation found that the ulcer relapse rate following the treatment of duodenal ulcer was reduced in patients who participated in hypnotherapy. The reduced relapse rate among those who received hypnotherapy in combination with an H_2 blocker is similar to that which has been reported in the literature utilizing bismuth therapy.*

78. Andersen LP: Cytoprotective agents and *C. pylori* associated acid peptic diseases. *Scand J Gastroenterol* 1988; 23(suppl 142):110–113. *This article reviews the "cytoprotective" agents used in the treatment of duodenal ulcer.*

79. Lambert JR, Borromeo M, Eaves ER, et al: Efficacy of different dosage regimens of bismuth in eradicating *Campylobacter pylori. Gastroenterology* 1988; 94:A248. *This is one of many reports which indicate that the clearance of C. pylori with bismuth and/or antibiotics rarely represents true eradication; recolonization is common following the completion of treatment.*

80. Goodwin CS, Marshall BJ, Blincow ED, et al: Prevention of nitroimidazole resistance in *Campylobacter pylori* by coadministration of colloidal bismuth subcitrate: Clinical and in vitro studies. *J Clin Pathol* 1988; 41:207–210. *These authors address the issue of the development of antibiotic resistance in isolates of C. pylori previously treated with antibiotics.*

81. Rauws EAJ, Langenberg W, Widjojokusumo A, et al: Molecular epidemiology of *Campylobacter pylori* colonization. *Gastroenterology* 1988; 94:A369. *This abstract is an extension of the work published by these authors in reference 9. Again, they find that cases of recolonization of C. pylori following treatment represent recrudescence of the same organism that was present prior to treatment.*

Rebuttal: Affirmative
James S. Barthel, M.D.

Drs. Karnes and Guth incant the tenets of the theory of etiological heterogeneity:

1. Excess acid production does not cause all duodenal ulcers.
2. Additional undefined aggressive factors must play a role in the etiology of duodenal ulcers.
3. Additional undefined defective defensive factors must play a role in the etiology of duodenal ulcers.

The reader is then asked to believe on the basis of faith that these unknown aggressive and defective defensive factors are extremely important in the causation of duodenal ulcer disease, but to exercise skepticism toward a role for *Campylobacter pylori* in the etiology of duodenal ulcer disease because gaps exist in our understanding of the pathophysiology! Drs. Karnes and Guth, of course, make no further explanation of the mysterious aggressive or defective defensive factors, presumably because they are unknown — a gap in our understanding infinitely more fundamental than the one which exists concerning the pathophysiology of *C. pylori.*

John Tukey's[1] observation that, "better an approximate answer to the right question than an exact answer to the wrong question" applies to the issue at hand. We have an approximate answer to the right question: Is *C. pylori* a significant etiological agent in peptic ulcer disease? The approximate answer based on the available data is probably yes. A more exact answer will be obtained by pursuing questions which relate to causation rather than questions which relate to pathophysiological mechanisms. From a teleologic standpoint it seems illogical to pursue mechanism before establishing causation (although this does not bother some). As Sir Austin Bradford Hill has pointed out:

...the decisive question is whether the frequency of the undesirable event B will be influenced by a change in the environmental feature A. How such a change exerts that influence may call for a great deal of research. However, before deducing "causation" and taking action we shall not invariably have to sit around awaiting the results of that research.[2]

If the undesirable event B is equated with duodenal ulcer and the environmental features A is equated with the presence of *C. pylori,* then causation can be explored within the context of the Bradford-Hill criteria (Table 1). Thus, a definite direction for the immediate future of research on the

---

TABLE 1.
The Bradford-Hill Criteria

Strength
Consistency
Specificity
Temporality
Biological gradient
Plausibility
Coherence
Experiment
Analogy

---

relationship between *C. pylori* and duodenal ulcer disease can be obtained. There is no need to await the results of research into such obscure questions as the reason why ulcer disease and *C. pylori* seropositivity are rare in Australian aborigines before deducing causation.

With respect to the relationship between *C. pylori* and duodenal ulcer disease, the Bradford-Hill criteria have not been fully satisfied. There are gaps in our proof of causation. The criteria of temporality and experiment have not been adequately met. In these areas, I find myself in agreement with Drs. Karnes and Guth. The concept of temporality refers to the "which came first, the chicken or the egg" question. The concept of experiment refers to the effect of the intentional removal of the offending environmental features. Does the disease go away? A cohort study of the incidence of ulcers detected endoscopically in patients with and without *C. pylori* in which the use of nonsteroidal anti-inflammatory agents is strictly controlled would address the question of temporality most directly. A vigorous effort is underway to develop an antimicrobial regimen which can eradicate *C. pylori* in vivo and thus address the issue of experiment. Preliminary studies indicate that the eradication of *C. pylori* does produce an impressive drop in the recurrence rate of duodenal ulcers.[3]

In conclusion, it appears that the time has arrived to abandon theories of ulcerogenesis based on acid hypersecretion, polygenetic inheritance, and etiological heterogeneity. These theories do not adequately explain both old and new observations concerning the phenomenon of peptic ulcer disease and, thus, they cannot be defended. We must avoid further wandering among alleged pathophysiological mechanisms unguided by any provable theory of causation. The immediate direction of research into the relationship between *C. pylori* and duodenal ulcer disease should address the remaining questions concerning causation in humans.

References

1. Tukey JW: Some thoughts on clinical trials, especially problems of multiplicity. *Science* 1977; 198:679–84.
2. Bradford Hill A: The environment and disease: Association or causation? *Proc R Soc Lond [Biol]* 1965; 58:295–300.
3. Coghlan JG, Humphries H, Dooley C, et al: *Campylobacter pylori* and recurrence of duodenal ulcers — a 12 month follow-up study. *Lancet* 1987; ii:1109–1111.

Rebuttal: Negative

William E. Karnes, M.D.
Paul Guth, M.D.

This debate serves to educate clinicans regarding the present state of the hypothesis that *Campylobacter pylori* is an important etiological factor in duodenal ulcer disease. *C. pylori* can now be added to the long list of other physiological and psychological factors which share varying degrees of association with duodenal ulcer disease. Association, however, does not imply causality.

Gastric acid secretion remains the only factor associated with duodenal ulcer disease which clearly plays an etiological role; ulcers heal when acid is removed, and marked hypersecretors of acid (e.g., Zollinger-Ellison syndrome patients) develop ulcers. Furthermore, Wormsley's statement quoted in Dr. Barthel's counter-debate that "...there is really no evidence that ... gastric juice is ever aggressive towards normal alimentary mucosa" is wrong. Gastrojejunostomy without vagotomy frequently causes marginal ulcers.[2]

The importance of *C. pylori* in the pathogenesis of duodenal ulcer disease has not been determined. From an historical context, as elegantly presented in Dr. Barthel's counter-debate, *C. pylori* offers an appealing explanation for many of the remaining mysteries of duodenal ulcer disease and excites our expectations that duodenal ulcers can be cured someday. However, history also teaches us that nature is not simple; we have been misled before by our tendency to believe naive hypotheses.

The importance of properly testing clinically relevant hypotheses cannot be disputed at any level. Our impulse to accept sensible but unproven theory fuels imaginative therapeutic decisions which may be harmful to our patients. While it is true that *C. pylori* is associated with duodenal ulcer disease, we must remain cognizant the *C. pylori* has not been shown through rigorous studies to be an etiological factor. Observed associations and historical inference are not enough.

References

1. Wormsley KG: Duodenal ulcer: Does pathophysiology equal aetiology. *Gut* 1983; 24:775–780. *A critique of the theory of etiological heterogenetity is presented.*
2. Menguy RB: Stomach, Schwartz SI (ed): *Principles of Surgery.* New York, McGraw-Hill Book Company, 1979, pp 1142–1143. *This is a brief review of the evolution of surgical procedures for duodenal ulcer disease with a rationale for vagotomy.*

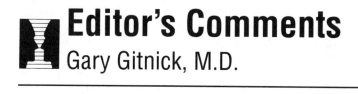

Editor's Comments
Gary Gitnick, M.D.

Are we ready for a new theory of ulcerogenesis? Dr. Barthel thinks that the time and the data have arrived. He takes us through an elegant historical review of the theories of ulcer development. He then points out that despite great advances in our ability to test acid concentrations and despite the availability of continuous pH monitoring, "a consistent association between duodenal ulcer and acid hypersecretion has not been demonstrated." He sums up the world's acid literature with this quotation by Wormsley:

> Pathophysiologic disturbances, like the gastric hypersecretion which occurs in one sixth to one third of patients with duodenal ulcer, are changes from the usual physiological situation and that is all they are. There is no evidence whatsoever that these variant reactions are anything other than that, or that they are in any way ulcerogenic.

He concludes that there is no evidence that acid causes ulcers.

After spending two thirds of his argument attacking the theory of acid ulcerogenesis, Barthel introduces another theory of ulcerogenesis. He turns first to Warren and Marshall's 1983 report describing the isolation of *Campylobacter pylori* from antral mucosal biopsies in patients with gastritis. Reproducible culturing of the organism together with a variety of supporting serological studies "suggested a pathogenetic role for the organism." After two human ingestion experiments fulfilling Koch's postulates were performed, an etiological relationship was established.

The same investigators reported an association between *C. pylori* gastritis and duodenal ulcer disease; this was confirmed. However, *C. pylori* could not be found in duodenal mucosa even though it was present in gastric mucosa. Eventually it was reported to be found in the foci of gastric metaplasia within the duodenum. Barthel suggests that these foci represent areas of "diminished acid resistance where peptic ulceration beings." Where is the proof? He then quotes a variety of forms of tangential evidence: *C. pylori* causes thinning of the mucus layer which returns to normal thickness following the eradication of the organism. *C. pylori* secretes a protease that is able to degrade gastric mucus and that also produces a toxin which causes cytopathic change in vitro. He advances a circuitous argument suggesting that the absence of hyperacidity in a signficant number of duodenal ulcer patients indicates that acid plays only an adjunctive role in ulceropathogenesis when the mucosa is already infected and inflamed. When this occurs, any acid, not necessarily excess acid, can cause mucosal damage. Where is the proof?

Drs. Karnes and Guth vehemently disagree with Dr. Barthel's assertions. They point out that "in an attempt to fulfill Koch's postulates two cases of self-inoculation resulted in acute gastritis but not ulcers." They admit that the argument that *C. pylori* causes gastric mucosal disease is compelling, but assert that it may not pertain to duodenal ulcers. They also point out that most people who harbor *C. pylori* are symptom-free and have normal endoscopic examinations. Though *Campylobacter* may be present, there is no gastritis or ulcer disease. They propose that *Campylobacter* chronically colonizes human stomachs and may produce chronic superficial antral gastritis often of unknown clinical significance. Although *C. pylori* is found in the majority of patients with duodenal ulcers, a cause and effect relationship has not been established. Indeed, ulcers are found only in a small number of those who are colonized with *C. pylori*. Although most patients with duodenal ulcers have antral gastritis and most patients with antral gastritis harbor *C. pylori,* there is no evidence that *C. pylori* is the cause of ulcers, only that it is associated with them. They point out that true eradication with antibiotics, bismuth, or combinations is rare and they argue further that long-term follow-up studies are needed to differentiate clearance from eradication.

Thus, they argue that published studies have not shown a clear causal relationship between *C. pylori* and duodenal ulcer, nor have they shown that therapies designed specifically to eradicate or clear *C. pylori* are superior to the acute and maintenance therapies currently established and proven safe. They argue that the scientific community should develop an effective and safe means of eradicating *C. pylori*. Thereafter, prospective long-term studies should be undertaken to compare this form of treatment to established therapies in order to assess the healing of acute ulcers and the recurrence of ulcer disease in a large group of *C. pylori*–positive and –negative cases. Finally, the long-term effects of eradication should be studied thoroughly to ensure that the result is not the elimination of a commensal organism which may be serving an unrecognized benefit to the host.

In this instance the editor will agree with both debators. Dr. Barthel is quite correct that the cause of ulcer disease remains unknown and the role of acid is unclear in spite of the exceptional sums of money devoted to investigating the pathogenesis of ulcer disease. Drs. Karnes and Guth are also correct in stating that a cause and effect relationship between *C. pylori* and peptic ulcer disease has not been established by the published literature. Both groups give good advice on directions for future research. Hopefully, that advice will be heeded.

Index

YEAR BOOK READY-ACCESS CARD!

[**✗**] Yes! I'd like to keep current. Please send me a *free* 30-day examination copy of the Year Book(s) checked below:

[ ] *Year Book of Anesthesia*® (AN)	$54.95
[ ] *Year Book of Cardiology*® (CV)	$54.95
[ ] *Year Book of Critical Care Medicine*® (16)	$51.95
[ ] *Year Book of Dermatology*® (10)	$51.95
[ ] *Year Book of Diagnostic Radiology*® (9)	$54.95
[ ] *Year Book of Digestive Diseases*® (13)	$51.95
[ ] *Year Book of Drug Therapy*® (6)	$54.95
[ ] *Year Book of Emergency Medicine*® (15)	$51.95
[ ] *Year Book of Endocrinology*® (EM)	$54.95
[ ] *Year Book of Family Practice*® (FY)	$51.95
[ ] *Year Book of Geriatrics and Gerontology* (GE)	$51.95
[ ] *Year Book of Hand Surgery*® (17)	$54.95
[ ] *Year Book of Hematology*® (24)	$51.95
[ ] *Year Book of Infectious Diseases*® (19)	$51.95
[ ] *Year Book of Infertility* (IN)	$51.95
[ ] *Year Book of Medicine*® (1)	$51.95
[ ] *Year Book of Neonatal-Perinatal Medicine* (23)	$51.95
[ ] *Year Book of Neurology and Neurosurgery*® (8)	$54.95
[ ] *Year Book of Nuclear Medicine*® (NM)	$54.95
[ ] *Year Book of Obstetrics and Gynecology*® (5)	$51.95
[ ] *Year Book of Oncology* (CA)	$54.95
[ ] *Year Book of Ophthalmology*® (EY)	$51.95
[ ] *Year Book of Orthopedics*® (OR)	$54.95
[ ] *Year Book of Otolaryngology – Head and Neck Surgery*® (3)	$54.95
[ ] *Year Book of Pathology and Clinical Pathology*® (PI)	$54.95
[ ] *Year Book of Pediatrics*® (4)	$51.95
[ ] *Year Book of Plastic and Reconstructive Surgery*® (12)	$54.95
[ ] *Year Book of Psychiatry and Applied Mental Health*® (11)	$49.95
[ ] *Year Book of Pulmonary Disease*® (21)	$51.95
[ ] *Year Book of Sports Medicine*® (SM)	$51.95
[ ] *Year Book of Surgery*® (2)	$54.95
[ ] *Year Book of Urology*® (7)	$54.95
[ ] *Year Book of Vascular Surgery*® (20)	$54.95

*All Year Books are published annually. For the convenience of its customers, Year Book enters each purchaser as a subscriber to future volumes and sends annual announcements of each volume approximately 2 months before publication. The new volume will be shipped upon publication unless you complete and return the cancellation notice attached to the announcement and it is received by Year Book within the time indicated (approximately 20 days after your receipt of the announcement). You may cancel your subscription at any time. The new volume may be examined on approval for 30 days, may be returned for full credit, and if returned Year Book will then remove your name as a subscriber. Return postage is guaranteed by Year Book to the Postal Service.

NAME/ACCT. NO.

ADDRESS

CITY/STATE/ZIP   CODE: EBF1

Prepaid orders are shipped postage free; add $3.50 per order to cover handling. Other orders will be billed a shipping and handling charge. IL, MA, TN residents are billed appropriate sales tax. Prices quoted in U.S. dollars. Canadian orders will be billed in Canadian funds at the current exchange rate. All prices subject to change without notice.

Mosby-Year Book, Inc. • 200 North LaSalle Street • Chicago, Illinois 60601